WMR3J

Language Lateralization
and Psychosis

Language Lateralization and Psychosis

Edited by

Iris E. C. Sommer

René S. Kahn

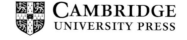

CAMBRIDGE UNIVERSITY PRESS
Cambridge, New York, Melbourne, Madrid, Cape Town, Singapore, São Paulo, Delhi

Cambridge University Press
The Edinburgh Building, Cambridge CB2 8RU, UK

Published in the United States of America by Cambridge University Press, New York

www.cambridge.org
Information on this title: www.cambridge.org/9780521882842

First published 2009

Printed in the United Kingdom at the University Press, Cambridge

A catalog record for this publication is available from the British Library

ISBN 978-0-521-88284-2 hardback

Contents

Color plate section is between pages 118 and 119.

Contributors

Marian Annett Ph.D., D.Sc.
Reader Emeritus, School of Psychology, University of Leicester, Leicester, United Kingdom

Sherry Aw B.S.
Graduate student, Biological and Biomedical Sciences Program Harvard Medical School, and Forsyth Center for Regenerative and Developmental Biology, Forsyth Institute Boston, MA, USA

Kelly Diederen M.Sc.
Researcher at the Neuroscience Department, University Medical Center Utrecht, The Netherlands

Sonia Dollfus M.D., Ph.D
Professor of Psychiatry and Head of the Department of Psychiatry, Centre Hospitalier et Universitaire and UMR 6232 CNRS CEA Universités de Caen et René Descartes, Centre d'Imagerie-Neurosciences et d'Applications aux Pathologies, Caen, France

Clyde Francks M.A., D.Phil.
Wellcome Trust Centre for Human Genetics, University of Oxford, Oxford, United Kingdom

Onur Güntürkün Dipl. Psych., Dr. Phil.
Biopsychologist, Faculty of Psychology, Ruhr University Bochum, Bochum, Germany

René S. Kahn M.D., Ph.D.
Psychiatrist and Head of the Neuroscience Department, University Medical Center Utrecht, The Netherlands

Tilo Kircher M.D., Ph.D.
Professor of Psychiatry, Depatment of Psychiatry,
RWTH Aachen University, Aachen, Germany

Stefan Knecht M.D.
Department of Neurology, University of Münster,
Germany

Michael Levin Ph.D.
Senior Member of the Staff, Forsyth Center for
Regenerative and Developmental Biology, Forsyth
Institute, and Associate Professor, Harvard School of
Dental Medicine, Boston, MA, USA

Olivier Maïza M.D.
Psychiatrist, Department of Psychiatry, Centre
Hospitalier et Universitaire and UMR 6232 CNRS
CEA Universités de Caen et René Descartes,
Centre d'Imagerie-Neurosciences et d'Applications
aux Pathologies, Caen, France

**I. C. McManus M.D., Ph.D., F.R.C.P., F.R.C.P.Ed., F.Med.
Sci.**
Professor of Psychology and Medical
Education, University College London, London,
United Kingdom

Alexander Rapp M.D.
Clinical Psychiatrist and Researcher, Department of
Psychiatry, University of Tübingen, Germany

Annick Razafimandimby Ph.D.
Researcher, UMR 6232 CNRS CEA Universités de Caen
et René Descartes, Centre d'Imagerie-Neurosciences et
d'Applications aux Pathologies, Caen, France

Metten Somers M.D.
Psychiatry Resident and researcher at the Neuroscience
Department, University Medical Center Utrecht, The
Netherlands

Iris E. C. Sommer M.D., Ph.D.
Psychiatrist and researcher at the Neuroscience
Department, University Medical Center Utrecht,
Netherlands

Bianca Stubbe-Dräger M.D.
Department of Neurology, University of Münster,
Germany

Carin Whitney M.A.
Department of Psychiatry, RWTH Aachen University,
Aachen, Germany

Preface

We tend to perceive ourselves as one person, with one consciousness, one mind. Yet, even a coarse inspection of the human brain tells us otherwise. Our brains consist of two separate hemispheres, connected by the fibers of the corpus callosum. How these hemispheres cooperate to form one thinking personality has fascinated brain researchers for centuries. Another mystery of the brain is that the degree to which the hemispheres share certain tasks (i.e., the degree of lateralization) can vary grossly between individuals. In general, even small alterations in the brain lead to devastating clinical symptoms. Cerebral lateralization obviously is an exception to this rule. Individuals may tolerate a partial or total reversal of functional differentiation between the hemispheres without loss of neurological or cognitive functions. On the other hand, differences in cerebral lateralization do lead to subtle differences in the way of thinking and, indeed, may predispose for psychosis.

The normal development of bodily asymmetry and lateralization of the brain is explained in the first section of the book. This section discusses the variation that occurs in language lateralization, its association with hand preference, genetic aspects, geographical differences and the influence of sex.

In the second section, research is reviewed on the association between language lateralization and psychosis. A more equal distribution of tasks between the hemispheres, allowing more language functions in the right hemisphere, appears to predispose for psychotic symptoms. The "additional" language from the right hemisphere may lead to psychotic symptoms such as auditory verbal hallucinations and formal thought disorder.

This book illustrates the important fundamental aspects of cerebral lateralization and integrates this knowledge to explain how decreased language lateralization can facilitate psychotic symptoms in the human brain.

Asymmetry, handedness and language lateralization

Molecular mechanisms establishing consistent left–right asymmetry during vertebrate embryogenesis

Sherry Aw and Michael Levin

Summary

The physiology and behavior of all animals are strongly dependent on the large-scale structure of the body plan. While many animals are fundamentally bilaterally symmetric, vertebrates and many invertebrates exhibit a consistently oriented left–right (LR) asymmetry of the heart, viscera, and brain. The biased asymmetry of LR patterning is distinct from environmentally determined asymmetry or the random developmental noise that gives rise to fluctuating asymmetries. How the LR axis is oriented in a world in which no macroscopic force distinguishes left from right is a profound puzzle linking evolutionary, developmental, and cell biology to cognitive science and perhaps even to quantum parity violations. Embryonic LR patterning includes a sequential process of symmetry breaking (likely on the intracellular level), consistent axis orientation, amplification to diverse multicellular targets, and restriction via the midline. Key questions include the timing of the first LR-asymmetric computation during embryonic development, the molecular nature of mechanisms underlying each of the necessary steps, and the degree of conservation of these mechanisms among taxa.

The field of LR asymmetry has made striking progress over the last two decades, uncovering a plethora of molecular details in a wide range of model organisms. Here, we present an overview of what is known about the phases of asymmetry initiation, physiological/biophysical signaling upstream of asymmetric gene expression cascades, and ultimate morphogenesis of the asymmetric organs. While the transcriptional programs specific to the left and right sides universally feed into the signaling protein *Nodal*, the degree of evolutionary conservation of various upstream mechanisms is more controversial.

The two major directions in the field are defined by models focusing on ciliary motion vs. physiological signaling. The former hold that asymmetry is bootstrapped from the biochemical structure of cilia via rotary motion that redistributes an extracellular morphogen or activates asymmetric Ca^{++} signaling in sensory cilia. In this scheme, most thoroughly explored in mouse and zebrafish embryos, asymmetry is generated fairly late – during gastrulation. In contrast, work in the frog and chick embryo identified modules based on ion transport, serotonin gradients, and gap junctional communication. The earliest steps (asymmetric localization of maternal ion transporter proteins) occur in the cleavage stage embryo (shortly after fertilization) and rely on cytoskeletal (intracellular) asymmetries that appear to be an evolutionarily ancient mechanism for generating chirality, although they have not been explored in mammals.

Future experiments must address whether cilia are primary to asymmetry or a mid-pathway step, and whether physiological mechanisms are relevant in mammals. The early steps of asymmetry in human development are still poorly understood. It is clear that clinical data must be integrated in this field, because of key phenomena that are not predicted by any of the current theoretical constructs derived from model species. These include unilateral presentation of genetic syndromes, cryptic functional asymmetries in anatomically symmetrical structures, conservation of hair whorl direction and other characteristics in monozygotic twins, and normal handedness (brain asymmetry) in patients of fully inverted body laterality. Future work in this fascinating field will have wide-ranging implications for basic biology, psychology, and clinical medicine.

Introduction

Most vertebrates, including man, appear to exhibit bilateral symmetry, whereby body parts on the left and right sides are approximate reflections of each

Language Lateralization and Psychosis, ed. Iris E. C. Sommer and René S. Kahn. Published by Cambridge University Press.
© Cambridge University Press 2009.

other across a midline plane stretching from head to toe (hence bilateral symmetry is also called plane or mirror symmetry). However, this external bilateral symmetry belies the consistently biased, internal left–right asymmetry in placement and shape of both unpaired (e.g., liver and heart) and paired organs (e.g., left and right lungs), as well as asymmetries in organ function (e.g., unilateral ovulation, brain hemisphere specialization). Left–right asymmetry, or laterality, consistent among individuals within a population, results from the execution of precisely orchestrated developmental programs during embryonic development.

Why are animals asymmetric? In paired organs, asymmetry can result in an increase in complexity that can be achieved with division of labor, compartmentalization, and specialization (e.g., different compartments in the heart for separating oxygenated blood that is to be circulated to the rest of the body from blood that is to be directed to the lungs) (Nerurkar *et al.*, 2006). Moreover, an asymmetric body plan necessarily results from the bending of tubular organs, which may have significant physiological advantages such as increased compaction from coiling and the maximizing of surface area (e.g., for absorption in the intestines). However, there seems to be no obvious benefit to have this asymmetry be maintained in *one specific* direction within a population (*situs solitus*). Indeed, the small percentage of humans whose internal organs are completely mirror-image of the norm (*situs inversus*), are usually very healthy. Yet, all vertebrate populations, instead of being a racemic (50%–50%) mix of the two body plans, are usually highly skewed towards one "enantiomer". This bias is well-conserved across a wide range of taxa (Cooke, 2004). This presents a fascinating problem, not only in developmental biology, but also in medicine, evolution, and cell biology.

Perturbations in normal left–right patterning (*situs solitus*) can result in several classes of laterality defects with varying degrees of clinical manifestations. The first, *situs inversus*, a complete mirror-image reversal of *situs*, has already been mentioned, and these individuals generally do not exhibit the severe clinical symptoms related to individual organ reversal, although there are now indications that the discordance between large-scale morphological reversal and

the normal underlying filament chirality may predispose patients to congenital heart disease (Delhaas *et al.*, 1993; Delhaas *et al.*, 2004; Layton, 1978; Ramsdell, 2005).

In individuals with *situs ambiguus*, however, only some organs are left–right reversed, in a random manner, which has significant health implications for the patient. The organ that seems particularly sensitive to aberrant left–right signaling is the heart, as many children with *situs ambiguus* exhibit complex cardiac defects, including atrioventricular discordance, pulmonary atresia, and aberrant placement and displacement of heart tubes such as the aorta or the great arteries (Kosaki & Casey, 1998). Defects in other organs include reversal of the position of the spleen, reversal of the left and right lobes of the liver, right-sided stomach, and gastrointestinal malrotation (Kosaki & Casey, 1998).

A third category is isomerism, where left–right asymmetry is lost. For example, individuals with Ivemark syndrome exhibit bilateral right-sidedness, where their organs on the right side are duplicated on the left (Krzelj *et al.*, 2000). Many individuals with *situs ambiguus* may exhibit a mixture of organ reversal and organ isomerism, e.g. midline liver, and lung right (tri-lobed) or left (bi-lobed) isomerism. It is worthwhile to note that most known modulators of left–right asymmetry produce a population of individuals with *heterotaxia* when disrupted, where individuals may be either *situs solitus*, *situs inversus totalis* or *situs ambiguus*.

Additional defects may arise as indirect effects of improper positioning, e.g. hypoplasia (underdevelopment or incomplete development of organs, e.g. smaller or missing gall bladders), aplasia (complete loss of an organ, e.g. asplenia), and atresia (regression of an organ). Others are midline defects such as the failure of the neural tube to properly close, resulting in defects such as anencephaly and meningomyelocele, and hindgut malformations such as anal atresia (Bisgrove *et al.*, 2003; Kosaki & Casey, 1998). As the midline has been shown to play an important role in asymmetry (Danos & Yost, 1995; Lohr *et al.*, 1997), some midline defects might be a cause of laterality disturbances. Because of the prominence of these teratologies in human medicine, developmental biologists have long turned to model species to try to understand normal left–right patterning.

A wonderful survey of animal asymmetries by Neville shows the fascinating variety of asymmetries in various body plan types throughout the animal kingdom (Neville, 1976). These include both random or fluctuating asymmetries (small, stochastic differences between the left and right sides) due to random developmental noise (Bowyer *et al.*, 2001), and environmentally determined asymmetries, such as in lobster claws, where the sidedness of the major, large crusher is dictated by usage (Govind, 1992; Palmer, 2004), in addition to consistently biased asymmetries such as the species-specific direction of snail shell coiling (chirality) and asymmetries of the heart and viscera. While behavioral asymmetries such as hand preference have fascinated psychologists for well over a century, the molecular details of how morphological asymmetries arise have begun to be elucidated relatively recently, in comparison to the much greater volume of work on anterior–posterior (AP) and dorsal–ventral (DV) axial patterning. A brief survey of early work involving unilateral drug effects and the genetics of snail shell coiling are given in Levin (1997).

A major early influence on how investigators thought about the patterning of left–right asymmetry was the identification of genetic mutants. In particular, the *iv* (*situs inversus viscerum*) mutation in the mouse has been extremely important in formulating models by which left–right asymmetry is patterned. Homozygous *iv* mice exhibit 50% *situs inversus* (Layton, 1976; McGrath *et al.*, 1992). Therefore the wild type allele permits bias, but is not necessary to the breaking of symmetry, nor for conveying the direction of bias to downstream steps. This is in contrast to mutations that cause *situs ambiguus*, where there is a loss of concordance and each organ appears to make an individual decision as to which side of the body it will occupy. The *iv* mouse suggests that the patterning of left–right asymmetry is a multistep process (Fig. 1.1a): there needs to be a process by which asymmetry is set up between the left and right sides, as well as a biasing mechanism to orient the direction of asymmetry (Brown & Wolpert, 1990a).

Much of the thinking about the initial symmetry breaking steps in left–right development was influenced by a model put forth by Brown and Wolpert (Brown & Wolpert, 1990b). They proposed a chiral "*F*" molecule (but in three dimensions) that would biologically occur only in one enantiomer, as is true of many compounds (Pasteur, 1860). This subcellular component can dictate left vs. right direction within a cell, when tethered consistently along the anterior–posterior and dorso–ventral axes. Though purely theoretical at the time, this model was crucial because it provided the only plausible mechanism that could determine LR direction *de novo*. It led naturally to the question of when the embryo first makes this computation, and to investigation of mechanisms that link this process to the placement and shape of the organs (which requires conversion of direction information into location with respect to the midline (Figs. 1.1b–c')).

The molecular LR pathway: the conserved latter part of left–right patterning

The patterning of the left–right axis can conceptually be broken down into several distinct steps (Fig. 1.1) that have served as a working model for the field (Brown & Wolpert, 1990b; Levin, 2006). In Step 1, the embryo orients the left–right axis with respect to the dorsal–ventral and the anterior–posterior axes, hence being able to "tell its left from its right". Next, the embryo must set up a stable biophysical or molecular difference between the left and right sides, which can be imposed upon multicellular fields as the embryo divides (so that cells can determine position with respect to the midline, not merely direction). Third, cell fields on the left and right sides execute transcriptional cascades that set up differential gene expression patterns impinging on organ primordia. Fourth, the various organs make use of this asymmetric information as they undergo asymmetric morphogenesis.

The best characterized part of this process is the distinct right- and left-sided transcriptional cascades that propagate asymmetric information on either side of the embryo. The deliberate induction and repression of side-specific gene expression through cell fields on the two sides in time (as the embryo develops, different sets of genes are turned on and off) and space

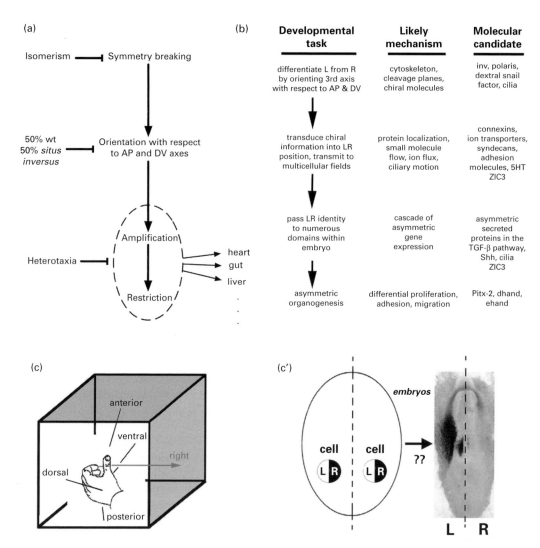

Figure 1.1 Fundamental steps in left–right patterning: one possible model.

(a) Consistent large-scale asymmetry likely requires several sequential steps: breaking of initial left–right symmetry, orientation of the LR axis with respect to the other two orthogonal axes (to ensure consistent asymmetry rather than fluctuating asymmetry), amplification of this information to communicate position to remote cells, and restriction of this information (to prevent its inappropriate cross over past the midline). The last two steps are a module that provides laterality cues to asymmetric organs. Blocking each of these steps results in different classes of laterality defects: (i) isomerism results from a failure to break asymmetry; (ii) blocking the orientation of the LR axis results in the *iv* phenotype, where 50% of the offspring are *situs solitus* and 50% are *situs inversus*; (iii) it is likely that a single locus of orientation is amplified into numerous downstream pathways; interference with mechanisms downstream of the unified steps results in heterotaxia, or a loss of concordance among individual organs.

(b) Schematic of the sequential steps and likely mechanisms that underlie these transitional events during left–right patterning. See (Levin, 2005) for a detailed description of each component.

(regulated gene expression occurs in distinct, specific regions on either side of the embryo), lays down the genetic instructions for sidedness in the subsequent organogenesis and morphogenesis steps.

Despite the controversy surrounding the nature and conservation of "Step 1", left–right determination appears to converge, during the transcriptional cascade steps, on Nodal signaling following interactions between molecules from the hedgehog, FGF, EGF-CFC, BMP, and other families (Burdine & Schier, 2000; Levin, 1998). Nodal, a TGFβ family member, propagates a left-sided gene cascade from the node to the left lateral plate meso-derm (Whitman & Mercola, 2001). Several components of this pathway have now been identified as human loci responsible for laterality birth defects, and, indeed, the fleshing out of this set of cascades immediately shed light on the mechanisms of birth defects of laterality.

Inversions of internal organs have been observed in one of a pair of human conjoined twins (Aird, 1959; Burn, 1991; Cuniff et al., 1988; Kapur et al., 1994; Torgersen, 1950; Winer-Muram, 1995). The spatial characterization of the molecular signals propagated by asymmetric gene expression in chick embryos allowed a partial understanding of this phenomenon. Analysis of spontaneous twins of chick embryos in various orientations suggests that laterality defects in one twin may be induced by cross-over of LR morpho-gen molecules from the adjacent twin, and this model predicts reasonably well the data on inversions in human conjoined twins (Levin et al., 1996).

In view of the fact that "leftness" and "rightness" are a consequence of distinct signaling cascades with complex feedback and suppressive interactions, and that nodal likely positively upregulates its own expression (Meno

et al., 1999), it is essential that there be some sort of barrier between the two sides to prevent spillover of signals from one side to the other, that might interfere with the sided transcriptional programs. Such a midline barrier would explain the laterality defects caused by either genetic or microsurgical interference with midline patterning (Lohr et al., 1997) but the nature of the barrier for many of the early signals (e.g., the left and right domains of Sonic hedgehog, separated by only the thin width of Hensen's node in the chick) is still unknown.

A few midline-expressing genes are likely candidates for this function at later stages. The best studied of these are the lefty proteins, divergent ligand members of the TGFβ superfamily (Meno et al., 1996). These findings led to the formation of the midline barrier model where lefty in the midline and LPM is upregulated by nodal, and antagonizes nodal by a negative feedback mechanism (Bisgrove et al., 1999), preventing nodal signals from crossing the midline. Indeed impressive recent efforts have led to the development of a mathematical model of these processes in the mouse (Nakamura et al., 2006).

These signaling mechanisms provide different infor-mation to the tissues on the left and right sides in the developing embryo, and ultimately culminate in asym-metric organ morphogenesis that produces the left–right asymmetric anatomical body plan. Anatomical asymme-try can be generated through several general processes (Ramsdell, 2005; Shiratori & Hamada, 2006). Directional looping occurs in organs that begin in a tube shape, such as the heart and the gut. Bending and rotational movements establish both structural and positional asymmetry. Unilateral regression and/or persistence of an initially bilateral structure occurs in the venous system, where structures on one side of the body

---

Figure 1.1 (cont.)

(c) Schematic of the "right-hand rule" as a way of aligning the LR axis in three-dimensional space. This illustrates the class of models known as the "F-molecule" theory (Brown & Wolpert, 1990a), according to which a cell can nucleate asymmetry by orienting a molecular entity that occurs in only one form or enantiomer.

(c′) Illustration of a major conversion of information that must occur during LR patterning: chiral molecules' orientation, which tells a cell which *direction* is L vs. R, must be transduced into *true positional information with respect to the midline*, in order for left- and right-sided cells to drive different genetic cascades and undergo different morphogenetic programs. The panel on the right is a chick embryo (with midline indicated by dashed line) showing two domains of expression of the left-sided gene *Nodal* (Levin et al., 1995), indicating that by this stage, the mesoderm cells clearly know whether they are on the left (express *Nodal*) or the right (do not express *Nodal*) of the midline.

completely regress, or in the spleen, where only the tissues on the left-side develop completely (Patterson *et al.*, 2000). Finally, asymmetrical development or branching occurs in structures such as the lung, in which an initially symmetric structure goes on to develop lateralization. The mechanisms underlying these anatomical asymmetries include differential cell death, migration, differentiation, growth and elongation, and tensile forces (Miller & White, 1998; Voronov *et al.*, 2004); however, the molecular players, their molecular mechanisms, and their conservation, both among tissues and across species, are still poorly understood.

Early biophysical components of laterality: ciliary and physiological mechanisms

The most interesting aspect of left–right patterning is arguably "Step 1", or the symmetry breaking and orientation point. It should be pointed out that most models in the field assume that this process confers asymmetry on a bilaterally symmetrical background, although this is challenged by arguments from paleontological data (Jefferies *et al.*, 1996), and recent work on the role of retinoic acid signaling in symmetrizing an initially asymmetric somite patterning process (Vermot & Pourquie, 2005). The identity of Step 1 is still highly controversial (Levin & Palmer, 2007; Tabin, 2005), and the field is currently split into two paradigms centered around the choice of model systems and focused on different molecular components.

The first paradigm focuses on a set of models involving the movement of cilia on the cells of the node during gastrulation. The first clue that cilia may play a role in left–right patterning came from Kartagener's syndrome. These patients have immotile sperm and malfunctioning cilia in respiratory airways, as well as laterality defects. Ultrastructural analysis showed their cilia to lack dynein arms (Afzelius, 1985). Further, mouse knockouts of two members of the kinesin superfamily (KIFs) of microtubule-dependent molecular motors, KIF3-A and KIF3-B, resulted in half the mutant mice exhibiting reverse heart loops and bilateral or absent *Lefty2* expression, indicating that the role of

the kinesins is upstream of known asymmetric gene expression in the mouse (Marszalek *et al.*, 1999; Nonaka *et al.*, 1998). Additional clues about the role of cilia came when the mutations for the *inversus viscerum* (*iv*) and *legless* (*lgl*) allelic mouse mutants, spontaneous mutants that exhibit *situs inversus* in half of the offspring (Lowe *et al.*, 1996; Schreiner *et al.*, 1993; Singh *et al.*, 1991), were positionally cloned and found to be located in an axonemal dynein gene, *left–right dynein* (*lrd*) (Supp *et al.*, 1997).

Examination of the ventral node cells of wildtype versus KIF3-A and KIF3-B knockout mouse embryos, as well as *iv* mouse embryos, yielded insight into the possible mechanistic role of cilia. In wildtype embryos, the monocilia in the ventral node rotate vigorously clockwise (Nonaka *et al.*, 1998; Takeda *et al.*, 1999). However, the ventral nodes of KIF3-A and KIF3-B knockout mice either have very short cilia or lack cilia completely, while the *iv* mice have stationary cilia (Okada *et al.*, 1999). A series of elegant experiments using fluorescent beads placed into the extra-embryonic space showed that the beating leads to a localized net fluid flow from the right to the left (Nonaka *et al.*, 1998; Okada *et al.*, 1999; Takeda *et al.*, 1999). Modeling showed that the rotational beating is able to generate a leftward flow, and not a circular vortex, due to a 40-degree tilt (from the vertical) of the cilia to the posterior (Nonaka *et al.*, 2005; Okada *et al.*, 2005).

There are currently two non-exclusive models for how ciliary flow sets up left–right patterning. The first posits that the asymmetric leftward flow leads to the setting up of a chemical morphogen gradient and accumulation of this morphogen preferentially on one side of the node (the left side), causing asymmetric downstream effects. This idea has recently gained traction with the discovery of nodal vesicular particles (NVPs) – membrane-sheathed particles that bud from node cells and that appear to be transported leftward in the nodal flow (Tanaka *et al.*, 2005). The particles contain retinoic acid and Shh, both of which have been implicated in left–right patterning (Schilling *et al.*, 1999; Tsukui *et al.*, 1999; Wang *et al.*, 2004). The second model, known as the two-cilia model, posits that there are two populations of cilia: motile, flow-generating rotating cilia in the center of the node, expressing both LRD and the cation channel polycystin-2 (PKD2), and immotile, mechanosensory cilia around the periphery expressing only PKD2. The immotile cilia sense the nodal flow, causing a downstream asymmetric calcium signal (McGrath *et al.*, 2003; Tabin & Vogan, 2003). This second model may explain the different phenotypes exhibited by embryos with immotile cilia and those with no cilia at all, and is also supported by the fact that laterality defects are observed in humans with polycystic kidney disease (PKD), caused by mutations in genes involved in environmental sensing in cilia (Pennekamp *et al.*, 2002).

The presence of beating cilia at the embryonic node has since been found to be conserved to fish and frog (Essner *et al.*, 2005; Schweickert *et al.*, 2007), in addition to mice. This elegant class of models is attractive because it bootstraps organismal asymmetry from the biochemical structure of the cilia themselves. A key feature of this hypothesis is that asymmetry is first decided fairly late – during gastrulation. At least in mammals, this is plausible since normal mice appear to result when the cells of earlier embryos are experimentally mixed (Brown *et al.*, 1991), and no one has yet reported any consistently asymmetric transcripts prior to the formation of the node. However, a number of mechanisms have now been discovered that function much earlier in several other vertebrates, giving rise to a different class of models based on intracellular events.

This second class of models, based on work in the chick and frog, but later extended to zebrafish and several invertebrates (Adams *et al.*, 2006; Duboc *et al.*, 2005; Hibino *et al.*, 2006; Levin, 2005; Raya *et al.*, 2004; Shimeld & Levin, 2006), comprises two modules: a system of intracellular motor proteins and cytoskeletal structures that establishes asymmetric distribution of ion transporters in the cleavage-stage embryo, and resulting in voltage gradients that electrophoretically redistribute a left–right morphogen that in turn activates asymmetric gene expression (Fukumoto *et al.*, 2005a; Fukumoto *et al.*, 2005b; Levin *et al.*, 2006).

Counter to the later necessity of isolated left and right compartments, it was found that in the early embryo, the left and right sides must communicate to decide left and right identity of lateral tissue. In both frog and chick, this communication takes place via gap junctions (protein conduits that allow direct cell-to-cell transfer of small molecules and current). A path of gap junctional communication (GJC) between cells occurs around a zone of junctional isolation that lies at the embryonic midline (Guthrie, 1984; Levin & Mercola, 1998; Olson *et al.*, 1991). In chick and frog, interrupting the circumferential contiguity of the gap junctional path, or inducing GJC across the zone of isolation, both lead to specific perturbations in left–right patterning (Levin & Mercola, 1998; Levin & Mercola, 1999). The role of gap junctional communication in both pathways lies upstream of known asymmetrical transcription.

Subsequent work revealed that the zone of isolation was a "battery": it contains an asymmetric distribution of several ion transporters, which establishes an electric field, consistently aligned with LR polarity, across the zone of isolation by differential exchange of ions with the outside medium (reviewed in Levin *et al.*, 2006). Two of the transporters are ion pumps: the H/K-ATPase and the V-ATPase (Adams *et al.*, 2006; Levin *et al.*, 2002). In the frog, maternal mRNA and protein subunits of both pumps are asymmetrically localized during the first two cell divisions, or within two hours post-fertilization, demonstrating that the frog embryo knows its left from its right long before cilia appear. Pharmacological or molecular–genetic blockade of the transporters, or modulation of the transmembrane voltage gradient by independent means, specifically cause heterotaxia and perturb downstream asymmetric gene expression, demonstrating an early role in left–right determination.

The data have been synthesized into a quantitative model (Esser *et al.*, 2006) whereby asymmetric ion flux and pH gradients across the midline generate an electrophoretic force for the movement of small molecules such as serotonin (Levin *et al.*, 2006; Fukumoto *et al.*, 2005a; Fukumoto *et al.*, 2005b), inositol phosphates (Sarmah *et al.*, 2005), or even ions such as calcium, leading to the accumulation of such effectors on one side of the midline, and asymmetric downstream signaling effects.

The gap junction and ion transporter data motivated the search for a putative morphogen-like signal, small enough to pass through gap junctions, charged to migrate directionally in an electric field, and associated with an intracellular system of receptors and effectors able to cause downstream signaling effects. One hypothesis was that such a molecule could traverse the circumferential gap junctional path down a voltage gradient, and accumulate preferentially on one side of the midline (Fukumoto *et al.*, 2005a; Fukumoto *et al.*, 2005b). A pharmacological screen using well-characterized blockers of various components of the serotonin signaling system implicated serotonin receptors R3 and R4, as well as the serotonin degradation enzyme monoamine oxidase (MAO) in left–right patterning in both chick and frog, functioning at very early stages prior to the appearance of cilia at the node. Indeed, the localization of maternal serotonin is dynamic, at first being uniformly distributed in the embryo during the first few cell divisions, and finally accumulating in the right side of the battery (by the 32-cell stage) in a voltage- and gap-junction-dependent process. Interestingly, several aspects of this pathway are targeted by drugs currently in widespread use as psychiatric medication (SSRIs, MAOIs, etc.). While the relevance of this pathway to mammals is not yet clear, it is possible that these may be able to affect asymmetry in human fetal development.

In the chick, the situation is less tidy. A battery at the center of an isolation zone (the primitive streak), and a region of gap-junctional communication around the battery, both exist and are required for normal LR patterning, just like in the frog. And, the same components of the serotonin pathway are required for correct left–right determination (serotonin itself, the MAO enzyme, the R3 and R4 family of receptors, and the membrane serotonin transporter SERT). However, the pattern of 5HT localization does not directly support the same sort of circumferential transport model, suggesting that either another (as yet undiscovered) small molecule takes the place of serotonin in a chick, or that asymmetric serotonin signaling in the chick is driven by a non-electrophoretic mechanism. In general, the reuse of molecular components in different ways in animals with different gastrulation architectures suggests that surprises may yet await in the earlier stages of mammalian LR patterning, since probing these pathways is not straightforward and has not

been conclusively carried out. For example, genetic deletion of single connexin genes may not be informative since other members of the family (or maternal components, Cote *et al.*, 2007) can compensate and thus mask LR-relevant phenotypes. The same would be true of many ion transporters, whose large families can guarantee redundancy.

Although no H^+ or K^+ transporters have been implicated in asymmetry in mammals, the Ca^{++} channel polycystin-2 (PKD2) likely plays an important role in left–right patterning in the mouse. In the two-cilia hypothesis described above, it has been proposed that leftward fluid flow sensed by mechanosensory immotile cilia expressing PKD2 leads to asymmetric calcium signaling to the left of the gastrulation organizing center in mice, frogs, and fish. Intriguingly, the asymmetric function of H/K-ATPase in the chick has been demonstrated to function through downstream asymmetric calcium and Notch signaling (Raya *et al.*, 2004). It is possible that the different symmetry-breaking steps in mouse versus frog and chick are a consequence of their vastly different gastrulation modes that impose biophysical constraints on when symmetry can be broken, but all species regardless use ion channels to finally attain asymmetric calcium signaling to the downstream *Nodal*-mediated transcriptional cascade (Speder *et al.*, 2007).

In fish, where both ion flux and nodal flow appear to be important in establishing left–right pattern, the relationship between the two is unclear. Inhibition of the H/K-ATPase during cleavage stages caused reversed heart-looping and randomization of asymmetric markers without affecting *LRD* expression, cilia distribution or size, or fluid flow (Kawakami *et al.*, 2005) suggesting the two pathways function in parallel; however, inhibition of V-ATPase led to fewer and shorter cilia (Adams *et al.*, 2006), suggesting that early pattern by ion flux affects downstream nodal flow. Further experiments will need to be done to tease apart the relationships between these two novel and exciting patterning mechanisms, and the issue of conservation is discussed in detail in Levin (2006).

The asymmetric early distribution of ion transporter proteins naturally pushes back the question of what lies upstream to produce this asymmetry. The data implicate the cytoskeleton of the very early embryo as having a causal role (Adams *et al.*, 2006; Yost, 1991), as well as suggesting novel intracellular functions for the molecules commonly interpreted in terms of ciliary roles, such as LRD, KIF3B, INV, etc. (Levin & Palmer, 2007; Qiu *et al.*, 2005). As the cytoskeleton of the fertilized *Xenopus* egg has been shown to contain intrinsic chiral properties (Danilchik *et al.*, 2006), and its organization is required for correct asymmetric localization of ion pump proteins, the components of the cytoskeleton (tubulin and actin as well as molecular motors such as kinesin and dynein) may fulfill the role of the symmetry-breaking *F* molecule in this model. In this proposal, genetic disruption of motor proteins (as has been performed in several mouse mutants) has consequences for cilia as a byproduct, and its primary role in LR randomization is by changes in intracellular transport roles. The association between laterality defects and kidney disease likewise is possibly a result of changes in cell polarity mechanisms that affect the LR axis and epithelial function as parallel byproducts. However, recent data convincingly demonstrated that a change of viscosity around the nodal cilia in a minimally perturbed system does indeed randomize asymmetry (Schweickert *et al.*, 2007), so a functional role is likely.

How can ciliary and physiological models be reconciled? While the latter model, based on fundamental aspects of cytoskeletal cell polarity, has the advantage that it is applicable to organisms as diverse as plants, snails, *Caenorhabditis elegans*, and birds (Oviedo & Levin, 2007), the cilia model is appealing because it identifies a specific molecular component as Step 1 (the motile cilium), whereas the physiological model still has yet to specifically characterize the cytoskeletal organizing center responsible for orienting the LR axis within the planar and apical-basal polarities of the early blastomeres. Our current suggestion is that the cilia are a middle step in the pathway, having appeared around the time of the fish to canalize or amplify the LR information produced by earlier steps (Levin & Palmer, 2007). Mice may or may not have dispensed with the earlier mechanisms entirely, and it remains to be seen whether human asymmetry is more like that of the chick (since most mammals gastrulate as a blastoderm like birds) or like that of the mouse (which has adapted its mechanisms to a highly derived cylindrical gastrulation).

Links between clinical data and molecular developmental biology, in the field of asymmetry

Aside from direct laterality defects, there are three other main areas in which clinical data and the molecular embryology of model species intersect to enrich the understanding of asymmetry. The first concerns the issue of laterality in monozygotic twins.

Non-conjoined monozygotic twins, while not exhibiting the kinds of visceral laterality defects that occur in conjoined twins, appear to manifest many subtler kinds of mirror-image asymmetry ("bookend" or enantiomer twin pairs). Pairs of such twins have been noted to present mirror asymmetries in hand preference, hair whorl direction, tooth patterns, unilateral eye and ear defects, cleft lip, cleft palate, supernumerary teeth, limb abnormalities, and even tumor locations and undescended testicles (Beere *et al.*, 1990; Carton & Rees, 1987; Gedda *et al.*, 1981; Morison *et al.*, 1994; Opitz & Utkus, 2001; Potter & Nance, 1976; Rife, 1933; Sommer *et al.*, 1999; Sommer *et al.*, 2002; Yager, 1984).

This phenomenon has not been investigated in sufficient detail (especially with respect to documentation of cases that do not match the bookend pattern). However, this is a very important but poorly understood issue. First, since almost all bookending phenomena in healthy twins involve features of the head, this may reveal the existence of separate embryonic organizers for the head and body (Meinhardt, 2002), that use different mechanisms to determine laterality (Harland & Gerhart, 1997). This theme is echoed in the discordance between brain and body *situs* discussed below.

Moreover, most healthy, non-conjoined twins presumably result from separation of cleavage, morula, or early blastocyst stage embryos (James, 1983). Thus, some chiral information may be present in the very early mammalian embryo, later manifesting as hair whorls, etc. if the cells are separated at an early stage. This is of great significance because it speaks to the timing at which asymmetry is first decided in the human embryo. The asymmetry of the major body organs seems to be unspecified (or plastic enough to be respecified) at those stages, and is developed correctly for both monozygotic twins. This may be related

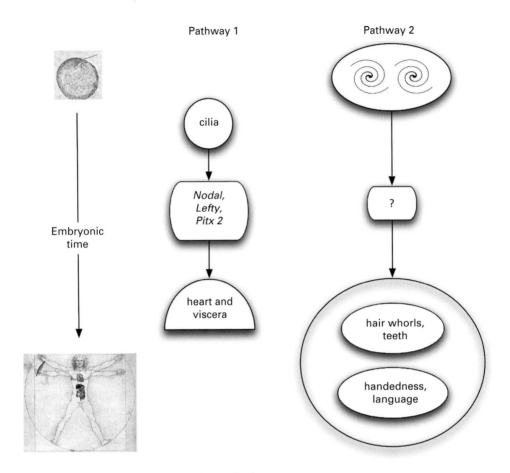

Figure 1.2 Two pathways of asymmetry in human development.

It appears that asymmetry may be elaborated by two distinct pathways in human embryogenesis. Though these two pathways may share a common origin (details are very poorly understood), clinical data suggest that one set of mechanisms controls the laterality of the heart and visceral organs through asymmetric gene expression, while another set controls asymmetry of the brain and subtle features such as hair whorls through unknown intermediary steps.

to the fact that heterotaxic reversals in hair whorls and tooth patterns would not be expected to be disadvantageous, while discordant *situs* for internal organs clearly is subject to negative evolutionary pressure. Crucially, there is yet no animal model system in which this phenomenon can be studied directly. Analysis of laterality in human twins produced by splitting of embryos during in vitro fertilization procedures may provide important clues. Likewise, the recent discovery of a role for planar polarity machinery in hair whorl patterns (Guo *et al.*, 2004; Wang

et al., 2006; Wang & Nathans, 2007) suggests molecular entry points into the fascinating link between fundamental cell polarity (anatomical and physiological) and the left–right axis (Levin, 2006).

The second major issue is the linkage between brain and body asymmetry. Interestingly, it has been found that brain asymmetry does not correlate with visceral asymmetry (Kennedy *et al.*, 1999; Tanaka *et al.*, 1999). For example, *situs inversus totalis* individuals still have the same language lateralization that is seen in right-handed normal *situs* individuals (Kennedy *et al.*, 1999), and the incidence of left-handedness is the same in *situs inversus* individuals as in the rest of the population (Cockayne, 1938; Torgersen, 1950). This suggests that mechanisms establishing the laterality of the brain are, at some early point in the LR pathway, different from those that determine the siddedness of visceral organs (Fig. 1.2). Moreover, human patients with classical primary ciliary dyskinesia (and the attendant randomization) do not exhibit reversals in the normal prevalence of right-handedness (McManus *et al.*, 2004), suggesting that at least some aspects of laterality in humans are indeed upstream of mutations affecting ciliary function, supporting the view that ciliary motion may not initiate asymmetry *de novo* during embryogenesis. While the zebrafish has enabled some progress into the molecular genetics of brain asymmetry (Bisgrove *et al.*, 2000; Concha *et al.*, 2000; Essner *et al.*, 2000; Liang *et al.*, 2000), it is not clear whether this model system will allow the investigation of human brain laterality since in the fish, brain asymmetry *is* tightly linked to body asymmetry and controlled by some of the same molecules (this appears not to be the case in human beings). This question is likely to be advanced by the identification of asymmetric gene expression (Sun *et al.*, 2006; Sun *et al.*, 2005; Sun & Walsh, 2006) and protein localization (Rodriguez-Medina *et al.*, 2002) in the mammalian brain.

Finally, clinical data have indicated a cryptic asymmetry in anatomically symmetrical structures. Most of the experimental work in the LR field has naturally addressed the mechanisms controlling the *situs* of morphologically asymmetric organs. However, several lines of evidence suggest that one member of a pair of bilateral complex structures (e.g., half of the face, one shoulder joint) can be affected in the absence of an effect on the other. Sometimes, as in the case of unilateral drug effects, the bias for one side is consistent (reviewed in Levin, 1997). The same is true in some genetic conditions (Delaney & Boyd, 2007; Paulozzi & Lary, 1999), such as Holt–Oram syndrome (Tbx5-related), which presents upper limb malformations that are much more common on the left side (Bruneau *et al.*, 1999; Hatcher *et al.*, 2000; Newbury-Ecob *et al.*, 1996; Smith *et al.*, 1979), while fibular a/hypoplasia affects the right side more often (Lewin & Opitz, 1986). In normal human beings, the feet are consistently different in size, with the larger foot being the right one in males, and the left one in females (Levy & Levy, 1978). In contrast, other phenomena are not LR-asymmetric but instead indicate that the left and right members of a symmetrical paired structure may respond differently to a systemic cue. This is most obvious in hemihypertrophy syndromes, in which a large number of tissues (e.g., the entire right leg), all on one side of the body, resume growth in adulthood (Clericuzio, 1993; Fraumeni *et al.*, 1967; Kloeppel *et al.*, 2002; Leung *et al.*, 2002; Sarkar *et al.*, 1992; Stalens *et al.*, 1993). The consistent LR asymmetries in the placement of male and female organs in hermaphrodites are striking and not at all understood (Mittwoch, 2001) but it is clear that there is a link between sex determination and LR asymmetry (Gebbia *et al.*, 1997). These data indicate that seemingly identical paired structures may in fact harbor subtle molecular differences conferring positional information along the LR axis, and that this information may persist well into adulthood. Future work must characterize novel molecular differences between paired structures and address the functional significance of this asymmetric gene expression. Identification of LR signals in locales other than overtly asymmetric organs, and an understanding of the temporal extent of LR information after completion of embryogenesis, is likely to have important implications for biomedicine and basic developmental biology.

Conclusion

The field of left–right asymmetry is currently at an exciting point, with a considerable body of genetic and cell-biological data elucidating dozens of mechanisms in a range of vertebrate and invertebrate model species. However, it is split by a central controversy between two paradigms (Levin, 2004; Tabin, 2005). One view holds that ciliary mechanisms initiate and orient asymmetry at gastrulation in all mammals (Hirokawa *et al.*, 2006). The other proposes that cytoskeletal asymmetries driving physiological processes are the initiating mechanism conserved throughout phyla and that cilia, in those species that utilize them, are a middle component of the pathway (Levin & Palmer, 2007). In any case, the LR axis is a fascinating example of how cellular polarity can be transduced into polarity on the scale of an entire organismal axis.

Fundamental questions facing the field include the following.

(1) Is the ultimate origin of asymmetry a frozen accident of evolution or does it follow from some aspect of quantum parity violation (reviewed in Levin, 1997)?

(2) Which of the mechanisms that have been discovered (Levin, 2006) apply to human laterality?

(3) What is the nature of the mechanisms involved in brain asymmetry in human development?

(4) What are the genetic endpoints that give rise to laterality defects and how many of them are compatible with otherwise normal development in human beings?

(5) What environmental and pharmacological (medical drug) factors can influence critical steps during human embryogenesis (e.g., the frequent use of Prozac[tm](fluoxetine), that targets a known element of the LR-relevant serotonin signaling)?

(6) What is the initiating event ("Step 1") of asymmetry and when does this molecular mechanism act during development? Is it the same in human embryos as other mammals, or even more widely conserved?

(7) Are symmetrical structures (arms, eyes, etc.) really different with respect to a molecular marker and does this have implications for human health?

Consistent asymmetry in a world in which no macroscopic force distinguishes left from right is a question that spans quantum parity violations, biochemistry, physiology, developmental biology, evolutionary mechanisms, and cognitive science. Advances in molecular embryology of left–right patterning in animal model systems must be integrated with insight gained from the unique contributions of clinical medicine in human patients. Continued progress in this fascinating field will shed light not only on the fundamental issues of evolutionary and cell biology, but also on the biomedical problem of prevention, detection, and repair of birth defects of laterality.

ACKNOWLEDGMENTS

We thank Chris McManus, Ann Ramsdell, and other members of the left–right asymmetry community for many useful discussions. This work was supported by NIH grants GM-067227 and GM-07742, and American Heart Association Established Investigator Grant #0740088N to Michael Levin. and the A*STAR overseas Ph.D. scholarship from the Agency for Science and Technology (Singapore) to Sherry Aw. Part of this manuscript was written in a Forsyth Institute facility renovated with support from Research Facilities Improvement Grant Number CO6RR11244 from the National Center for Research Resources, National Institutes of Health.

REFERENCES

Adams, D. S., Robinson, K. R., Fukumoto, T. *et al.* (2006). Early, H$^+$-V-ATPase-dependent proton flux is necessary for consistent left–right patterning of non-mammalian vertebrates. *Development*, **133**, 1657–71.

Afzelius, B. A. (1985). The immotile-cilia syndrome: a microtubule associated defect. *CRC Crit Rev Biochem*, **19**, 63–87.

Aird, I. (1959). Conjoined twins. *B Med J*, **1**, 1313–15.

Beere, D., Hargreaves, J., Sperber, G. & Cleaton-Jones, P. (1990). Mirror image supplemental primary incisor teeth in twins: case report and review. *Pediatr Dent*, **12**, 390–2.

Bisgrove, B. W., Essner, J. J. & Yost, H. J. (1999). Regulation of midline development by antagonism of lefty and nodal signaling. *Development*, **126**, 3253–62.

Bisgrove, B. W., Essner, J. J. & Yost, H. J. (2000). Multiple pathways in the midline regulate concordant brain, heart and gut left-right asymmetry. *Development*, **127**, 3567–79.

Bisgrove, B. W., Morelli, S. H. & Yost, H. J. (2003). Genetics of human laterality disorders: insights from vertebrate model systems. *Annu Rev Genomics Hum Genet*, **4**, 1–32.

Bowyer, R., Stewart, K. M., Kie, J. G. & Gasaway, W. C. (2001). Fluctuating asymmetry in antlers of Alaskan moose: size matters. *J Mammal*, **82**, 814–24.

Brown, N., McCarthy, A. & Wolpert, L. (1991). Development of handed body asymmetry in mammals. *CIBA Found Symp*, **162**, 182–96.

Brown, N. & Wolpert, L. (1990). The development of handedness in left/right asymmetry. *Development*, **109**, 1–9.

Bruneau, B. G., Logan, M., Davis, N. *et al.* (1999). Chamber-specific cardiac expression of Tbx5 and heart defects in Holt–Oram syndrome. *Dev Biol*, **211**, 100–8.

Burdine, R. & Schier, A. (2000). Conserved and divergent mechanisms in left–right axis formation. *Genes Dev*, **14**, 763–76.

Burn, J. (1991). Disturbance of morphological laterality in humans. *CIBA Found Symp* **162**, 282–296.

Carton, A. & Rees, R. (1987). Mirror image dental anomalies in identical twins. *Br Dent J*, **162**, 193–4.

Clericuzio, C. L. (1993). Clinical phenotypes and Wilms tumor. *Med Pediatr Oncol*, **21**, 182–7.

Cockayne, E. (1938). The genetics of transposition of the viscera. *Quart J Med*, **31**, 479–93.

Concha, M. L., Burdine, R. D., Russell, C., Schier, A. F. & Wilson, S. W. (2000). A nodal signaling pathway regulates the laterality of neuroanatomical asymmetries in the zebrafish forebrain. *Neuron*, **28**, 399–409.

Cooke, J. (2004). The evolutionary origins and significance of vertebrate left–right organisation. *Bioessays*, **26**, 413–21.

Cote, F., Fligny, C., Bayard, E. *et al.* (2007). Maternal serotonin is crucial for murine embryonic development. *Proc Natl Acad Sci USA*, **104**, 329–34.

Cuniff, C., Jones, K., Jones, M. *et al.* (1988). Laterality defects in conjoined twins: implications for normal asymmetry in human embryogenesis. *Am J Med Genet*, **31**, 669–77.

Danilchik, M. V., Brown, E. E. & Riegert, K. (2006). Intrinsic chiral properties of the Xenopus egg cortex: an early indicator of left–right asymmetry? *Development*, **133**, 4517–26.

Danos, M. C. & Yost, H. J. (1995). Linkage of cardiac left–right asymmetry and dorsal–anterior development in Xenopus. *Development*, **121**, 1467–74.

Delaney, M. & Boyd, T. K. (2007). Case report of unilateral clefting: is sonic hedgehog to blame? *Pediatr Dev Pathol*, **10**, 117–20.

Delhaas, T., Arts, T., Bovendeerd, P. H., Prinzen, F. W. & Reneman, R. S. (1993). Subepicardial fiber strain and stress as related to left ventricular pressure and volume. *Am J Physiol*, **264**, H1548–59.

Delhaas, T., Decaluwe, W., Rubbens, M., Kerckhoffs, R. & Arts, T. (2004). Cardiac fiber orientation and the left–right asymmetry determining mechanism. *Ann NY Acad Sci*, **1015**, 190–201.

Duboc, V., Rottinger, E., Lapraz, F., Besnardeau, L. & Lepage, T. (2005). Left–right asymmetry in the sea urchin embryo is regulated by nodal signaling on the right side. *Dev Cell*, **9**, 147–58.

Esser, A. T., Smith, K. C., Weaver, J. C. & Levin, M. (2006). Mathematical model of morphogen electrophoresis through gap junctions. *Dev Dyn*, **235**, 2144–59.

Essner, J. J., Amack, J. D., Nyholm, M. K., Harris, E. B. & Yost, H. J. (2005). Kupffer's vesicle is a ciliated organ of asymmetry in the zebrafish embryo that initiates left–right development of the brain, heart and gut. *Development*, **132**, 1247–60.

Essner, J. J., Branford, W. W., Zhang, J. & Yost, H. J. (2000). Mesendoderm and left–right brain, heart and gut development are differentially regulated by pitx2 isoforms. *Development*, **127**, 1081–93.

Fraumeni, J. F., Jr., Geiser, C. F. & Manning, M. D. (1967). Wilms' tumor and congenital hemihypertrophy: report of five new cases and review of literature. *Pediatrics*, **40**, 886–99.

Fukumoto, T., Blakely, R. & Levin, M. (2005a). Serotonin transporter function is an early step in left–right patterning in chick and frog embryos. *Dev Neurosci*, **27**, 349–63.

Fukumoto, T., Kema, I. P. & Levin, M. (2005b) Serotonin signaling is a very early step in patterning of the left–right axis in chick and frog embryos. *Curr Biol*, **15**, 794–803.

Gebbia, M., Ferrero, G. B., Pilia, G. *et al.* (1997). X-linked situs abnormalities result from mutations in ZIC3. *Nat Genet*, **17**, 305–8.

Gedda, L., Brenci, G., Franceschetti, A., Talone, C. & Ziparo, R. (1981). Study of mirror imaging in twins. *Prog Clin Biol Res*, **69A**, 167–8.

Govind, C. K. (1992). Claw asymmetry in lobsters: case study in developmental neuroethology. *J Neurobiol*, **23**, 1423–45.

Guo, N., Hawkins, C. & Nathans, J. (2004). Frizzled6 controls hair patterning in mice. *Proc Natl Acad Sci USA*, **101**, 9277–81.

Guthrie, S. C. (1984). Patterns of junctional communication in the early amphibian embryo. *Nature*, **311**, 149–51.

Harland, R. & Gerhart, J. (1997). Formation and function of Spemann's organizer. *Annu Rev Cell Dev Biol*, **13**, 611–67.

Hatcher, C. J., Goldstein, M. M., Mah, C. S., Delia, C. S. & Basson, C. T. (2000). Identification and localization of TBX5 transcription factor during human cardiac morphogenesis. *Dev Dyn*, **219**, 90–5.

Hibino, T., Ishii, Y., Levin, M. & Nishino, A. (2006). Ion flow regulates left–right asymmetry in sea urchin development. *Dev Genes Evol*, **216**, 265–76.

Hirokawa, N., Tanaka, Y., Okada, Y. & Takeda, S. (2006). Nodal flow and the generation of left–right asymmetry. *Cell*, **125**, 33–45.

James, W. (1983). Twinning, handedness, and embryology. *Percept Mot Skills*, **56**, 721–2.

Jefferies, R. P. S., Brown, N. A. & Daley, P. E. J. (1996). The early phylogeny of chordates and echinoderms and the origin of chordate left–right asymmetry and bilateral symmetry. *Acta Zool (Stockholm)*, **77**, 101–22.

Kapur, R., Jack, R. & Siebert, J. (1994). Diamniotic placentation associated with omphalopagus conjoined twins. *Am J Med Genet*, **52**, 188–95.

Kawakami, Y., Raya, A., Raya, R. M., Rodriguez-Esteban, C. & Belmonte, J. C. (2005). Retinoic acid signalling links left–right asymmetric patterning and bilaterally symmetric somitogenesis in the zebrafish embryo. *Nature*, **435**, 165–71.

Kennedy, D., O'Craven, K., Ticho, B. *et al.* (1999). Structural and functional brain asymmetries in human situs inversus totalis. *Neurology*, **53**, 1260–5.

Kloeppel, R., Rothe, K., Hoermann, D. *et al.* (2002). Proteus syndrome. *J Comput Assist Tomogr*, **26**, 262–5.

Kosaki, K. & Casey, B. (1998). Genetics of human left–right axis malformations. *Semin Cell Dev Biol*, **9**, 89–99.

Krzelj, V., Kragic, I., Glavina-Durdov, M. *et al.* (2000). Ivemark syndrome: asplenia with kidney collecting duct cysts and polysplenia with cerebellar cyst. *Turk J Pediatr*, **42**, 234–8.

Layton, W. M., Jr. (1976). Random determination of a developmental process: reversal of normal visceral asymmetry in the mouse. *J Hered*, **67**, 336–8.

Layton, W. M., Jr. (1978). Heart malformations in mice homozygous for a gene causing situs inversus. *Birth Defects Orig Artic Ser*, **14**, 277–93.

Leung, A. K., Fong, J. H. & Leong, A. G. (2002). Hemihypertrophy. *J R Soci Health*, **122**, 24–7.

Levin, M. (1997). Left–right asymmetry in vertebrate embryogenesis. *Bioessays*, **19**, 287–96.

Levin, M. (1998). Left–right asymmetry and the chick embryo. *Semin Cell Dev Biol*, **9**, 67–76.

Levin, M. (2004). The embryonic origins of left–right asymmetry. *Crit Rev Oral Biol Med*, **15**, 197–206.

Levin, M. (2005). Left–right asymmetry in embryonic development: a comprehensive review. *Mech Dev*, **122**, 3–25.

Levin, M. (2006). Is the early left–right axis like a plant, a kidney, or a neuron? The integration of physiological signals in embryonic asymmetry. *Birth Defects Res C Embryo Today*, **78**, 191–223.

Levin, M., Buznikov, G. A. & Lauder, J. M. (2006). Of minds and embryos: left–right asymmetry and the serotonergic controls of pre-neural morphogenesis. *Dev Neurosci*, **28**, 171–85.

Levin, M., Johnson, R., Stern, C., Kuehn, M. & Tabin, C. (1995). A molecular pathway determining left–right asymmetry in chick embryogenesis. *Cell*, **82**, 803–14.

Levin, M. & Mercola, M. (1998). Gap junctions are involved in the early generation of left–right asymmetry. *Dev Biol*, **203**, 90–105.

Levin, M. & Mercola, M. (1999). Gap junction-mediated transfer of left–right patterning signals in the early chick blastoderm is upstream of Shh asymmetry in the node. *Development*, **126**, 4703–14.

Levin, M. & Palmer, A. R. (2007). Left–right patterning from the inside out: widespread evidence for intracellular control. *Bioessays*, **29**, 271–87.

Levin, M., Roberts, D., Holmes, L. & Tabin, C. (1996). Laterality defects in conjoined twins. *Nature*, **384**, 321.

Levin, M., Thorlin, T., Robinson, K. R., Nogi, T. & Mercola, M. (2002). Asymmetries in H$^+$/K$^+$-ATPase and cell membrane potentials comprise a very early step in left–right patterning. *Cell*, **111**, 77–89.

Levy, J. & Levy, J. M. (1978). Human lateralization from head to foot: sex-related factors. *Science*, **200**, 1291–2.

Lewin, S. O. & Opitz, J. M. (1986). Fibular a/hypoplasia: review and documentation of the fibular developmental field. *Am J Med Genet Suppl*, **2**, 215–38.

Liang, J. O., Etheridge, A., Hantsoo, L. *et al.* (2000). Asymmetric nodal signaling in the zebrafish diencephalon positions the pineal organ. *Development*, **127**, 5101–12.

Lohr, J. L., Danos, M. C. & Yost, H. J. (1997). Left–right asymmetry of a nodal-related gene is regulated by dorsoanterior midline structures during Xenopus development. *Development*, **124**, 1465–72.

Lowe, L. A., Supp, D. M., Sampath, K. *et al.* (1996). Conserved left–right asymmetry of nodal expression and alterations in murine situs inversus. *Nature*, **381**, 158–61.

Marszalek, J. R., Ruiz-Lozano, P., Roberts, E., Chien, K. R. & Goldstein, L. S. (1999). Situs inversus and embryonic ciliary morphogenesis defects in mouse mutants lacking the KIF3A subunit of kinesin-II. *Proc Natl Acad Sci USA*, **96**, 5043–8.

McGrath, J., Horwich, A. L. & Brueckner, M. (1992). Duplication/deficiency mapping of situs inversus viscerum (*iv*), a gene that determines left–right asymmetry in the mouse. *Genomics*, **14**, 643–8.

McGrath, J., Somlo, S., Makova, S., Tian, X. & Brueckner, M. (2003). Two populations of node monocilia initiate left–right asymmetry in the mouse. *Cell*, **114**, 61–73.

McManus, I. C., Martin, N., Stubbings, G. F., Chung, E. M. & Mitchison, H. M. (2004). Handedness and situs inversus in primary ciliary dyskinesia. *Proc R Soc Lond B Biol Sci*, **271**, 2579–82.

Meinhardt, H. (2002). The radial–symmetric hydra and the evolution of the bilateral body plan: an old body became a young brain. *Bioessays*, **24**, 185–91.

Meno, C., Gritsman, K., Ohishi, S. *et al.* (1999). Mouse Lefty2 and zebrafish antivin are feedback inhibitors of nodal signaling during vertebrate gastrulation. *Mol Cell*, **4**, 287–98.

Meno, C., Saijoh, Y., Fujii, H. *et al.* (1996). Left–right asymmetric expression of the TGF beta-family member lefty in mouse embryos. *Nature*, **381**, 151–5.

Miller, S. & White, R. (1998). Right–left asymmetry of cell proliferation predominates in mouse embryos undergoing clockwise axial rotation. *Anat Rec*, **250**, 103–8.

Mittwoch, U. (2001). Genetics of mammalian sex determination: some unloved exceptions. *J Exp Zool*, **290**, 484–9.

Morison, D., Reyes, C. V. & Skorodin, M. S. (1994). Mirror-image tumors in mirror-image twins. *Chest*, **106**, 608–10.

Nakamura, T., Mine, N., Nakaguchi, E. *et al.* (2006). Generation of robust left–right asymmetry in the mouse embryo requires a self-enhancement and lateral-inhibition system. *Dev Cell*, **11**, 495–504.

Nerurkar, N. L., Ramasubramanian, A. & Taber, L. A. (2006). Morphogenetic adaptation of the looping embryonic heart to altered mechanical loads. *Dev Dyn*, **235**, 1822–9.

Neville, A. C. (1976). *Animal Asymmetry*. London: Edward Arnold.

Newbury-Ecob, R. A., Leanage, R., Raeburn, J. A. & Young, I. D. (1996). Holt–Oram syndrome: a clinical genetic study. *J Med Genet*, **33**, 300–7.

Nonaka, S., Tanaka, Y., Okada, Y. *et al.* (1998). Randomization of left–right asymmetry due to loss of nodal cilia generating leftward flow of extraembryonic fluid in mice lacking KIF3B motor protein. *Cell*, **95**, 829–37.

Nonaka, S., Yoshiba, S., Watanabe, D. *et al.* (2005). De novo formation of left–right asymmetry by posterior tilt of nodal cilia. *PLoS Biol*, **3**, e268.

Okada, Y., Nonaka, S., Tanaka, Y. *et al.* (1999). Abnormal nodal flow precedes situs inversus in iv and inv mice. *Mol Cell*, **4**, 459–68.

Okada, Y., Takeda, S., Tanaka, Y., Belmonte, J. C. & Hirokawa, N. (2005). Mechanism of nodal flow: a conserved symmetry breaking event in left–right axis determination. *Cell*, **121**, 633–44.

Olson, D. J., Christian, J. L. & Moon, R. T. (1991). Effect of wnt-1 and related proteins on gap junctional communication in Xenopus embryos. *Science*, **252**, 1173–6.

Opitz, J. M. & Utkus, A. (2001). Comments on biological asymmetry. *Am J Med Genet*, **101**, 359–69.

Oviedo, N. J. & Levin, M. (2007). Gap junctions provide new links in left–right patterning. *Cell*, **129**, 645–7.

Palmer, A. R. (2004). Symmetry breaking and the evolution of development. *Science*, **306**, 828–33.

Pasteur, L. (1860). Researches on molecular asymmetry. Alembic Club Reprint 14.

Patterson, K. D., Drysdale, T. A. & Krieg, P. A. (2000). Embryonic origins of spleen asymmetry. *Development*, **127**, 167–75.

Paulozzi, L. J. & Lary, J. M. (1999). Laterality patterns in infants with external birth defects. *Teratology*, **60**, 265–71.

Pennekamp, P., Karcher, C., Fischer, A. *et al.* (2002). The ion channel polycystin-2 is required for left–right axis determination in mice. *Curr Biol*, **12**, 938–43.

Potter, R. H. & Nance, W. E. (1976). A twin study of dental dimension. I. Discordance, asymmetry, and mirror imagery. *Am J Phys Anthropol*, **44**, 391–5.

Qiu, D., Cheng, S. M., Wozniak, L. *et al.* (2005). Localization and loss of function implicates ciliary proteins in early, cytoplasmic roles in left–right asymmetry. *Dev Dyn*, **234**, 176–89.

Ramsdell, A. F. (2005). Left–right asymmetry and congenital cardiac defects: getting to the heart of the matter in vertebrate left–right axis determination. *Dev Biol*, **288**, 1–20.

Raya, A., Kawakami, Y., Rodriguez-Esteban, C. *et al.* (2004). Notch activity acts as a sensor for extracellular calcium during vertebrate left–right determination. *Nature*, **427**, 121–8.

Rife, D. C. (1933). Genetic studies of monozygotic twins, III: mirror-imaging. *J Hered*, **24**, 443–6.

Rodriguez-Medina, M. A., Reyes, A., Chavarria, M. E. *et al.* (2002). Asymmetric calmodulin distribution in the hypothalamus: role of sexual differentiation in the rat. *Pharmacol Biochem Behav*, **72**, 189–95.

Sarkar, S., Prakash, D., Marwaha, R. K., Samujh, R. & Rao, K. L. (1992). Congenital hemihypertrophy and Wilms' tumor. *Indian Pediatr*, **29**, 1160–2.

Sarmah, B., Latimer, A. J., Appel, B. & Wente, S. R. (2005). Inositol polyphosphates regulate zebrafish left–right asymmetry. *Dev Cell*, **9**, 133–45.

Schilling, T. F., Concordet, J. P. & Ingham, P. W. (1999). Regulation of left–right asymmetries in the zebrafish by Shh and BMP4. *Dev Biol*, **210**, 277–87.

Schreiner, C. M., Scott, W. J., Jr., Supp, D. M. & Potter, S. S. (1993). Correlation of forelimb malformation asymmetries with visceral organ situs in the transgenic mouse insertional mutation, legless. *Dev Biol*, **158**, 560–2.

Schweickert, A., Weber, T., Beyer, T. *et al.* (2007). Cilia-driven leftward flow determines laterality in Xenopus. *Curr Biol*, **17**, 60–6.

Shimeld, S. M. & Levin, M. (2006). Evidence for the regulation of left–right asymmetry in *Ciona intestinalis* by ion flux. *Dev Dyn*, **235**, 1543–53.

Shiratori, H. & Hamada, H. (2006). The left–right axis in the mouse: from origin to morphology. *Development*, **133**, 2095–104.

Singh, G., Supp, D. M., Schreiner, C. *et al.* (1991). Legless insertional mutation: morphological, molecular, and genetic characterization. *Genes Dev*, **5**, 2245–55.

Smith, A. T., Sack, G. H., Jr. & Taylor, G. J. (1979). Holt–Oram syndrome. *J Pediatr*, **95**, 538–43.

Sommer, I., Ramsey, N., Bouma, A. & Kahn, R. (1999). Cerebral mirror-imaging in a monozygotic twin. *Lancet*, **354**, 1445–6.

Sommer, I. E., Ramsey, N. F., Mandl, R. C. & Kahn, R. S. (2002). Language lateralization in monozygotic twin pairs concordant and discordant for handedness. *Brain*, **125**, 2710–18.

Speder, P., Petzoldt, A., Suzanne, M. & Noselli, S. (2007). Strategies to establish left/right asymmetry in vertebrates and invertebrates. *Curr Opin Genet Dev*, **17**(4), 351–8.

Stalens, J. P., Maton, P., Gosseye, S., Clapuyt, P. & Ninane, J. (1993). Hemihypertrophy, bilateral Wilms' tumor, and clear-cell adenocarcinoma of the uterine cervix in a young girl. *Med Pediatr Oncol*, **21**, 671–5.

Sun, T., Collura, R. V., Ruvolo, M. & Walsh, C. A. (2006). Genomic and evolutionary analyses of asymmetrically expressed genes in human fetal left and right cerebral cortex. *Cereb Cortex*, **16** Suppl 1, i18–25.

Sun, T., Patoine, C., Abu-Khalil, A. *et al.* (2005). Early asymmetry of gene transcription in embryonic human left and right cerebral cortex. *Science*, **308**, 1794–8.

Sun, T. & Walsh, C. A. (2006). Molecular approaches to brain asymmetry and handedness. *Nat Rev Neurosci*, **7**, 655–62.

Supp, D. M., Witte, D. P., Potter, S. S. & Brueckner, M. (1997). Mutation of an axonemal dynein affects left–right asymmetry in inversus viscerum mice. *Nature*, **389**, 963–6.

Tabin, C. (2005). Do we know anything about how left–right asymmetry is first established in the vertebrate embryo? *J Mol Histol*, **36**(5), 317–23.

Tabin, C. J. & Vogan, K. J. (2003). A two-cilia model for vertebrate left–right axis specification. *Genes Dev*, **17**, 1–6.

Takeda, S., Yonekawa, Y., Tanaka, Y. *et al.* (1999). Left–right asymmetry and kinesin superfamily protein KIF3A: new insights in determination of laterality and mesoderm induction by kif3A-/- mice analysis. *J Cell Biol*, **145**, 825–36.

Tanaka, S., Kanzaki, R., Yoshibayashi, M., Kamiya, T. & Sugishita, M. (1999). Dichotic listening in patients with situs inversus: brain asymmetry and situs asymmetry. *Neuropsychologia*, **37**, 869–74.

Tanaka, Y., Okada, Y. & Hirokawa, N. (2005). FGF-induced vesicular release of Sonic hedgehog and retinoic acid in leftward nodal flow is critical for left–right determination. *Nature*, **435**, 172–7.

Torgersen, J. (1950). Situs inversus, asymmetry and twinning. *Am J Hum Genet*, **2**, 361–370.

Tsukui, T., Capdevila, J., Tamura, K. *et al.* (1999). Multiple left–right asymmetry defects in Shh(-/-) mutant mice unveil a convergence of the shh, and retinoic acid pathways in the control of Lefty-1. *Proc Natl Acad Sci USA*, **96**, 11376–81.

Vermot, J. & Pourquie, O. (2005). Retinoic acid coordinates somitogenesis and left–right patterning in vertebrate embryos. *Nature*, **435**, 215–20.

Voronov, D. A., Alford, P. W., Xu, G. & Taber, L. A. (2004). The role of mechanical forces in dextral rotation during cardiac looping in the chick embryo. *Dev Biol*, **272**, 339–50.

Wang, S., Yu, X., Zhang, T. *et al.* (2004). Chick Pcl2 regulates the left–right asymmetry by repressing Shh expression in Hensen's node. *Development*, **131**, 4381–91.

Wang, Y., Badea, T. & Nathans, J. (2006). Order from disorder: self-organization in mammalian hair patterning. *Proc Natl Acad Sci USA*, **103**, 19800–5.

Wang, Y. & Nathans, J. (2007). Tissue/planar cell polarity in vertebrates: new insights and new questions. *Development*, **134**, 647–58.

Whitman, M. & Mercola, M. (2001). TGF-beta superfamily signaling and left–right asymmetry. *Sci STKE*, **2001**(64), RE1.

Winer-Muram, H. (1995). Adult presentation of heterotaxic syndromes and related complexes. *J Thorac Imaging*, **10**, 43–57.

Yager, J. (1984). Asymmetry in monozygotic twins. *Am J Psychiatry*, **141**, 719–20.

Yost, H. J. (1991). Development of the left–right axis in amphibians. *Ciba Found Symp*, **162**, 165–76.

2

Cerebral lateralization in animal species

Onur Güntürkün

Summary

For a very long time, human cerebral asymmetries were thought to be unique. This view consequently requires that stable left–right differences of brain and behavior only emerged within the last few million years in the lineage leading to modern man. This assumption contrasts with a large number of recent reports on various asymmetries in animals. These data necessitate a completely new interpretation of the evolutionary events that resulted in the final pattern of human left–right differences of brain and behavior. This chapter attempts to provide an overview of animal asymmetries of handedness, spatial orientation, and communication. The aim of this review is twofold.

First, it will be shown that left–right differences are not only widespread among mammals but also among many other vertebrates. Thus, cerebral asymmetry is a ubiquitous phenomenon that possibly is not the exception but the rule. Second, the overview tries to reveal that in all three reviewed areas of asymmetry research the observations follow a consistent pattern. One aspect of this pattern is the fact that functional asymmetries mostly occur at the population level such that the majority of individuals are skewed into one direction. A further aspect of the consistent pattern becomes especially visible for asymmetries of communication: here, with few exceptions, a left hemispheric dominance can be seen that reaches from frog to man. Thus, not only cerebral asymmetry as such, but a certain pattern of left–right differences emerged during the evolution of vertebrates and is still visible in many species, including humans.

This overview makes it likely that cerebral asymmetries of anatomy and function have a history that stretches back at least several hundred million years. A brain architecture that is so old and can be found in so many different functional systems and forms of life must provide a solid selection advantage. The challenge of the future of the comparative analyses of asymmetry research will be to discover what this selection advantage is.

Introduction

Charles Darwin made a strong argument for continuity across species in both physical and psychological characteristics (Darwin, 1859; 1871). Around the same time, Pierre Paul Broca (1865) crucially advanced the principle of localization of function in the nervous system when he proposed that cerebral control for speech as well as for right-handedness lay in the left hemisphere. In combination, these two developments lent new significance to the possibility of animal laterality. Although both speech and handedness were seen as reaching their pinnacle of expression in humans, laterality itself ought not to be uniquely human. Thus, Broca (1877) assumed asymmetry to be possible in animals, noting that left–right differences of gyrification were very pronounced in man, but that "there is a less but still very evident degree of dysymmetry in the great apes" (p. 527) (Harris, 1989).

The general assumption of those times was that of a *scala naturae* – the natural staircase. Within this framework of thinking, evolution heads towards the more sophisticated, complex, intelligent, advanced representatives of the animal kingdom, leaving the clumsy previous forms behind. This long haul of nature finally culminates in humans. The less successful previous versions of life may survive in niches and can still be studied like specimens in a museum to testify to the inaptness of life before the arrival of *Homo sapiens*. Within this theoretical position, the presence of lateralized neural systems in humans makes cerebral asymmetries necessarily an advanced feature. According to the same logic, if non-human asymmetries exist, they

Language Lateralization and Psychosis, ed. Iris E. C. Sommer and René S. Kahn. Published by Cambridge University Press.
© Cambridge University Press 2009.

should be less profound and may be present in chimpanzees, our closest relatives. Since apes don't speak, only handedness remains as a tool to discover these lighter versions of left–right differences. As outlined below, the search for human-like handedness in apes was unsuccessful over a long period of time. The result of this frustrating search was the erroneous assumption that cerebral asymmetries must be a trait unique to humans. In bolder versions of this thought, asymmetries were even regarded as the critical evolutionary event that enabled us to achieve those cognitive abilities that truly separate us from the rest of life on our planet. In these theories that are still partly discussed today, the *scala naturae* persists.

The concept of the *scala naturae* is in its essence non-Darwinian and simply wrong (Hodos & Campbell, 1969). But as a consequence of this kind of thinking, studies on animal asymmetries halted for nearly a century, until the landmark paper of Nottebohm (1970) on song lateralization in chaffinches appeared. In 1985, Terry Robinson still soberly wrote: "With the exception of Nottebohm's … work on birdsong, research on behavioral and brain asymmetries in nonhuman animals is just in its infancy" (Robinson *et al.*, 1985, p. 187). Now, about 20 years after this sentence, the situation radically differs. We can now overlook a rich tapestry of studies that more and more begin to create a larger picture (Vallortigara & Rogers, 2005). Obviously, it is not possible to review this whole field within a book chapter. For readers interested in further details, the book of Rogers and Andrew (2002) is an excellent choice. Given the limited space, I will concentrate on three topics, handedness, spatial orientation, and vocalization. For all three systems, we have detailed knowledge on the behavioral and neural asymmetries in humans. In the end I will try to capture the details into a wider framework of cerebral asymmetries in animals, including humans.

Handedness

John Daniel led a life full of luxury at the end of the British Empire. During parties at his home in 15 Sloane Street, London, he was known for his perfect manners;

at 5 o'clock he never missed drinking a cup of tea and after dinner he always asked for a coffee. Apart from that he was known to be right-handed. This aspect of him was, probably, noted by his contemporaries only because John Daniel was not a human being but a gorilla (Güntürkün, 2002). The description of the life and death of John Daniel (Cunningham, 1921) is typical for a period of handedness research in animals that produced many anecdotes but fewer truly scientific papers. Additionally, since the preponderance of one hand, paw, or foot over the other during reaching or scratching is possibly the most easily observed aspect of laterality, most reports concentrated on these simple behavioral acts, ignoring that also in humans these behaviors produce, if at all, only a very mild handedness bias (Marchant *et al.*, 1995). However, a large number of sophisticated studies and major meta-analyses have been meanwhile published on this subject. As will be shown in the next paragraphs, these studies testify that many animals have limb preferences that partly resemble human handedness.

Handedness in primates

Great apes

Chimpanzees and bonobos from the genus *Pan* are our closest relatives. The orang-utan (genus *Pongo*) and the gorilla (genus *Gorilla*) are more distantly related. This genetic proximity was the reason why the handedness of these animals was studied so often. However, decades of observations that produced dozens of papers could until recently not produce conclusive evidence. While all observations were able to reveal individual asymmetries (most animals prefer one hand but the number of left- and right-handed individuals is about equal), a population level asymmetry (most animals prefer the same hand) was often not observed. Examples of these kinds of data are the studies on simple reaching in chimps ($n = 30$; Finch, 1941) and gorillas ($n = 31$; Annett & Annett, 1991). A further battlefield has been the distinction of apes in captivity and those in the wild. While an overview of a large data set gave evidence for population-level right-handedness in chimpanzees (Hopkins & Cantalupo, 2005), data from chimps in the wild were far less clear. Consequently, several authors argued that animals under captivity may copy the right-handedness of their caretakers, thus producing an arbitrary data pattern (McGrew & Marchant, 1997; Palmer, 2002). A third area of dispute is the behavior under study. In humans many activities with the hands involve simple behaviors such as picking or holding that do not show a pronounced right-sided bias (Marchant *et al.*, 1995). Similarly, analyzing only these simple activities in great apes could result in an underestimation of a possibly existing population asymmetry. Fourth, handedness in humans is hereditary for direction and strength (Carter-Saltzman, 1980), while in mice it was found to be only genetically transmitted for strength (Collins, 1985).

A recent meta-analysis that involved reports on 1524 great apes could clarify a good part of these open questions (Hopkins, 2006). This analysis revealed that, overall, great apes show population-level right-handedness. However, there were two important caveats. First, there were clear species differences with chimpanzees and bonobos displaying a significant right-hand preference, while orang-utans and gorillas showed no population-level asymmetry. Second, the overall effect size was relatively small. This could explain why smaller samples from previous reports were usually unable to reveal population asymmetries. Importantly, both captive and wild great apes were significantly right-handed; although asymmetry was more pronounced in captive animals (see also Lonsdorf & Hopkins, 2005). Thus, in the genus *Pan*, population-level asymmetry of hand use is not as pronounced as in humans, but it exists and is not an effect of simply copying the behavioral patterns of caretakers.

The picture becomes more interesting when looking into the details. Usually, many simple behavioral patterns that can most easily be observed (e.g., hit, hold, scratch, pluck, touch, etc.) were not lateralized. Significant right-handed asymmetries were instead mostly evident in more complex and fine-tuned behaviors such as throwing, bimanual feeding, grooming, pulling food out of a tube, and gesturing (Fig. 2.1). Thus, the failure of many studies to find asymmetries of hand use was probably mostly due to an over-representation of simple behavioral units in the data

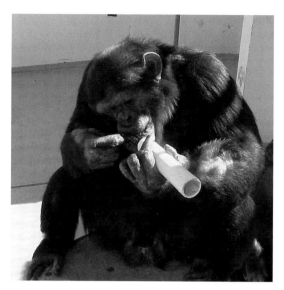

Figure 2.1 Chimpanzee during the coordinated bimanual tube task in which peanut butter is smeared on the inside of the tube. Most animals use the right hand to remove the peanut butter (courtesy of William D. Hopkins).

sample. Additionally, both in chimpanzees and bonobos strength and direction of hand preferences seem to run in families (Hopkins, 2006).

The population-level right-handedness in chimpanzees is associated with brain asymmetries. Hopkins *et al.* (2007a) discovered that chimpanzees show a population level leftward bias of their cortical gyrification that is modulated by handedness. In right-handed individuals this gyrification is even more geared towards the left hemisphere, while no left–right differences in the extent of cortical folding are present in non-right-handed chimps. Sherwood *et al.* (2007) additionally analyzed the fine structure of the primary motor cortex of 18 chimpanzees tested on a coordinated bimanual task before death. They found a higher neuronal density of layer II/III cells on the left side. Interestingly, Hopkins *et al.* (2007b) additionally revealed that the asymmetries in the homologs to Broca's and Wernicke's areas are associated with tool use. These results go along with similar data in humans (Steinmetz *et al.*, 1991) and may suggest that the neural substrate for tool use has served as a preadaptation for the evolution of language.

Monkeys

The situation in monkeys is probably comparable to that in great apes. In 1987 MacNeilage *et al.* published a target article in which they supposed that the early condition in the primate lineage consisted of a left-hand specialization for visually guided movements and a right-hand dominance for postural control and finer manipulation. In humans, they supposed, did the left-side reaching preference disappear while the right hand became dominant for all unimanual tasks. A few years later, Fagot and Vauclair (1991) published a new interpretation of the data from the literature and organized their review around the distinction between simple manual behaviors (picking, plucking, etc.) and more complex ones (adjusting an object into a frame, catching fish, etc.). Simple behaviors displayed individual- but no population-level asymmetry, while most of the more complicated ones evoked asymmetries at individual and population levels. When monkeys had to adjust their hand movements precisely to accomplish a fine-motor spatial task (object alignment in baboons: Fagot & Vauclair, 1988; haptic discrimination in rhesus macaques: Brown & Ettlinger, 1983; catching live goldfish in squirrel monkeys: King *et al.*, 1987; manipulation of a joystick in baboons: Vauclair & Fagot, 1993) a left-hand preference emerged. However, when monkeys had to extract food from a narrow tube (capuchin monkey: Spinozzi *et al.*, 1998; olive baboons: Vauclair *et al.*, 2005) or were gesturing towards other monkeys (olive baboons: Meguerditchian & Vauclair, 2006) a strong right-hand prevalence was recorded. This is similar to humans who also are more adept in fine spatial adjustments or haptic discriminations with the left hand (Fagot *et al.*, 1997), while being right-handed for other fine-motor tasks or for gesturing (Kimura, 1973).

Non-primate mammals

The issue of pawedness is far less settled in non-primate mammals. Tsai and Maurer (1930) were probably the first to analyze pawedness in rats. They described that virtually all animals had a preferred side but that no population bias towards one side was discernible. Collins (1985) revealed a similar pattern in mice. Other studies using more sophisticated techniques, however, could observe a population level right-pawedness both in rats (Güven *et al.*, 2003) and some strains of mice (Bianki, 1981; Maarouf *et al.*, 1999). The relation of pawedness to brain asymmetries was mostly studied by spreading depression, a potassium ion mediated self-propagating wave of cellular depolarization that is confined to a single hemisphere. Spreading depression of the left hemisphere is seen to result in larger motor decrements than that of the right hemisphere in mice (Bianki, 1981). Aydinlioglu *et al.* (2000) could additionally reveal in dogs that paw preferences were significantly related to the size of the isthmus of the corpus callosum, a finding that resembles the human pattern described by Witelson (1985). The studies of Tan (1987) and Wells (2003) make it additionally clear that dogs have population-level asymmetries of paw use that is sex dependent and additionally correlates with immune measures (Quaranta *et al.*, 2004). While males prefer the left paw, females go with the right.

Overall, several non-primate mammalian species have been shown to prefer one paw over the other in activities such as reaching or scratching. Different from the view prevailing in the 1980s (Walker, 1980), these issues of sidedness can not only be found at the individual but also at the population-level. The population level bias, however, is usually small.

Birds

Birds make counter-clockwise full body turns to escape the egg during hatching. The major force during this act is exerted by the right foot. Subsequent to hatching, domestic chicks, bobwhite, and Japanese quail chicks preferentially use the right foot to initiate ground scratching while searching for food (Rogers & Workman, 1993; Casey, 2005). Since ground scratching involves forceful behaviors, it is likely that the initially stronger foot is used. This population asymmetry of footedness persists into adulthood in several species of birds of prey that also have to strike by exerting strong forces (Csermely, 2004).

The situation is different for fine movement patterns. Friedman and Davies (1938) and Rogers (1980) revealed

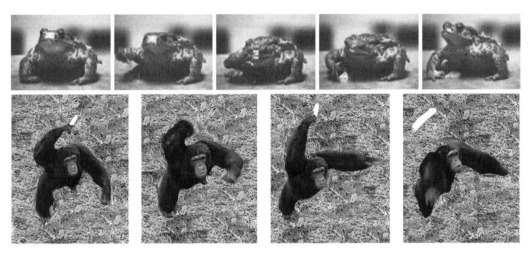

Figure 2.2 Above: video sequence of a toad (*Bufo bufo*) using the right claw to remove a sticky tape from the snout (courtesy of Giorgio Vallortigara). Below: picture sequence of a chimpanzee throwing a tube with the right hand (courtesy of William D. Hopkins).

a left-footed population asymmetry for food holding in 14, and a right-footed asymmetry in 2 Australian and South American parrot species. This result is reminiscent of an old report from Ogle (1871), who observed 86 parrots in the London Zoological Garden and reported that 63 of them preferred their left foot to hold and rotate a food item. Unfortunately, Ogle (1871) did not identify the species, such that his observation is of limited scientific value (Harris, 1989). Left-footedness was also observed for goldfinches when they are trained to manipulate doors to obtain a food reward (Dücker *et al.*, 1986). A further point where birds need fine movement control is during landing. Consequently, Davies and Green (1991) showed pigeons to strongly prefer their left foot when landing from flight.

Absence of footedness in birds has been obtained when testing the animals in tasks where no naturally specialized movement pattern is involved. For example, individual- and population-level footedness is absent in pigeons and budgerigars for removing adhesive tapes from the beak (Güntürkün *et al.*, 1988; Rogers & Workman, 1993).

Taken together, nearly two dozen avian species show a clear population asymmetry of footedness. The occurrence of this motor bias seems to depend on the need to either exert strong forces (right foot) or to use fine manipulations (left foot).

Amphibia

Some species of anurans use their front paws during feeding. Bisazza *et al.* (1997) used this behavioral pattern to test for pawedness by either wrapping a balloon around the head of the animals or by sticking a paper strip across the mouth. Toads of the species *Bufo bufo* tried to remove these objects preferentially with their right paws (Fig. 2.2), while no significant population level asymmetry was observed in *Bufo viridus*. A third anuran species tested, *Bufo marinus*, showed no population asymmetry in the ballon/paper-test but a population asymmetry for the right paw for righting when overturned on their back (Bisazza *et al.*, 1998). Thus, population-level right-pawedness exists in some anuran species for some tasks.

Summary of handedness studies with animals

Studying handedness in humans, Healey *et al.* (1986) discovered two kinds of lateralized behavior that seem to be controlled by different neural systems: (1) simple tasks such as reaching and carrying that require limited fine motor skills and have a relatively weak, or non-existent, lateralized bias at the individual or the population level, and (2) complex tasks such as throwing and writing that require considerably finer motor skills and have a relatively strong lateralized bias across the population. Summing up the evidence for limb dominances in animals it becomes evident that the distinction of Healey et al. (1986) describes not only the human condition but the pattern throughout the animal kingdom.

If species only use their extremities for locomotion or if they are tested with extremely simple tasks, only weak individual asymmetries without a population bias can be observed. The more demanding the motor output has to be, the more individual asymmetries with a clear population bias emerge. Presently it is unclear if there is a common motor theme that explains the different kinds of sidedness discovered in vertebrates. Equally likely, motor specialization could have independently evolved several times during evolution, such that, for example, the avian pattern has nothing in common with the primate condition.

Especially the need for fast, precise and strong actions (such as in striking or throwing) or fine and spatially guided manipulations (such as in pulling food out of crevices or in grooming) seems to promote the emergence of diverse hand or foot asymmetries. Within such a scenario, a species such as Homo sapiens naturally could not go without handedness including a clear population bias. If indeed the human condition does not differ in kind but only in quantity from the pattern of great apes, the question is, whether the extreme right-handedness of the human population is a true biological difference or the result of cultural evolution. Marchant et al. (1995) could not reveal much of an overall right-handed population bias when observing individuals of three preindustrial cultures. Right-handedness was only visible if the data pattern were analyzed for fine manipulations. Thus, it is in principle possible that cultural evolution created increasing demands for fine manipulation, thereby promoting right-handedness during ontogeny. By a snowballing effect that is also known from monkey hand use (Warren, 1977), increased right-hand use could have promoted the extreme right-sided population bias that characterizes Homo.

Asymmetries for spatial orientation

After Pierre Paul Broca (1865) published his landmark observations, the view of the major and the minor hemisphere was born. Since handedness and speech, the only known lateralized functions in those days, were both under left hemispheric control, Broca was interpreted as assuming a major role for this side of the brain. By default, the right hemisphere had to be the minor twin. According to Eling (1986), Broca himself was against such a view since he saw handedness and language as independent functions that were by chance both left-hemisphere based. But a lack of fluency in French prevented British, American, and German scientists reading Broca's writings in the original, paving the way to the century-long misunderstanding of the left brain side being the major hemisphere.

In 1917, Riddoch described the case of a British Captain who was wounded by a bullet that destroyed his right hemisphere when trying to attack the Turkish lines at the battle of Gallipoli. "His ability to orientate in space things he sees quite well is almost entirely lost..." (Riddoch, 1917, S. 45). At the same time German scientists made identical observations on the other side of the front. "...so ist sogar die Vermutung möglich, daß rechtshirnige Herde bei den Störungen der Raumbildung ein Übergewicht haben"; *It is even possible to conceive a dominance of right brain lesions for malfunctions of space conception* (Pötzl, 1928, S. 267–268, Poppelreuter, 1917). Today a general right hemispheric superiority in spatial functions is firmly established (Hugdahl & Davidson, 2002). However, spatial cognition is, like language, a toolbox with diverse functions and it is important to differentiate these and then try to map them onto the hemispheres. Indeed, Kosslyn (1987) suggested a dissociation of two kinds of spatial representations: categorical and coordinate, the former being computed by the left and the latter by the right hemisphere. In addition, with practice, a "categorization" of the coordinate computation was assumed to appear. This basic dichotomy has been expanded in the last years to cover further left and right hemispheric processes (Laeng *et al.*, 2003). In the following, I will review studies with diverse animal species that make functional asymmetries for spatial cognition likely, although not necessarily revealing a pattern like that proposed by Kosslyn (1987).

Mammals

Only a few spatial laterality studies with non-human primates are available. Unfortunately, none of them has tested spatial orientation during navigation but concentrated on visual pattern discriminations that contain a spatial component. Jason *et al.* (1984) tested macaques in a discrimination task between two squares, one containing a centered, the other an off-centered dot of varied amplitude. Then the splenium was transected along with a unilateral ablation of the left or right occipital lobe. Only monkeys with a left lesion were unable to discriminate small eccentricities. Dépy *et al.* (1999) conducted a similar task with baboons and also found a left-hemisphere advantage. This is clearly different from the expected right-hemisphere advantage in a visuospatial task. However, the monkeys could also use a category-based strategy ("centered" vs. "non-centered"), which also in humans would result in a left-hemisphere advantage (Kosslyn, 1987). This is different for the studies of Hamilton and Vermeire (1988) and Vogels *et al.* (1994) who showed that monkeys were better with the left hemisphere in discriminating between lines differing in orientation. Here, the data are truly discrepant to comparable results with humans (Corballis *et al.*, 2002). Within the framework of Kosslyn's theory, however, even these discrepant data between humans and monkeys can be reconciled if the vast differences in training time are considered. Usually, more than 1000 training trials were needed for the monkeys to meet the training criterion, while humans learned in less than 100 trials. The long training could facilitate categorical procedures for which the left hemisphere appears to be predominant. No study in humans has so far employed so many trials. The practice effect and its resulting hemispheric shift can be observed in some human studies after just a few dozen trials (e.g., Kosslyn *et al.*, 1989). In macaques

such a shift has also been demonstrated after extensive training (Doty *et al.*, 1999).

A completely different approach was taken by different authors when using haptic exploration studies. For example, Agnès Lacreuse gave capuchin monkeys sunflower seeds hidden in crevices of various objects that could not be seen but haptically explored. Humans are superior in exploring the spatial details of unseen objects with the left hand (Fagot *et al.*, 1997). The same is true for capuchin (Lacreuse & Fragaszy, 1996), spider (Laska, 1996), and rhesus monkeys (Fagot *et al.*, 1991). Chimpanzees, however, depart from this result pattern and show higher performance measures with the right hand (Lacreuse *et al.*, 1999).

If rats are handled during the first weeks of life, a functional asymmetry in emotionality and spatial cognition emerges (Cowell *et al.*, 1999). Handled rats have a tendency to first turn left when being placed in an open field (Sherman *et al.*, 1980). This may indicate a right-hemispheric bias for spatial behavior, but it could also result from other lateralized processes. The experiment of Cowell *et al.* (1997) makes a spatial asymmetry more likely. Here, handled rats were tested in the Morris water maze with either the left or the right eye covered by a patch. Since more than 90% of the optic fibers cross at the optic chiasm in rats, most of the visual information from one eye crosses to the contralateral hemisphere. Cowell *et al.* (1997) discovered that male subjects with a right patch outperformed those with a patch on the left side. This result points to a right-hemispheric superiority of spatial navigation in male rats. For females, no clear left–right differences were discernable.

LaMendola and Bever (1997) showed that spatial navigation in rats is constituted by complementary specializations of both hemispheres. In their experiment they tested the effect of anesthetizing the left or the right whiskers. For rats, whiskers are an important source of information; they use whisker information to learn new pathways and to discriminate textures. By abolishing input from the left or the right whisker system it was shown that the left hemisphere of rats accesses a map-like representation during foraging, whereas the right hemisphere enables a rote path of a previously learned environment.

Birds

In birds, the optic nerves are nearly completely crossed. This anatomical condition enables the use of eye caps to study the performance of the animals with sight restricted to one eye, and so mainly the contralateral hemisphere. Different species of birds display right-eye (left-hemisphere) superiority during the discrimination of visual patterns (Güntürkün, 2002). In contrast to the left-hemispheric superiority in pattern learning, many studies could reveal a right-hemispheric advantage in spatial tasks. This was first shown by Rashid and Andrew (1989) who trained chicks to find food buried under sawdust at certain areas in an arena. When the chicks were tested monocularly, birds searched with their left eye in the critical areas, while those seeing with the right eye searched randomly.

The lateralized role of different spatial and non-spatial cues can be elegantly studied in food-storing birds during cache localization. Marsh tits store food in many caches, which they can retrieve days later with astounding accuracy (Shettleworth, 1990). To study lateralization of food storing and cache retrieval under controlled conditions, Clayton and Krebs (1994) used a room with four feeders that were distinguishable by their location and by markings that made them visually unique. Birds tested with eye caps were given parts of a nut in one of these feeders and were then removed for five minutes. During this interval, the location of the correct feeder was swapped with an empty one so that spatial and object cues could be dissociated. Then the animals were allowed to re-enter and to retrieve the rest of the nut. With the left eye (right hemisphere), marsh tits searched at the correct spatial location, while they relied on object specific cues using the right eye (left hemisphere).

Vallortigara and colleagues were able to uncover further details of spatial cognitive asymmetry in chicks. First, chicks were trained to find food in the center of a square-shaped arena by ground-scratching under sawdust. The position of the food was indicated by two different cues. The first, was the geometric position of the arena center. The second, was that conspicuous landmarks were placed somewhere in the arena, or provided as panels hung to some of the walls. By changing the form or the size of the arena, geometric orientation (room shape) could be tested. By altering the position of the landmarks and panels, orientation according to visual objects could be analyzed. Both geometry and landmarks turn out to be utilized for spatial memory (Tommasi & Vallortigara, 2004; Gray *et al.*, 2004) (Fig. 2.3). During geometric coding relations of objects (in this case the walls) have to be utilized. Landmark coding utilizes a conspicuous object and guides the search to a defined spot in space. Now let us consider what such studies on the asymmetry of these cognitive strategies have revealed in birds (see Vauclair *et al.* 2006 for a detailed review).

Geometric coding

Most studies reveal the relative predominance of the right hemisphere in utilizing the shape (geometry) of the environment (Kahn & Bingman, 2004; Vallortigara *et al.*, 2004; but see Nardi & Bingman, 2007). If the size of the arena is altered (Tommasi & Vallortigara, 2001), or if object and geometric cues contradict each other (Vallortigara *et al.*, 2004), chicks still search in the center with their left eye and therefore rely on room shape

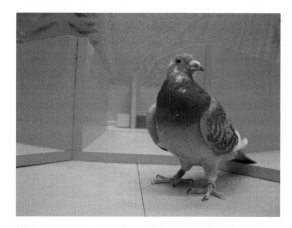

Figure 2.3 Pigeon tested in a radial maze where object cues (colors of the food containers visible at the end of an arm) and spatial cues (position of the arms within the room) are tested simultaneously (from Prior & Güntürkün, 2001). The cardboard fir tree at the back serves as one of the distant cues that is used to properly orient in the room.

with their right hemisphere. If pigeons are tested in complex, very large-scale arenas, alterations of the position of diverse landmarks do not interfere with orientation as long as the animals are using the left eye, indicating also in pigeons a right-hemispheric geometric processing of major room cues (Prior *et al.*, 2002). Hippocampal lesion studies in chicks reveal that encoding of global information actually occurs only in the right hippocampus (Tommasi *et al.*, 2003; Kahn & Bingman, 2004). Since hippocampal lesions are known to interfere with homing performance (Bingman *et al.*, 2003), it is possible that right hippocampal mechanisms aid homebound flights by using the relational position of stable and reliable spatial cues to construct a map-like representation (Vargas *et al.*, 2004; Kahn & Bingman, 2004; but see Nardi & Bingman, 2007).

Landmark coding

Chicks (Vallortigara *et al.*, 2004) as well as pigeons (Colombo & Broadbent, 2000; Prior & Güntürkün, 2001) can utilize various landmarks or other objects to guide their search for food. When geometric and landmark cues are brought into conflict, left-hemisphere chicks rely on landmarks (Tommasi & Vallortigara, 2001; Vallortigara *et al.*, 2004). Similarly, right-eye pigeons significantly reduce their searching speed when major landmarks have been removed (Prior *et al.*, 2002). Unilateral forebrain lesions reveal that landmark coding seems to be mainly a property of the left hemisphere (Tommasi *et al.*, 2003; but see Nardi & Bingman, 2007). Although the hippocampus plays an important role in spatial navigation, birds are able to guide their search according to landmarks also without a functional hippocampus (Tommasi *et al.*, 2003).

When pigeons home from a distant release site over known territory to the loft, they display a clear right-eye advantage (Ulrich *et al.*, 1999), which does not seem to be due to a visual memory-based snapshot tracking that pursues visual features along their pre-learned route (Prior *et al.*, 2004). Wiltschko *et al.* (2002) could also show a right-eye superiority in magnetic orientation in robins. In birds, magnetic compass orientation is based on intraocular light-dependent processes involving photon absorption to singlet-excited states that form radical pairs (Ritz *et al.*, 2000).

As a result, a bird looking in different directions might "see" the magnetic field vector as a visual pattern on its retina that points into a constant direction. Thus, the magnetic field could be a true landmark that therefore is primarily analyzed by the visual system of the left hemisphere (Heyers *et al.*, 2007).

Plasticity of cerebral asymmetries

In birds, the ontogenetic plasticity of visual asymmetry can easily be reconstructed. Embryos of virtually all avian species bend forward in the egg and keep their head turned to the right, so that the right eye is exposed to light that is shining through the translucent shell, while the left eye is occluded by the body. Since brooding parents regularly turn their eggs and often leave their nests for short time periods, the embryo's right eye has a high probability to be stimulated by light before hatching (Buschmann *et al.*, 2006). Thus, it is conceivable that asymmetry of light stimulation is the key event leading to visual lateralization. Indeed dark incubation of chick and pigeon eggs prevents the establishment of visual lateralization in discrimination tasks (Rogers, 1982; Skiba *et al.*, 2002). It is even possible to reverse the direction of the behavioral and anatomical asymmetry by withdrawing the head of the chicken embryo from the egg before hatching, occluding the right eye and exposing the left to light (Rogers, 1990).

Since pigeons are altricial animals, the developmental plasticity of their visual pathways is prolonged and extends far into posthatching time (Manns & Güntürkün, 1997). Therefore covering the right eye of newly hatched pigeons for ten days reverses behavioral and anatomical asymmetries as tested up to three years later (Manns & Güntürkün, 1999). Thus, light stimulation asymmetry during a critical ontogenetic time span seems to be the trigger for avian visual asymmetry. Visual asymmetry in birds seems to be mediated through left–right differences in brightness between the eyes. These brightness differences are probably coded by mere activity differences between the left and right retinal ganglion cells since blocking retinal activity changes asymmetry (Prior *et al.*, 2004). The differences in retinal activity are probably translated at a central level in a lateralized release of growth hormones (Manns *et al.*, 2005).

These data reveal two different important aspects. First, the establishment of a functional asymmetry can proceed with the same principles of synaptic plasticity that are well known from other sensory or motor systems. Second, the key event of the avian visual asymmetry, namely the right-turn of the head during embryogenesis, is mediated by mechanisms outside of the visual system. Thus, avian visual asymmetry results from an epigenetic event during ontogenesis.

Summary of spatial orientation studies with animals

The studies reviewed in this chapter show that the hemispheres of mammals and birds contribute differentially to spatial cognition, although both sides are to some degree able to utilize the strategy of the other. The situation in primates is rather patchy and less settled compared to birds. Several studies revealed a role of the left hemisphere in visual discriminations involving a spatial component. This is contrary to what would be expected from humans. However, the monkey data might reflect a left hemisphere categorical strategy that emerges after intensive training. Experiments with primates during haptic discriminations mostly indicate a right-hemispheric advantage in stereognosis. This resembles the human pattern. Also studies with rats point to a dominance of the right hemisphere in spatial navigation.

The experiments with bird species show that spatial navigation requires different computational strategies of the left and right brain. The left hemisphere is mostly specialized to orient according to landmarks. The right hemisphere, on the other side, is able to utilize the shape of the room or the spatial relation of major objects to locate the goal. Both strategies work and probably both hemispheres complement each other during normal search bouts (Prior & Güntürkün, 2001) or non-spatial visual tasks (Yamazaki et al., 2007). But depending on certain circumstances, one strategy can be more useful than the other. In this case, we have to assume that a single hemisphere can temporarily be solely in charge of generating spatial orientation.

Asymmetries of communication

Soon after Broca's seminal contributions, some authors wondered if animals might have an asymmetry resembling human speech. Obviously, only humans are able to speak, but most animals communicate and they might do so asymmetrically. Cunningham (1892) studied the Sylvian fissure in humans, apes, and monkeys and discovered similar left–right differences in all of them. Kalischer (1905) decided on a different approach. He taught 60 parrots phrases like "Eins zwei drei, Hurra!" and then lesioned their left or right hemisphere. To his disappointment, lesion groups did not differ. Most of these initial attempts were soon forgotten and replaced by the assumption that cerebral asymmetries are uniquely human. Several generations later, studies on the asymmetry of non-human communication restarted after Nottebohm's (1970) demonstration of song asymmetry in chaffinches. The following account gives an overview on the results gathered since then.

Mammals

Primates

Several lines of evidence make a left-hemispheric superiority in the analysis and production of species-specific vocalizations in primates likely. Petersen et al. (1978) tested the ability of Japanese macaques to discriminate a communicatively relevant acoustic feature of their "coo" sound. This is a brief, very tonal sound that occurs during affinitive, contact-seeking behavior. Several kinds of coo-sounds exist. The smooth early high variant is mostly produced by estrous females soliciting males, while the smooth late high variant is used by all individuals for general contact-seeking. Japanese macaques were significantly better in discriminating these two variants with their right ear. A left-ear advantage emerged when the animals had to discriminate pitch as an orthogonal (and non-communicative) feature of the same vocalizations. In other monkey species for which the coo-sound is not part of their species-specific communication, no asymmetry was present. The results of Heffner and Heffner

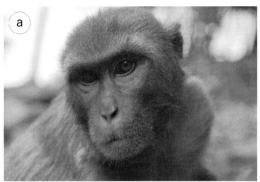
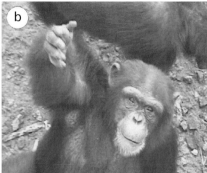

Figure 2.4 (a) Rhesus monkey turning its head towards the right side to listen to a species-typical call from the back (courtesy of Marc Hauser); (b) chimpanzees gesture more with the right hand, especially when vocalizing (courtesy of William D. Hopkins).

(1984) support these results by showing that lesions of the left, but not the right, temporal lobe reduce the ability of Japanese macaques to discriminate coo-sounds. Similarly, Poremba *et al.* (2004) showed that the left, but not the right, pole of the dorsal temporal cortex increased its local cerebral metabolic activity when the animals were listening to macaque-specific calls.

Hauser and Andersson (1994) tested 80 adult free-ranging rhesus monkeys squatting in front of an apparatus where they could obtain food. Occasionally sounds of either their own species-specific repertoire or from turnstones, a local seabird, were played from the back. Sixty-one of the eighty animals turned their right ear towards the loudspeaker when hearing sounds from the own repertoire, but favored the left ear when listening to turnstones (Fig. 2.4a). Infants less than a year old displayed no asymmetry. A further piece of evidence for left-hemispheric communication asymmetries comes from studies in baboons. These animals quickly and repetitively rub or slap their hand on the ground to threaten or intimidate other individuals. Baboons never do so without a social partner. Meguerditchian and Vauclair (2006) showed that mainly the right hand is used for this activity, and that right-handedness increases when the animals signal towards other baboons instead of towards humans. However, not all primates tested up to now have displayed a left-hemispheric dominance for communicative

sounds. Gil-da-Costa and Hauser (2006) showed that vervet monkeys display a left-ear (right-hemisphere) advantage for listening to species-specific vocalizations. Thus, an asymmetry of brain organization for communicative processes seems to be a general feature in primates, but not all species follow a left-hemispheric dominance.

The situation in chimpanzees is similar. Language-trained chimps only show a right visual field (left-hemisphere) advantage when being primed by a warning stimulus with a communicative meaning (Hopkins *et al.*, 1992). Like humans, they also gesture more with the right hand (Hopkins *et al.*, 2005) (Fig. 2.4b). This is especially evident when these gestures are accompanied by a vocalization. Even more interesting is the observation that the left inferior frontal gyrus (probably a homolog to Broca's area) is enlarged in those individuals that reliably employ their right hand for gestures (Taglialatela *et al.*, 2006). In chimpanzees, the equivalent of Wernicke's area is larger on the left side (Gannon *et al.*, 1998). The same is true for Broca's area in chimpanzees, bonobos, and gorillas (Cantalupo & Hopkins, 2001). Thus, brain areas that in humans are lateralized and language related show morphological asymmetries in non-speaking species. This probably implies that human language asymmetry results from a precursor that already had anatomical and functional asymmetries related to communication in a broad sense.

Non-primate mammals

A left-hemispheric superiority for communication is no primate specificity. Mice decrease their reactions to pups' ultrasound vocalizations when the right auditory meatus is closed (Ehret, 1987). Geissler and Ehret (2004) could show that the extent of activation of the auditory cortex of mice mothers listening to wriggling calls of mouse pups is larger on the left side. This difference was largely due to the labeling of an auditory association field that probably integrates call recognition with maternal responsiveness.

Böye *et al.* (2005) tested Californian sea lions with an experimental approach as used in monkeys. When the animals were resting on a platform at the pool, conspecific or non-conspecific calls were delivered from behind. Adult, but not infant, sea lions consistently turned their heads to the right when hearing conspecific calls. Control sounds did not evoke any consistent bias. Taken together, a left-hemispheric superiority in the analysis of communicatory sounds seems to be present in many mammals and can be shown in representatives of primates, rodents, and pinnipeds.

Birds

The modern era of lateralization studies in animals started with the landmark paper of Nottebohm (1970) on the asymmetry of song production in chaffinches. Songbirds have to learn their song from adult conspecifics within a critical period in early ontogeny. The song is produced by the flow of air past the elastic membranes of the syrinx. In chaffinches normal song consists of a series of notes, some of which regularly are combined to form distinct syllables. Motor input to the syrinx is provided bilaterally by the hypoglossal nerve. If the left hypoglossal nerve is sectioned in adult chaffinches, 81% of song elements disappear or are produced in a highly altered way. Right transsections produce effects only in 26% of the units (Nottebohm, 1970). This basic observation has been reproduced in canaries of the Waterschlager strain, Bengalese finches, as well as white-crowned, white-throated, and Java sparrows (Nottebohm & Nottebohm, 1976; Seller, 1979; Okanoya & Yoneda, 1995).

Lesions of central parts of the left forebrain song system disrupt singing much more than comparable lesions of the right side (Nottebohm *et al.*, 1976). That this asymmetry is not only due to the production of song but also its perception has been shown by Okanoya *et al.* (2001). They trained Bengalese finches to discriminate songs of Bengalese and zebra finches. Subsequent lesions of the left-hemisphere song system had a higher impact on discrimination ability than right-sided lesions. However, courtship singing involves not only song but also display, and involves a visually guided interaction with the other bird. Consequently, George *et al.* (2006) discovered that male zebra finches had higher levels of activated immediate early genes on the left side of their visual tectofugal system when singing to a female companion. Additionally, the hypoglossal nucleus, which contains the motor neurons that innervate the syrinx, is larger on the left side in canaries (DeVoogd *et al.*, 1991).

Up to now, the situation seems to indicate a straightforward pattern of left-hemisphere dominance for singing in song birds. Looking in greater detail, however, reveals a higher complexity. If not the Waterschlager strain of domestic canaries are chosen as experimental subjects but outbred strains from common canaries, no strong asymmetries are visible (Suthers *et al.*, 2004). This is partly due to the specialization of the left and right halves of the syrinx to lower and higher frequencies, respectively. Since Waterschlager canaries specialize in low frequencies due to a hereditary hearing loss, they rely more on left syringeal song production (Suthers *et al.*, 2004). Similarly, left- or right-sided lesions of the forebrain song system reduce the capacity to produce low or high frequencies, respectively (Halle *et al.*, 2003). Three conclusions can be drawn from these results. First, strain differences can importantly alter asymmetries. Second, part of the observed asymmetries in song production are due to simple peripheral factors in syrinx functions. Third, both left and right halves of the song system can specialize in different aspects of song production, although the contribution of the left side is still more important even in outbred common canaries.

This last conclusion does not fully apply to zebra finches. Here, lesions on the right side produce more pronounced asymmetries (Floody & Arnold, 1997), although both sides of the song system differentially contribute to the final song pattern (Cynx *et al.*, 1992). Similarly, left- and right-hemispheric song systems in starlings seem also to involve a specialization to long- or short-distance communication, respectively (George *et al.*, 2005). Also non-songbirds show a left-hemispheric bias when being confronted with conspecific vocalizations. When captive juvenile harpy eagles, aerial predators in the neotropics, are given conspecific or other sounds, they only turn their head to the right when hearing conspecifics (Palleroni & Hauser, 2003).

Amphibia

Bauer (1993) induced vocalizations in northern leopard frogs by clasping the animals behind the forelimbs. Animals with lesions in the neural vocalization system on the left produced less vocalizations than those with equivalent lesions on the right side.

Summary of studies on communication asymmetries in animals

Experiments on asymmetries in the perception and production of communicatory signals cover a wide range of species from chimpanzees to frogs. With few exceptions, most of these studies show a predominance of left-hemispheric mechanisms. This goes along with anatomical brain asymmetries in neural systems. Additionally, in several studies, a larger number of right-sided gestures could be observed that accompany vocalizations. While this picture holds for most animals studied, a few species are less lateralized (common canary) or even show a reversed asymmetry (vervet monkey, zebra finch). Such a rather consistent pattern that reaches from man to frog is highly unlikely to occur by chance. Instead, it points to common heritage with a long history that possibly dates back several hundred million years. Although human language is unique, its asymmetry probably is not.

Overall résumé

(1) Non-human animals have asymmetries of brain and behavior at the population level. This has been shown in *c.* 1000 scientific publications that were conducted on more than 50 different species. Human cerebral asymmetries with their typical population bias are in no way unique.

(2) At least some of the asymmetries reviewed above show a rather consistent pattern. This is especially visible for communication asymmetries. With more caution, this is to some extent also true for handedness and spatial orientation. This distribution can be used to trace certain asymmetries back in time. If the left dominance for vocalization in frogs is included in such an analysis, communication/vocalization asymmetries with left-hemisphere dominance have a history of at least 350 million years (Carroll, 1988). If only mammalian and avian data are considered, their common history dates back to a time between 250 million and 280 million years. In any case, we as a species have inherited a pattern of cerebral asymmetries to then develop our species-typical mechanisms of language, manual control, etc. onto this asymmetrical fundament. Theories that assume that first a human-unique asymmetry pattern had to occur before we could develop our species-typical neural functions are certainly wrong, at least for the systems discussed.

(3) There is no *scala naturae* of cerebral asymmetries. If it were to exist, we would expect apes to consistently show more clear-cut examples of functional and/or anatomical lateralizations than monkeys. Monkeys should be more asymmetric than non-primate mammals; and mammals should leave birds behind. This is not the case. The extent of population asymmetry in the preference of one limb over the other is larger in parrots than in apes. The data for communication asymmetries are equally compelling in birds and primates. The clearest evidences for asymmetries of spatial cognition do not come from chimpanzees but from domestic chicks and pigeons. The *scala naturae* is a pre-scientific, Aristotelian assumption. It has no place in today's enquiries on the structure and evolution of cerebral asymmetries.

REFERENCES

Annett, M. & Annett, J. (1991). Handedness for eating in gorillas. *Cortex*, **27**, 269–85.

Aydinlioglu, A. A., Arslanirli, K. A. & Riza, E. M. A. *et al.* (2000). The relationship of callosal anatomy to paw preference in dogs. *European Journal of Morphology*, **38**, 128–33.

Bauer, R. H. (1993). Lateralisation of neural control for vocalization by the frog (*Rana pipiens*). *Psychobiology*, **21**, 243–8.

Bianki, V. L. (1981). Lateralizations of functions in the animal brain. *International Journal of Neuroscience*, **15**, 37–47.

Bingman, V. P., Hough, G. E. 2nd, Kahn, M. C. & Siegel, J. J. (2003). The homing pigeon hippocampus and space: in search of adaptive specialization. *Brain, Behavior, Evolution*, **62**, 117–27.

Bisazza, A., Cantalupo, C., Robins, A., Rogers, L. J. & Vallortigara, G. (1997). Pawedness and motor asymmetries in toads. *Laterality*, **2**, 49–64.

Bisazza, A., Rogers, L. J. & Vallortigara, G. (1998). The origins of cerebral asymmetry: a review of evidence of behavioural and brain lateralization in fishes, reptiles and amphibians. *Neuroscience and Biobehavioral Reviews*, **22**, 411–26.

Böye, M., Güntürkün, O. & Vauclair, J. (2005). Right ear advantage for conspecific calls in adults and subadults, but not infants, California sea lions (*Zalophus californianus*): hemispheric specialization for communication? *European Journal of Neuroscience*, **21**, 1727–32.

Broca, P. P. (1865). Sur la siege de la faculté de langage articulé. *Bulletin de la Société d'Anthropologie, Paris*, **6**, 377–93.

Broca, P. P. (1877). De l'inégalité dynamique des deux hemispheres cérébraux. *Bulletin de l'Académie de Médicine*, **6**, 508–39.

Brown, J. V. & Ettlinger, G. (1983). Intermanual transfer of mirror-image discrimination by monkeys. *Quarterly Journal of Experimental Psychology*, **35B**, 119–24.

Buschmann, J.-U., Manns, M. & Güntürkün, O. (2006). "Let there be light!" Pigeon eggs are naturally exposed to light during breeding. *Behavioural Processes*, **73**, 62–7.

Cantalupo, C. & Hopkins, W. D. (2001). Asymmetric Broca's area in great apes. *Nature*, **414**, 505.

Carroll, R. L. (1988). *Vertebrate Paleontology and Evolution*. W. H. Freeman and Company.

Carter-Saltzman, L. (1980). Biological and sociocultural effects on handedness: comparison between biological and adoptive families. *Science*, **209**, 1263–5.

Casey, M. B. (2005). Asymmetrical hatching behaviors: the development of postnatal motor laterality in three precocial bird species. *Developmental Psychobiology*, **47**, 123–35.

Clayton, N. S. & Krebs, J. R. (1994). Memory for spatial and object-specific cues in food-storing and non-storing birds. *Journal of Comparative Physiology A*, **174**, 371–9.

Collins, R. L. (1985). On the inheritance of direction and degree of asymmetry. In S. Glick, ed., *Cerebral Lateralization in Non-Human Species*. Academic Press, pp. 150–64.

Colombo, M. & Broadbent, N. (2000). Is the avian hippocampus a functional homologue of the mammalian hippocampus? *Neuroscience and Biobehavioral Reviews*, **24**, 465–84.

Corballis, P. M. Funnell, M. G., & Gazzaniga, M. S. (2002). Hemispheric asymmetries for simple visual judgements in the split brain. *Neuropsychologia*, **40**, 401–10.

Cowell, P. E., Fitch, R. H. & Denenberg, V. H. (1999). Laterality in animals: relevance to schizophrenia. *Schizophrenia Bulletin*, **25**, 41–62.

Cowell, P. E., Waters, N. S. & Denenberg, V. H. (1997). The effects of early environment on the development of functional laterality in Morris maze performance. *Laterality*, **2**, 221–32.

Csermely, D. (2004). Lateralisation in birds of prey: adaptive and phylogenetic considerations. *Behavioural Processes*, **67**, 511–20.

Cunningham, D. F. (1892). *Contribution to the Surface Anatomy of the Cerebral Hemispheres*. Royal Irish Academy.

Cunningham, D. J. (1921). A gorilla's life in civilization. *Zoological Society Bulletin*, **24**, 118–24.

Cynx, J., Williams, H. & Nottebohm, F. (1992). Hemispheric differences in avian song discrimination. *Proceedings of the National Academy of Sciences of the USA*, **89**, 1372–5.

Darwin, C. (1859). *On the Origin of Species by Means of Natural Selection*. London: John Murray.

Darwin, C. (1871). *The Descent of Man*. London: John Murray.

Davies, M. N. O. & Green, P. R. (1991). Footedness in pigeons or simply sleight of foot? *Animal Behaviour*, **42**, 311–12.

Dépy, D., Fagot, J. & Vauclair, J. (1999). Processing of above/below categorical spatial relations by baboons (*Papio papio*). *Behavioural Processes*, **48**, 1–9.

DeVoogd, T. J., Pyskaty, D. J. & Nottebohm, F. (1991). Lateral asymmetries and testosterone-induced changes in the gross morphology of the hypoglossal nucleus in adult canaries. *The Journal of Comparative Neurology*, **307**, 65–76.

Doty, R. W., Fei, R., Hu, S. & Kavcic, V. (1999). Long-term reversal of hemispheric specialization for visual memory in a split-brain macaque. *Behavioural Brain Research*, **102**, 99–113.

Dücker, G., Luscher, C. & Schulz, P. (1986). Problemlöseverhalten von Stieglitzen bei manipulativen Aufgaben. *Zoologische Beiträge*, **29**, 377–412.

Ehret, G. (1987). Left hemisphere advantage in the mouse brain for recognizing ultrasonic communication calls. *Nature*, **325**, 249–51.

Eling, P. (1986). Speech and the left hemisphere: what Broca actually said. *Folia Phoniatica*, **38**, 13–15.

Fagot, J., Lacreuse, A. & Vauclair, J. (1997). Role of sensory and post-sensory factors on hemispheric asymmetries in tactual perception. In S. Christman, ed., *Cerebral Asymmetries in Sensory and Perceptual Processing*. Elsevier, pp. 469–94.

Fagot, J. & Vauclair, J. (1988). Handedness and manual specialization in the baboon. *Neuropsychologia*, **26**, 795–804.

Fagot, J. & Vauclair, J. (1991). Manual laterality in nonhuman primates: a distinction between handedness and manual specialization. *Psychological Bulletin*, **109**, 76–89.

Finch, G. (1941). Chimpanzee handedness. *Science*, **94**, 117–18.

Floody, O. R. & Arnold, A. P. (1997). Song lateralization in the zebra finch. *Hormones and Behavior*, **31**, 25–34.

Friedman, H. & Davis, M. (1938). "Left-handedness" in parrots. *Auk*, **55**, 478–80.

Gannon, P. J., Holloway, R. L., Broadfield, D. C. & Braun, A. R. (1998). Asymmetry of chimpanzee planum temporale: human-like pattern of Wernicke's brain language area homolog. *Science*, **279**, 220–2.

Geissler, D. B. & Ehret, G. (2004). Auditory perception vs. recognition: representation of complex communication sounds in the mouse auditory cortical fields. *European Jornal of Neuroscience*, **19**, 1027–40.

George, I., Cousillas, H., Richard, H.-P. & Hausberger, M. (2005). State-dependent hemispheric specialization in the song bird brain. *Journal of Comparative Neurology*, **488**, 48–60.

George, I., Hara, E. & Hessler, N. A. (2006). Behavioral and neural lateralization of vision in courtship singing of the zebra finch. *Journal of Neurobiology*, **66**, 1164–73.

Gil-da-Costa, R. & Hauser, M. D. (2006). Vervet monkeys and humans show brain asymmetries for processing conspecific vocalizations, but with opposite patterns of laterality. *Proceedings of Biological Sciences*, **22**, 2313–18.

Gray, E. R., Spetch, M. L., Kelly, D. M. & Nguyen, A. (2004). Searching in the center: Pigeons (*Columba livia*) encode relative distance from walls of an enclosure. *Journal of Comparative Psychology*, **118**, 113–17.

Güntürkün, O. (2002a). Ontogeny of visual asymmetry in pigeons. In L. J. Rogers and R. Andrew, eds., *Comparative Vertebrate Lateralization*. Cambridge: Cambridge University Press, pp. 247–73.

Güntürkün, O. (2002b). Hemispheric asymmetry in the visual system of birds. In K. Hugdahl and R. J. Davidson, eds., *Brain Asymmetry*, 2nd edn. Cambridge, MA: MIT Press, pp. 3–36.

Güntürkün, O., Kesch, S. & Delius, J. D. (1988). Absence of footedness in pigeons. *Animal Behavior*, **36**, 602–4.

Güven, M., Elalmis, D. D., Binokay, S. & Tan, Ü. (2003). Population-level right paw preference in rats assessed by a new computerized food-reaching test. *International Journal of Neuroscience*, **113**, 1675–89.

Halle, F., Gahr, M. & Kreutzer, M. (2003). Effects of unilateral lesions of HVC on song patterns of male domesticated canaries. *Journal of Neurobiology*, **56**, 303–14.

Hamilton, C. R. & Vermeire, B. A. (1988). Complementary hemispheric specialization in monkeys. *Science*, **242**, 1691–4.

Harris, L. J. (1989). Footedness in parrots: three centuries of research, theory, and mere surmise. *Canadian Journal of Psychology*, **43**, 369–96.

Hauser, M. & Andersson, K. (1994). Left hemisphere dominance for processing vocalizations in adult, but not infant, rhesus monkeys: field experiments. *Proceedings of the National Academy of Sciences of the USA*, **91**, 3946–8.

Healey, J. M., Liederman, J. & Geschwind, N. (1986). Handedness is not a unidimensional trait. *Cortex*, **22**, 33–53.

Heffner, H. E. & Heffner, R. S. (1984). Temporal lobe lesions and perception of species-specific vocalizations by macaques. *Science*, **226**, 75–6.

Heyers, D., Manns, M., Luksch, H., Güntürkün, O. & Mouritsen, H. (2007). A visual pathway links brain structures active during magnetic compass orientation in migratory birds. *Public Library of Science: One*, **2**, e937.

Hodos, W. & Campbell, C. B. G. (1969). The *scala naturae*: Why there is no theory in comparative psychology. *Psychological Review*, **76**, 337–50.

Hopkins, W. D. (2006). Comparative and familial analysis of handedness in great apes. *Psychological Bulletin*, **132**, 538–59.

Hopkins, W. D. & Cantalupo, C. (2005). Individual and setting differences in the hand preferences of chimpanzees (*Pan troglodytes*): a critical analysis and some alternative explanations. *Laterality*, **10**, 65–80.

Hopkins, W. D., Cantalupo, C. & Taglialatela, J. (2007a). Handedness is associated with asymmetries in gyrification of the cerebral cortex of chimpanzees. *Cerebral Cortex*, **17**, 1750–6.

Hopkins, W. D., Morris, R. D., Savage-Rumbaugh, E. S. & Rumbaugh, D. M. (1992). Hemisphere priming by meaningful and nonmeaningful symbols in language-trained chimpanzees (*Pan troglodytes*): further evidence of a left hemisphere advantage. *Behavioral Neuroscience*, **106**, 575–82.

Hopkins, W. D., Russell, J. L. & Cantalupo, C. (2007b). Neuroanatomical correlates of handedness for tool use in chimpanzees (*Pan troglodytes*): implications for theories on the evolution of language. *Psychological Science*, **18**, 971-7.

Hopkins, W. D., Russell, J., Freeman, H., *et al.* (2005). The distribution and development of handedness for manual gestures in captive chimpanzees (*Pan troglodytes*). *Psychological Science*, **16**, 487-93.

Hugdahl, K. & Davidson, R. J. (2002). *Brain Asymmetry*, 2nd edn. MIT Press.

Jason, G. W., Cowey, A. & Weiskrantz, L. (1984). Hemispheric asymmetry for a visuo-spatial task in monkeys. *Neuropsychologia*, **22**, 777-84.

Kahn, M. C. & Bingman, V. P. (2004). Lateralization of spatial learning in the avian hippocampal formation. *Behavioral Neuroscience*, **118**, 333-44.

Kalischer, O. (1905). Das Großhirn der Papageien in anatomischer und physiologischer Beziehung. *Abhandlungen der Preussischen Akademie der Wissenschaften*. IV, **1**, 1-105.

Kimura, D. (1973). Manual activity during speaking. Part I: right-handers. *Neuropsychologia*, **11**, 45-50.

King, J. E., Landau, V. I., Scott, A. G. & Berning, A. L. (1986). Hand preference during capture of live fish by squirrel monkeys. *International Journal of Primatology*, **8**, 540.

Kosslyn, S. M. (1987). Seeing and imagining in the cerebral hemispheres: a computational approach. *Psychological Review*, **94**, 148-75.

Kosslyn, S. M., Koenig, O., Barrett, A., *et al.* (1989). Evidence for two types of spatial representations: hemispheric specialization for categorical and coordinate relations. *Journal of Experimental Psychology: Human Perception and Performance*, **15**, 723-35.

Lacreuse, A. & Fragaszy, D. M. (1996). Hand preferences for a haptic searching task by tufted capuchins (*Cebus paella*). *International Journal of Primatology*, **17**, 613-32.

Lacreuse, A., Parr, L. A., Smith, H. M. & Hopkins, W. D. (1999). Hand preferences for a haptic task in chimpanzees (*Pan troglodytes*). *International Journal of Primatology*, **20**, 867-81.

Laeng, B., Chabris, C. F. & Kosslyn, S. M. (2003). Asymmetries in encoding spatial relations. In K. Hugdahl and R. Davidson, eds., *The Asymmetrical Brain*. Cambridge, MA: MIT Press, pp. 303-39.

LaMendola, N. P. & Bever, T. G. (1997). Peripheral and cerebral asymmetries in the rat. *Science*, **278**, 483-6.

Laska, M. (1996). Manual laterality in spider monkeys (*Ateles geoffroyi*) solving visually and tactually guided food-reaching tasks. *Cortex*, **32**, 717-26.

Lonsdorf, E. V. & Hopkins, W. D. (2005). Wild chimpanzees show population-level handedness for tool use. *Proceedings of the National Academy of Sciences of the USA*, **102**, 12634-8.

Maarouf, F. D. L., Roubertoux, P. L. & Carlier, M. (1999). Is mitochondrial DNA involved in mouse behavioural laterality? *Behavioral Genetics*, **29**, 311-18.

MacNeilage, P. F., Studdert-Kennedy, M. G. & Lindblom, B. (1987). Primate handedness reconsidered. *Behavioral and Brain Sciences*, **10**, 247-303.

Manns, M. & Güntürkün, O. (1997). Development of the retinotectal system in the pigeon: a choleratoxin study. *Anatomy and Embryology*, **195**, 539-55.

Manns, M. & Güntürkün, O. (1999). Monocular deprivation alters the direction of functional and morphological asymmetries in the pigeon's visual system. *Behavioral Neuroscience*, **113**, 1-10.

Manns, M., Güntürkün, O., Heumann, R. & Blöchl, A. (2005). Photic inhibition of TrkB/Ras activity in the pigeon's tectum during development: impact on brain asymmetry formation. *European Journal of Neuroscience*, **22**, 2180-6.

Marchant, L. F., McGrew, W. C. & Eibl-Eibesfeldt, I. (1995). Is human handedness universal? Ethological analysis from three traditional cultures. *Ethology*, **101**, 239-58.

McGrew, W. C. & Marchant, L. F. (1997). On the other hand: current issues in and meta-analysis of the behavioural laterality of hand function in non-human primates. *Yearbook on Physical Anthropology*, **40**, 201-32.

Meguerditchian, A. & Vauclair, J. (2006). Baboons communicate with their right hand. *Behavioural Brain Research*, **171**, 170-4.

Nardi, D. & Bingman, V. P. (2007). Asymmetrical participation of the left and right hippocampus for representing environmental geometry in homing pigeons. *Behavioural Brain Research*, **178**, 160-71.

Nottebohm, F. (1970). Ontogeny of bird song. *Science*, **167**, 950-6.

Nottebohm, F. & Nottebohm, M. E. (1976). Left hypoglossal dominance in the control of canary and white-crowned sparrow song. *Journal of Comparative Physiology A*, **108**, 171-92.

Nottebohm, F., Stokes, T. F. & Leonard, C. M. (1976). Central control of song in the canary, Serinus canaries. *Journal of Comparative Neurology*, **165**, 457-86.

Ogle, W. (1871) On dextral pre-eminence. *Lancet*, **54**, 279-301.

Okanoya, K., Ikebuchi, M., Uno, H. & Watanabe, S. (2001). Left-side dominance for song discrimination in Bengalese finches (*Lonchura striata* var. domestica). *Animal Cognition*, **4**, 241-5.

Okanoya, K. & Yoneda, T. (1995). Effect of tracheosyringeal nerve section on sexually dimorphic distance calls in Bengalese finches (*Lonchura striata* var. domestica). *Zoological Science*, **12**, 801-5.

Palmer, A. R. (2002). Chimpanzee right-handedness reconsidered: evaluating the evidence with funnel plots. *American Journal of Physical Anthropology*, **118**, 191–9.

Palleroni, A. & Hauser, M. (2003). Experience-dependent plasticity for auditory processing in a raptor. *Science*, **299**, 1195.

Petersen, M. R., Beecher, M. D., Zoloth, S. R., Moody, D. B. & Stebbins, W. C. (1978). Neural lateralization of species-specific vocalizations by Japanese macaques (*Macaca fuscata*). *Science*, **202**, 324–7.

Poppelreuter, W. (1917). *Die psychischen Schädigungen durch Kopfschuss im Kriege 1914/16 mit besonderer Berücksichtigung der pathopsychologischen, pädagogischen, gewerblichen und sozialen Beziehungen. I. Die Störungen der niederen und höheren Sehleistungen durch Verletzungen des Okzipitalhirns.* Verlag von Leopold Voss.

Poremba, A., Malloy, M., Saunders, R. C. *et al.* (2004). Species-specific calls evoke asymmetric activity in the monkey's temporal poles. *Nature*, **427**, 448–51.

Pötzl, O. (1928). *Die Aphasielehre vom Standpunkte der klinischen Psychiatrie. I. Die optisch-agnostischen Agnosien (die verschiedenen Formen der Seelenblindheit).* Franz Deuticke Verlag.

Prior, H., Diekamp, B., Güntürkün, O. & Manns, M. (2004). Activity-dependent modulation of visual lateralization in pigeons. *NeuroReport*, **15**, 1311–14.

Prior, H. & Güntürkün, O. (2001). Parallel working memory for spatial location and object-cues in foraging pigeons. Binocular and lateralized monocular performance. *Learning and Memory*, **8**, 44–51.

Prior, H., Lingenauber, F., Nitschke, J. & Güntürkün, O. (2002). Orientation and lateralized cue use in pigeons navigating a large indoor environment. *Journal of Experimental Biology*, **205**, 1795–805.

Prior, H., Wiltschko, R., Stapput, K., Güntürkün, O. & Wiltschko, W. (2004). Visual lateralization and homing in pigeons. *Behavioural Brain Research*, **154**, 301–10.

Quaranta, A., Siniscalchi, M., Frate, A. & Vallortigara, G. (2004). Paw preference in dogs: Relations between lateralised behaviour and immunity. *Behavioural Brain Research*, **153**, 521–5.

Rashid, N. & Andrew, R. J. (1989). Right hemisphere advantage for topographic orientation in the domestic chick. *Neuropsychologia*, **27**, 937–48.

Riddoch, G. (1917). Dissociation of visual perceptions due to occipital injuries, with especial reference to appreciation of movement. *Brain*, **40**, 15–57.

Ritz, T., Adem, S. & Schulten, K. (2000). A model for photoreceptor-based magnetoreception in birds. *Biophysical Journal*, **78**, 707–18.

Robinson, T. E., Becker, J. B., Camp, D. M. & Mansour, A. (1985). Variation in the pattern of behavioral and brain asymmetries due to sex differences. In S. D. Glick, ed., *Cerebral Lateralization in Nonhuman Species*. New York: Academic Press, pp. 185–231.

Rogers, L. J. (1980). Lateralisation in the avian brain. *Bird Behaviour*, **2**, 1–12.

Rogers, L. J. (1982). Light experience and asymmetry of brain function in chickens. *Nature*, **297**, 223–5.

Rogers, L. J. (1990). Light input and the reversal of functional lateralization in the chicken brain. *Behavioural Brain Research*, **38**, 211–21.

Rogers, L. J. & Andrew, R. (2002). *Comparative Vertebrate Lateralization*. Cambridge: Cambridge University Press.

Rogers, L. J. & Workman, L. (1993). Footedness in birds. *Animal Behaviour*, **45**, 409–11.

Seller, T. J. (1979). Unilateral nervous control of the syrinx in Java sparrows. *Journal of Comparative Physiology: A*, **129**, 281–8.

Sherman, G. F., Garbanati, J. A., Rosen, G. D., Yutzev, D. A. & Denenberg, V. H. (1980). Brain and behavioral asymmetries for spatial preference in rats. *Brain Research*, **16**, 61–7.

Sherwood, C. C., Wahl, E., Erwin, J. M., Hof, P. R. & Hopkins, W. D. (2007). Histological asymmetries of primary motor cortex predict handedness in chimpanzees (*Pan troglodytes*). *Journal of Comparative Neurology*, **503**, 525–37.

Shettleworth, S. J. (1990). Spatial memory in food-storing birds. *Philosophical Transactions of the Royal Society of London B*, **329**, 143–51.

Skiba, M., Diekamp, B. & Güntürkün, O. (2002). Embryonic light stimulation induces different asymmetries in visuoperceptual and visuomotor pathways of pigeons. *Behavioural Brain Research*, **134**, 149–56.

Spinozzi, G., Castornina, M. G. & Truppa, V. (1998). Hand preferences in unimanual and coordinated-bimanual tasks by tufted capuchin monkeys (*Cebus apella*). *Journal of Comparative Psychology*, **112**, 183–91.

Steinmetz, H., Volkmann, J., Jäncke, L. & Freund, H. J. (1991). Anatomical left-right asymmetry of language-related temporal cortex is different in left- and right-handers. *Annals of Neurology*, **29**, 315–19.

Suthers, R. A., Vallet, E., Tanvez, A. & Kreutzer, M. (2004). Bilateral song production in domestic canaries. *Journal of Neurobiology*, **60**, 381–93.

Taglialatela, J. P., Canatalupo, C. & Hopkins, W. D. (2006). Gesture handedness predicts asymmetry in the chimpanzee inferior frontal gyrus. *NeuroReport*, **17**, 923–7.

Tan, Ü. (1987). Paw preference in dogs. *International Journal of Neuroscience*, **32**, 825–9.

Tommasi, L., Gagliardo, A., Andrew, R. J. & Vallortigara, G. (2003). Separate processing mechanisms for encoding of geometric and landmark information in the avian hippocampus. *European Journal of Neuroscience*, **17**, 1695–702.

Tommasi, L. & Vallortigara, G. (2001). Encoding of geometric and landmark information in the left and right hemispheres of the avian brain. *Behavioral Neuroscience*, **115**, 602–13.

Tommasi, L. & Vallortigara, G. (2004). Hemispheric processing of landmark and geometric information in male and female domestic chicks (*Gallus gallus*). *Behavioural Brain Research*, **155**, 85–96.

Tsai, L. S. & Maurer, S. (1930). "Right-handedness" in white rats. *Science*, **72**, 436–8.

Ulrich, C., Prior, H., Duka, T., *et al.* (1999). Left-hemispheric superiority for visuospatial orientation in homing pigeons. *Behavioural Brain Research*, **104**, 169–78.

Vallortigara, G., Pagni, P. & Sovrano, V. A. (2004). Separate geometric and non-geometric modules for spatial reorientation: evidence from a lopsided animal brain. *Journal of Cognitive Neuroscience*, **16**, 390–400.

Vallortigara, G. & Rogers, L. J. (2005). Survival with an asymmetrical brain: advantages and disadvantages of cerebral lateralization. *Behavioral and Brain Sciences*, **28**, 578–89.

Vargas, J. P., Petruso, E. J. & Bingman, V. P. (2004). Hippocampal formation is required for geometric navigation in pigeons. *European Journal of Neuroscience*, **20**, 1937–44.

Vauclair, J. & Fagot, J. (1993). Manual and hemispheric specialization in the manipulation of a joystick by baboons (*Papio papio*). *Behavioral Neuroscience*, **107**, 210–14.

Vauclair, J., Meguerditchian, A. & Hopkins, W. D. (2005). Hand preferences for unimanual and coordinated bimanual tasks in baboons (*Papio anubis*). *Cognitive Brain Research*, **25**, 210–16.

Vauclair, J., Yamazaki, Y. & Güntürkün, O. (2006). The study of hemispheric specialization for categorical and coordinate spatial relations in animals. *Neuropsychologia*, **44**, 1524–34.

Vogels, R., Saunders, R. C. & Orban, G. A. (1994). Hemispheric lateralization in rhesus monkeys can be task-dependent. *Neuropsychologia*, **32**, 425–38.

Walker, S. F. (1980). Lateralization of functions in the vertebrate brain: a review. *British Journal of Psychology*, **71**, 329–67.

Warren, J. M. (1977). Handedness and cerebral dominance in monkeys. In S. Harnad, R. W. Doty, L. Goldstein, J. Jaynes and G. Krauthamer, eds., *Lateralization in the Nervous System*. New York: Academic Press.

Wells, D. L. (2003). Lateralised behaviour in the domestic dog, *Canis familiaris*. *Behavioural Processes*, **61**, 27–35.

Wiltschko, W., Traudt, J., Güntürkün, O., Prior, H. & Wiltschko, R. (2002). Lateralization of magnetic compass orientation in a migratory bird. *Nature*, **419**, 467–70.

Witelson, S. F. (1985). The brain connection: the corpus callosum is larger in left handers. *Science*, **229**, 665–8.

Yamazaki, Y., Aust, U., Huber, L. & Güntürkün, O. (2007). Lateralized cognition: asymmetrical and complementary strategies of pigeons during discrimination of the "human" concept. *Cognition*, **104**, 315–44.

3

The history and geography of human handedness

I. C. McManus

Summary

About 90% of people are right-handed and 10% are left-handed. Handedness is associated with functional lateralization for cerebral dominance, and may also be associated with various types of psychopathology. Broadly speaking, the vast majority of humans seem to have been right-handed since the emergence of the genus *Homo*, some three to four million years ago. Likewise, in all societies studied, there is a large excess of right-handers. However, there have been few studies exploring the detailed history and geography of handedness, not least because adequate pre-twentieth-century historical data are difficult to find, and very large sample sizes with consistent measurement methods are required for geographical studies. This chapter overviews the various sets of data that provide insight into handedness's history and geography.

It is probable that about 8% to 10% of the population has been left-handed for at least the past 200 000 years or so. Detailed data only began to become available for those born in the nineteenth century, and there is growing evidence that the rate of left-handedness fell precipitously during the Victorian period, reaching a nadir of about 3% in about 1895 or so, and then rising quite quickly until an asymptote is reached for those born after about 1945 to 1950, with 11% to 12% of men and 9% to 10% of women typically being left-handed in Western countries. The sex ratio seems to remain constant, not only during historical changes but also with geographical differences, and is presumably the result of a biological rather than a cultural process.

Geographical differences in handedness are clearly apparent both between continents (as in Singh & Bryden's, 1994, comparison of Canada and India) and within continents: rates in Europe seeming to be highest in Britain, Holland, and Belgium, and falling away towards the east and south, and within countries, seen well in Stier's (1911) study of the German Army, in Leask and Beaton's (2007) study of the United Kingdom, and between the various states of the USA, in the very large Gilbert and Wysocki (1992) database.

Ethnic differences in handedness are related to geographical differences, with left-handedness generally being more common in White, Asian and Hispanic populations – a difference seen both in the UK, and historically in the United States, where the difference between ethnic groups has grown smaller during the twentieth century, but was still present even for those born in the 1970s. Migration studies in the UK show that the lower rate of left-handedness in those from the Indian sub-continent is similar in those born in the UK and those born outside the UK, implying that genes rather than environment are the primary source of the difference.

Different rates of left-handedness can reflect either environmental or genetic differences between societies, and rates alone cannot distinguish the two processes. However, a mathematical model shows that effects of different social pressure or gene frequencies can be distinguished if family data on handedness are available. That model suggests not only that geographical differences but also historical differences primarily reflect changes in gene frequency rather than direct social pressure.

Introduction

The important discoveries of Dax and Broca in the nineteenth century showed that human brains are functionally asymmetric, most people processing language in their left hemisphere (Finger, 1994; Finger & Roe, 1999). However, it soon also became clear that a minority of people process language with their right hemisphere (Harris, 1991; Harris, 1993a), so that language processing can be seen as what geneticists call a

Language Lateralization and Psychosis, ed. Iris E. C. Sommer and René S. Kahn. Published by Cambridge University Press.

polymorphism, there being two qualitatively different types, akin to human blood groups. Since at least the beginnings of recorded history, and probably long before, people have also noted that while most people are right-handed, a minority of individuals are the opposite way around, being left-handed. Handedness and language dominance also show a moderate correlation, although the pattern is somewhat counter-intuitive, about 5% to 6% of right-handers showing right hemisphere language dominance, compared with about 30% to 35% of left-handers.

Language dominance is not easy to assess reliably in large populations, with techniques such as functional Magnetic Resonance Imaging (fMRI) (Pujol *et al.*, 1999) or transcranial Doppler (Knecht *et al.*, 2000) requiring complex technology that is expensive and not particularly portable, while dichotic listening and tachistoscopic hemi-field studies are not particularly reliable within individuals. As a result, handedness, which is easily assessed by questionnaire or direct observation, has been studied both as an important lateralization in its own right, and also as a surrogate for language dominance. Handedness is thought by most researchers to be genetic in origin, although there are differences in the precise models (McManus & Bryden, 1992), and, perhaps crucially, most models also assume that the genes determining handedness also influence language dominance, making the study of handedness directly relevant to the study of language dominance. If left-handedness is under genetic control, as several theories suggest, then it is likely, as with other genetically determined biological characteristics, such as blood groups, that there will be geographical variation (or clines), because of some combination of genetic drift, founder effects, and selection, be it natural or artificial.

A simplifying assumption for many earlier studies of handedness, and here the present author is no exception (McManus, 2004), has been to regard either the rate of left-handedness itself, or the frequency of the underlying genes, as constant historically and geographically. However, neither proposition seems likely a priori, not least because almost all human polymorphisms vary geographically (see, e.g., Cavalli-Sforza, Menozzi & Piazza, 1994), and the frequency of some

polymorphisms, such as that of sickle-cell anemia, also varies historically in relation to changing selection pressures (Cavalli-Sforza & Bodmer, 1971). It therefore seems probable that left-handedness, and perhaps the genes underlying it, will also vary both geographically and historically. If historical and geographical variation has been little studied by researchers, it is mainly because of the difficulty of obtaining adequate, large-scale databases. Attempts at meta-analysis of multiple small-scale studies have generally been unsuccessful, mainly because methods of measurement vary almost as much between studies as do rates of handedness (Raymond & Pontier, 2004; Seddon & McManus, unpublished manuscript, 1991).

Geographical and historical variation in handedness also raises the possibility that language dominance will also vary geographically and historically, as perhaps will other traits related to handedness and language dominance, and here one might think of dyslexia, stuttering, autism, schizophrenia, etc., in each of which atypical cerebral lateralization has been implicated. This chapter will concentrate on handedness, mainly because there is extensive data concerning it, but throughout the sub-text will be that similar conclusions might apply more broadly to cerebral dominance and its correlates.

Historical differences in the rate of left-handedness

The previous two centuries

Historical data on left-handedness are surprisingly rare, to the extent that a museum curator attempting to curate an exhibition on handedness referred to left-handers as being "a people without a history" (Sadler, 1997). Although estimating historical rates of left-handedness might seem easy, until recent years there has been very little systematic data. Modern work asking whether the historical rate of left-handedness might have changed systematically probably begins with that of Brackenridge (1981). However, quite the most important modern source on rates of left-handedness is the vast study by Gilbert and Wysocki (1992), which although never intended as a study of handedness has emerged as a key resource. In 1986, *National Geographic* magazine published a special issue on olfaction (Gibbons, 1986), which was accompanied by a "scratch and sniff" card, which readers were encouraged to scratch, report what, if anything, they could smell, and then, after completing a brief demographic questionnaire, return the card. Over 1.4 million people did so (Gilbert & Wysocki, 1987; Gilbert & Wysocki, 1992; Wysocki & Gilbert, 1989; Wysocki, Pierce & Gilbert, 1991). The authors of the original study felt it was possible that handedness and olfaction were linked (perhaps through cerebral dominance), and therefore Gilbert and Wysocki included two questions on handedness: one on writing hand and the other on throwing hand. Subsequent analyses have found no relationship between olfactory acuity and handedness, and it seems reasonable therefore to regard the survey as unbiased in relation to handedness (even if it is potentially biased in other ways, such as in sex, age, ethnicity, and olfactory ability). Respondents of course also reflect the typical readership of the magazine, which is likely to be more educated and middle-class than the population as a whole, but that is unlikely to be a source of bias in relation to handedness, since other large-scale studies have shown handedness to be unrelated to social class or education (McManus, 1981; Perelle & Ehrman, 1994).

The Gilbert and Wysocki data show two key findings. First, men are about 25% more likely to be left-handed than women; there being about five left-handed men for every four left-handed women, a finding that was also found in a large-scale meta-analysis (McManus, 1991), and helps cross-validate the data. More interestingly, there was also a strong relationship of handedness to year of birth, only about 3% to 4% of those born before about 1920 being left-handed, compared with about 11% to 12% of those born after 1950, a three fold difference. It should also be emphasized that the relative extent of the sex difference, expressed as an odds ratio, remained constant for those born in the early or late twentieth century.

Figure 3.1 shows the Gilbert and Wysocki data in two versions. The original paper (Gilbert & Wysocki, 1992) contained only data from 1900 onwards (indicated by the vertical dashed line), and the solid line shows a constrained Weibull function, which has been fitted to

the data (see McManus *et al.*, in press a). A reasonable account of just these data might be that the rate of left-handedness was low in the nineteenth century, and then rose through the twentieth century, reaching its current asymptote in about 1950. Interpreting the finding is, however, not so straightforward, mainly because the data are not proper historical series, but instead are cross-sectional, so that cohort effects must be inferred from individuals of different ages. The group born in 1900 in the Gilbert and Wysocki data were therefore aged 86 when the study was carried out in 1986. One possibility, extensively discussed in the handedness literature, is that left-handers die earlier, which results in a lower rate of left-handedness in older individuals (Coren & Halpern, 1991; Halpern & Coren, 1988; Halpern & Coren, 1991). Subsequent analyses of other data have convincingly shown that there is little evidence for differential mortality of left-handers (Ellis *et al.*, 1998; Halpern & Coren, 1993; Harris, 1993b; Harris, 1993c; Marks & Williamson, 1991; Wolf, D'Agostino & Cobb, 1991), although there is one study that compellingly suggests a higher mortality of young left-handed males in World War I, perhaps due to having to use right-handed equipment (Aggleton *et al.*, 1994). An alternative explanation of the lower rate of left-handedness suggests that the elderly are more likely, because of social pressure, either to have been forced to shift from writing with the left hand to writing with the right hand, or they prefer to call themselves right-handed, because of a taboo against left-handedness (Hugdahl *et al.*, 1993; Hugdahl, 1996). Both this and the differential mortality explanation become unlikely when one looks at the entire Gilbert and Wysocki database, which included unpublished data on individuals born between 1887 and 1899 (see McManus *et al.*, in press a). These data on these very oldest respondents are shown in Fig. 3.1, and the heavy dotted line shows the fit of a mixture of two constrained Weibull functions. Now it is clear that the very oldest respondents have a *higher* rate of left-handedness than those who are somewhat younger, an effect which is significant (McManus *et al.*, in press a), and is utterly at odds with explanations due either to differential mortality or greater social pressure to be right-handed. The best account of the Gilbert and Wysocki data is that it

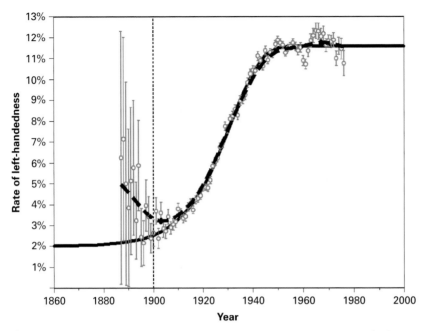

Figure 3.1 The overall rate of left-handedness in the data of Gilbert and Wysocki, 1992 (with permission), for those born from 1900 onwards (solid line); the fitted line is a constrained Weibull (for further details see McManus *et al.*, in press a). The data before 1900 (birth year 1887–99) are unpublished data from the Gilbert and Wysocki study, and are fitted by the dashed line, which is a mixture of two constrained Weibull functions.

directly reflects the actual rate of left-handedness in the population.

The additional Gilbert and Wysocki data implies that the rate of left-handedness might have been falling in those born in the last decade or so of the nineteenth century, and subsequently rose again in the twentieth century. Understanding the history of left-handedness in the nineteenth century therefore becomes important, although it is far from easy, adequate data sources being few and far between and not easy to interpret. The earliest scientific estimate of the rate of left-handedness is that of Ogle (1871), who asked 2000 consecutive patients at St George's Hospital whether they were right- or left-handed, 85 (4.25%) responded saying they were left-handed. Since these patients were adults in 1871, their mean year of birth was probably about 1835. Other somewhat later studies providing estimates of left-handedness rates for those born before 1900 include Lombroso (1884), Mayhew (see

Crichton-Browne, 1907), Crichton-Browne (1907), Stier (1911), and Schäfer (1911), and in addition Parson (1924) and Burt (1937) provide early twentieth-century estimates, which help to validate the broad picture shown by Gilbert and Wysocki. Two other sources have also been analyzed recently. In 1953, the BBC broadcasted an early television science programme called *Right Hand, Left Hand*, to which over 6000 people returned postcards describing their handedness and basic demographics (McManus *et al.*, in press b). Although biased, with left-handers being substantially over-represented among the respondents, it is nevertheless possible to estimate the true rate of left-handedness, which is of particular interest for the respondents born before 1900. Finally, rates of left-handedness have also been estimated from the early documentary films made by Mitchell and Kenyon between 1900 and 1906, the oldest participants of which were born before about 1850 (McManus & Hartigan, 2007).

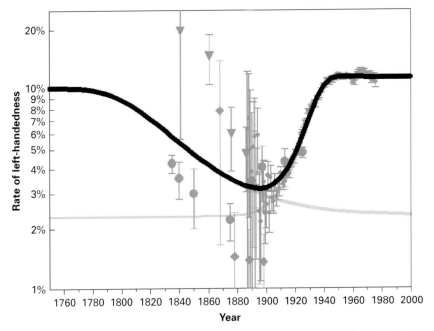

Figure 3.2 Summary of data from multiple studies on the rate of left-handedness during the nineteenth and twentieth centuries, from McManus *et al.* (McManus *et al.*, in press a). The solid black line is the fitted mixture of two constrained Weibull functions, which are shown separately as the two solid gray lines. Note that the ordinate is on a logarithmic scale.

The films showed large numbers of people waving at the camera, mostly with the right arm, and given modern data on the relationship between waving and hand preference, one can estimate the rate of left-handedness. Perhaps most striking is that left arm-waving is substantially more common among the *older* individuals, precisely the opposite pattern to that seen in the Gilbert and Wysocki data where left-handedness is most common in the *younger* individuals. The data from the Mitchell and Kenyon films are almost impossible to explain in terms of differential mortality or social pressure.

Figure 3.2 is a complex figure, taken from McManus *et al.* (in press a), which summarizes all of the historical data from the nineteenth and twentieth centuries. The solid black line consists of a mixture of two constrained Weibull functions, fitted using a maximum likelihood method, the two pale gray lines showing its components. The best statistical description of the recent history of handedness is that the rate was about 10% at the

end of the eighteenth century, the rate then fell throughout the nineteenth century, until it reached its nadir in about 1890–5, and then rose during the twentieth century, reaching its asymptote in about 1950, after which rates seem to have been unchanged.

The historical reasons for the nineteenth- and twentieth-century changes are unclear at present, but the nineteenth century changes may reflect an increasing visibility and stigmatization of left-handers, resulting from the Industrial Revolution, with large numbers of individuals using complex machinery in mills and factories, coupled with increasing rates of education and literacy (Stephens, 1990; Stone, 1969; West, 1978). In an agricultural society, left-handers are relatively invisible (except perhaps, as Thomas Carlyle noted, when a group of men is scything a field, see Pye-Smith, 1871). However, both complex machines and education would not only have made left-handers more visible, but left-handers may also have appeared less capable and more clumsy, as left-handed adults worked on machines that were almost certainly designed with right-handers in mind, and left-handed children were taught to write with steel dip pens that needed to be dragged across the paper from left to right by right-handers, and were not capable of being pushed across by the left hand without digging into the paper and making blots and stains. Whatever the mechanism, it seems undoubted that there was a general stigmatization and discrimination against left-handers at the end of the nineteenth century, which Bertrand (2001, pp. 88 and 91) refers to as "La haute époque de l'intolérance", such that there was "La gaucherie persécutée".

The distant past

The history of handedness before 1800 consists almost entirely of a few isolated points, which often are illuminated only briefly through indirect evidence that has to be treated with great care. Claims that, for instance, left-handedness was much more common in medieval than modern Britain (Steele & Mays, 1995), must be treated with caution, because they are based on bone asymmetries, which even in modern samples are inaccurate indicators of handedness, Steele (2000) pointing out how, "perplexingly ... left-handed subjects are equally likely to have a stronger grip in either hand" (p. 205). Likewise, although it is often hoped that cultural artifacts may provide insight into rates of handedness, interpretation is often difficult. For instance, although the twist of spun cotton or other fibers ("Z"- or "S"-twist) might at first seem to indicate handedness, the relationship of spinning direction to handedness seems to be weak (Minar, 2001), different fibers such as cotton and flax naturally twist in opposite directions (Batigne & Bellinger, 1953), there is evidence of communities of practice in different directions (Minar, 2001), and technological development can override pre-existing manual asymmetries (Crowfoot, Pritchard & Staniland, 2001).

No attempt will be made to be inclusive, although the broad picture that emerges, which is shown synoptically in Fig. 3.3, is fairly straightforward. Note in particular that the time axis for Fig. 3.3 is logarithmic, in terms of years before the present. The right-hand end

of the figure shows the last two centuries, with a modern rate of left-handedness of about 11% (section a). The rate was similar, at perhaps 8% to 10% at the end of the eighteenth century, but then fell to 3% or so during the nineteenth century, rising again in the first half of the twentieth century (sections b and c).

For the past 5000 years the best historical data are the elegant study by Coren and Porac (1977), which looked at five millennia of artistic representations of unimanual activity (such as playing board games, throwing spears, writing, etc.). Overall about 8% of paintings, drawing, and sculptures show the left hand being used, with little variation over the entire period of recorded history (section d in Figure 3.3). Specific written references to left-handedness are rare, with the intriguing exception of a use for left-handed workers in Roman stone mines, where a left-hander and a right-hander worked cooperatively on removing blocks of stone in the very confined spaces of a mine (see Steele & Uomini, 2005, p. 229 for an account of the various work of Röder, Bedon, and Monthel).

Data on handedness from the prehistoric period and pre-literate societies are necessarily indirect, take many forms, and can be difficult to interpret; see Steele and Uomini (2005) for an overview. Frustratingly, some data, such as one of the two arrows carried by the "Ice Man", Ötzi, which had been fletched in the left-handed manner (Spindler, 1994), undoubtedly indicate the presence of left-handers, but do not allow an accurate estimate of the rate. However, the study of Spenneman (1984), looking at stone and bone tools from the Neolithic period of about 4000 BP (before present), found a rate of left-handedness of between 6% (of 597 tools at Twann in Switzerland) and 19% (of 51 tools at Bodman in Germany). The data of Cahen *et al.* (1979), from the Upper Paleolithic period of about 9000 BP found one likely left-handed toolmaker among 22 (5%), with left-handed knapping and counterclockwise rotation marks. The study by Faurie and Raymond (2004) of silhouetted hand prints on the walls of Upper Paleolithic caves from about 30 000 to 10 000 BP also allows a proper estimate of the rate. About 77% of prints showed a left hand, a figure that the authors showed was almost identical to that provided by a modern group of 179 students carrying out

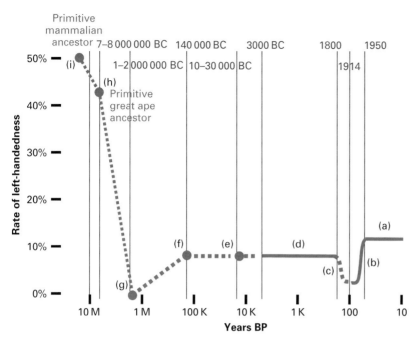

Figure 3.3 A synoptic map of the broad changes in the rate of left-handedness over the past ten million years. Note that the abscissa is logarithmic in terms of years before present.

the same task, 14 of whom were left-handed, implying a similar Upper Paleolithic rate of left-handedness to that of the modern period (point e in Fig. 3.3).

A study of a much earlier population by Fox and Frayer (1997), looked at tooth striations on Neanderthal teeth from about 130 000 BP (see also de Castro, Bromage & Jalvo, 1988). These striations probably come either from techniques for eating meat, or from the use of animal tendons or plant matter as primitive "dental floss" to remove interdental detritus. In the 20 specimens, the direction was compatible with right-handed use in 18 cases and left-handed use in 2 cases, giving an estimated rate, albeit not a particularly accurate one, of about 10% (point f in Fig. 3.3). Earlier than this, there is once again clear but isolated evidence of the presence of a left-hander who was knapping stone tools at the Boxgrove Site of about 500 000 BP (Roberts & Parfitt, 1999). Phillipson (1997) also looked at edge modification in 54 stone tools from the Lower Paleolithic period of about 500 000 to 1 000 000 years

BP at Kariandusi in Kenya, and suggested that 6 (11%) were compatible with left-hand use.

Undoubtedly the oldest data on human handedness are those of Toth (1985) (see also Ambrose, 2001) who looked at the flakes left by the stone tool making of *Homo habilis* at the site of Koobi Fora in the African Rift Valley, which is from about 1.5 million years BP. There was a modest excess of flakes typical of those produced by right-handers, which was entirely compatible with the rate of such flakes found in modern knappers who are known to be right-handed. The implication, albeit not a strong one, is that perhaps *all* humans at that time were right-handed (indicated as point g in Fig. 3.3). Without repeating the theoretical arguments again here, elsewhere (McManus, 1999) I have argued that handedness in humans is likely to have evolved in two stages, in the first of which was the evolution from an ancient C^* gene to what I call the D gene, when the majority of humans became right-handed, and a second, subsequent stage, with the evolution of the modern *C* gene, when a substantial minority of humans became left-handed, the polymorphism of *D* and *C* genes presumably being maintained by heterozygote advantage or some other mechanism.

Modern humans evolved from a primitive great ape ancestor, perhaps about 7 to 8 million years ago, and that primitive great ape ancestor must itself have derived from a primitive mammalian ancestor. The handedness of modern great apes is controversial, with some researchers believing that great apes do not show population level handedness (i.e., 50% are right-handed and 50% are left-handed (Annett & Annett, 1991; Marchant & McGrew, 1991; Marchant & McGrew, 1996). However, a meta-analysis by Hopkins (2006) suggested that perhaps 60% of bonobos and maybe 55% of chimpanzees and gorillas show right-handedness, although there are concerns that some of the difference from 50% may result from imitation learning in captive animals.

Geographical differences in the rate of left-handedness

People everywhere are mostly right-handed, as was recognized as long ago as 1837 by the English physician, Sir Thomas Watson, who wrote:

The employment of the right hand in preference to the left is universal throughout all nations and countries. I believe no people or tribe of left-handed persons has ever been known to exist. ... Among the isolated tribes of North America which have the most recently become known to the civilized world, no exception to the general rule has been met with. Captain Back has informed me that the wandering families of Esquimaux, whom he encountered in his several expeditions towards the North Pole, all threw their spears with the right hand, and grasped their bows with the left. (Watson, 1836)

Watson's strong theoretical position is still acceptable today, as also is Back's perception of the right-handedness of the "Esquimaux", Delacato (1963) reporting that in photographs of 46 Canadian and Greenland Inuit using "an arm for one purpose or another", 43 were using the right hand and only 3 (6.5%) were using the left hand. Likewise data from New Guinea (Connolly & Bishop, 1992), Amazonia

(Bryden, Ardila & Ardila, 1993) and Tristan da Cunha (McManus & Bryden, 1993) all support the universal predominance of right-handedness, but their small sample sizes usually preclude any other detailed comparison of rates and the drawing of any strong conclusions on mechanism and process.

Although Watson was correct that right-handers predominate in all human societies, the related question of whether *rates* of left-handedness vary between countries is much more open to contention. Despite there being many papers in the literature with titles such as "The rate of left-handedness in ....", such studies usually say little about whether countries differ because they typically use different methods to measure handedness, making it unclear whether differences are due to the method of measurement or a difference in the true rate of left-handedness. Indeed Raymond and Pontier (2004), after their long meta-analysis, could still only entitle their paper, "Is there geographical variation in human handedness?" The problem of finding geographical differences is compounded by the fact that sample sizes are typically small (and although several hundred individuals may seem reasonable, it is not). Detecting differences in small proportions of individuals between populations requires surprisingly large samples, as can be seen even with the seemingly straightforward question of sex differences in the rate of left-handedness. We now believe that there about five left-handed males for every four left-handed females, male to females ratios of 1.238, 1.211, 1.207, 1.343, and 1.273 being found in the very large studies of Gilbert and Wysocki (Ross *et al.* 1992), Halpern *et al.* (1998), Peters *et al.* (2006), Carrothers (1947), and the meta-analysis of Seddon and McManus (unpublished manuscript, 1991). However, to have an 80% chance of finding such a difference with a one-tailed test at the 5% significance level requires about 2500 males and 2500 females, a number that is far larger than in most of the studies that had looked at sex differences (and therefore, for instance, the conclusion of Erlenmeyer-Kimling *et al.* (2005), that 517 children of schizophrenic parents did not show the standard sex difference in rates of left-handedness, is very unsafe). Using a similar calculation, when the rate of left-handedness is 10% in one population, then to find a significant difference with 80% power at the 5% level when the true rate in a second population is 5%, 6%, 7%, 8%, or 9% requires samples in each population of 350, 600, 1100, 2500, and 11 000, making it unlikely that most studies will reliably be able even to find quite largish differences.

One of the clearest studies to look systematically for differences in handedness between countries was that of Singh and Bryden (1994), which used large samples of students in Canada and India, two countries expected to be very different in their rate of handedness, and it used the identical questionnaire in both countries. The rate of left-handedness was 9.8% in Canada compared with only 5.2% in India, a nearly twofold difference, with factor structure being very similar (see also Singh *et al.* 2001). A parallel study comparing Canada and Japan found an even larger difference, the rate of left-handedness in Japan being only 4.7% (Ida & Bryden, 1996). Another study finding clear differences between countries in the rate of left-handedness is the important study of Perelle and Ehrman (1994), which benefited both from a large sample size and a single consistent questionnaire translated for use in all the countries.

The very large sample sizes needed for proper geographical studies of handedness, which allow some form of mapping, are often only available when the data have been collected for some other purpose, with handedness being tagged on as an additional question (as for instance in the *National Geographic* study, described earlier). A similar situation exists in the case of a recent internet-based study of sexual behavior and attitudes, which was carried out under the auspices of the BBC (Reimers, 2007). The survey was live from February 2005 to May 2005, during which time more than half a million people provided some data and 255 116 individuals completed all six sections of the study. One of the questions asked, "Which is your natural writing hand?" (Peters *et al.* 2006). Overall there were sufficient respondents from Europe to allow a map to be drawn, although for the map shown in Fig. 3.4 it has been necessary to group together some countries as sample sizes were otherwise too small. However, a trend surface analysis, which is weighted by the sample size in each country, has no such problems, and from that it is clear that the highest rates of left-handedness in Europe are

in Britain, the Netherlands, and Belgium. To a first approximation the rate of left-handedness then declines as one moves away from those countries, be it west to Ireland, south-west to France and then the Iberian peninsula, north-east to Scandinavia, or east to Germany, Poland, the Baltic, and Russia, or south-east to the Balkans, Greece, Bulgaria, and Romania. The reasons for such geographical differences are not clear, although Medland *et al.* (2004) have suggested that countries with a more formal education system have lower rates of left-handedness than those with a more informal education system.

Somewhat surprisingly, it is sometimes easier to find evidence for geographical trends *within* countries rather than *between* them, in part because in national surveys the same survey methods are used in the same language for subjects. One of the biggest, and still one of the best, such studies is that of Ewald Stier (1911), who in 1909 surveyed the soldiers of the German Army. As expected the overall rate was much lower than in modern Europe, at about 3.9%, but the real interest comes in the details of his study, as in the map shown in Fig. 3.5, which shows how the rate of left-handedness was lowest for those from Eastern Prussia, and highest for those from southern Germany, around Stuttgart, where there were over twice as many left-handers as in the East. Comparing Fig. 3.5 with Fig. 3.4 suggests that many of the same trends can still be found today, with higher rates in Germany than in Poland and the Baltic States, and higher rates still towards the Swiss border. Other studies finding differences within countries are rare, but mention should be made of the study of Olivier (1978) in France, left-handedness being most frequent in the north, and of lowest frequency in Brittany and the Massif central, in Italy of Viggiano *et al.* (2001), where left-handedness was more frequent in the north of the country than the south (see also Salmaso & Longoni, 1983), and in Britain, where Leask and Beaton (2007) showed that within mainland Britain, left-handedness is less common in Scotland and Wales than in England (a trend that perhaps is hinted at in Fig. 3.4, where Ireland has a lower rate of left-handedness than the United Kingdom).

Another example of a large national survey finding geographical differences is the Gilbert and Wysocki

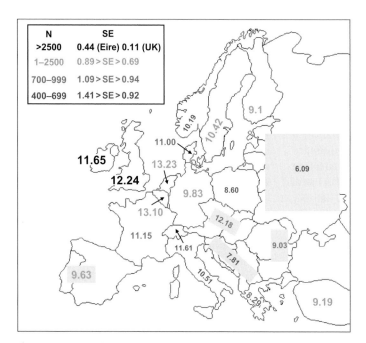

Figure 3.4 Rates of left-handedness in different European countries, based on data in the BBC internet survey (McManus & Peters, in press). Where sample sizes of contiguous countries are relatively low the countries are merged together, indicated by the gray boxes overlapping borders (e.g., Spain and Portugal were grouped together). The rate of left-handedness is shown as a percentage. The sample size and the approximate standard errors are shown by different sizes of numbers, the key being provided at the top left.

(1992) study, where the zip code for each US respondent was recorded in the database, but no further analyses were ever carried out on those data. However the Gilbert and Wysocki data reveal some fascinating trends, which are both geographical and historical (McManus & Wysocki, in press). Zip codes for each respondent can readily be translated into latitudes and longitudes, and handedness can then be mapped. Figure 3.6 shows the percentage of left-handers in White Americans born in 1950 and afterwards in each of the contiguous states of mainland United States. Even at this level of spatial resolution it can be seen that the highest rates of left-handedness are in the north-east, in Maine, Vermont, Massachusetts, and Connecticut, whereas the lowest rates are in the mid-West, in Wyoming and North Dakota. More detailed mapping suggests that left-handers are also more frequent in the north-east of the USA, as well as in Florida, and around the west coast cities of San Francisco, Portland, and Seattle. The causes of these differences are complex, but of particular interest is that as one looks at those born a generation and then two generations earlier, the geographical patterns shift, with left-handers then being more common in the agricultural areas of the United States, such as the mid-west and the south. The implication is that there may be differential migration of left-handers.

Finally, it should be mentioned that there must always be a worry about whether there are response biases in surveys, particularly those carried out using magazine readers or internet browsers. To respond to the BBC internet survey a respondent must have a computer, must understand English well, and must be aware of the survey, all of which may make biases possible. Having said that, similar trends are apparent to those in Stier's (1911) study, which used a conscripted sample, and was entirely in the subjects' native language, thereby providing a validation in principle of the method.

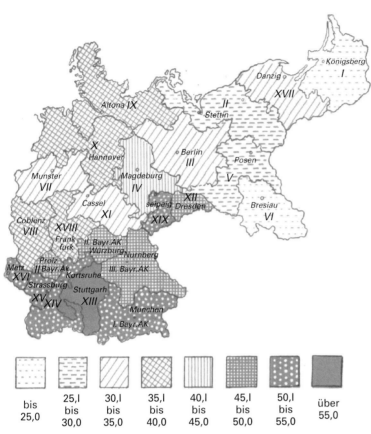

Figure 3.5 The rate of left-handedness in German soldiers in 1909 (plotted as left-handers per thousand) in relation to the area in which they were recruited (Stier, 1911).

Ethnicity and handedness

Analysis of handedness by ethnicity has been left until last, since in the modern world, ethnicity, which in some sense expresses the distant geographical origin of individuals, perhaps many generations previously, inevitably incorporates a historical component according to when an individual's family or ancestors migrated from one geographical region to another. Few studies have assessed ethnic differences in handedness, and the two sets of data presented here, one from the UK and the other from the USA, have both been prepared specially for this chapter.

Singh and Bryden (1994) showed that the rate of left-handedness was lower in the Indian sub-continent than in the West. A classic epidemiological method for distinguishing the effects of genes and culture is to observe migrants between two countries which differ in some characteristic. If migrants become like the society to which they have migrated then socio-cultural factors are probably responsible for the difference, whereas if the difference remains in the migrants then genes are probably responsible. The method can be used to look at handedness in applicants for medical education in the UK, considering only those who are either White or from the Indian sub-continent (Table 3.1; for further details of these studies see McManus *et al.*, 1995; McManus, Richards & Maitlis, 1989). The odds ratio for the difference between White and Asian (Indian sub-continent) applicants is

Table 3.1 Handedness of 4902 applicants to UK medical schools for admission in 1986 and 1991, comparing self-classified Indian sub-continent applicants with White applicants, with non-White applicants divided into those born in the UK and those not born in the UK. Logistic regression showed an overall effect of being male (OR = 1.387, $p < 0.001$), and a highly significant effect of being White (OR = 1.513, $p < 0.001$), but no significant effect of being born in the UK (OR = 1.218, $p = 0.117$). Restricting the analysis to those of Asian origin, there was still a significant effect of being male (OR = 1.558, $p = 0.017$), but no effect of being born in the UK (OR = 1.273, $p = 0.182$). Analyses comparing the 1986 and 1991 cohorts (not shown here) showed no significant differences.

Ethnic origin	Males	Females	Total
White	13.0% (302/2331)	9.6% (248/2581)	11.2% (550/4902)
Indian sub-continent	9.2% (92/995)	6.1% (47/769)	7.9% (139/1764)
Born in the UK	10.7% (57/534)	6.0% (26/430)	8.6% (83/964)
Not born in the UK	7.6% (35/461)	6.2% (21/339)	7.0% (56/800)

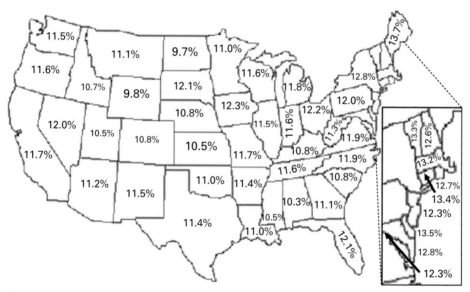

Figure 3.6 Rate of left-handedness of White respondents, born from 1950 onwards, in each of the contiguous states of the USA, based on the data of Gilbert and Wysocki (1992); for further details see McManus and Wysocki (in press). Sample sizes vary from 1197 for the District of Columbia to 52 081 for California, with a mean of 8427, median of 5267, and inter-quartile range of 2879–11 939. The standard error for a state of median size is about 0.4%.

1.513×, which is broadly similar to that observed in Singh and Bryden's (1994) comparison of Canada and India. Most importantly, though, there is no difference between the Asian applicants born in the UK and those born in the Indian sub-continent (and presumably reared outside of the UK for at least their early childhood), which suggests that socio-cultural factors are relatively unimportant in the origin of ethnic differences in handedness, and implies instead that genes may be more important in determining differences.

Ethnicity can also be looked at in the very large Gilbert and Wysocki (1992) study. Although 97% of

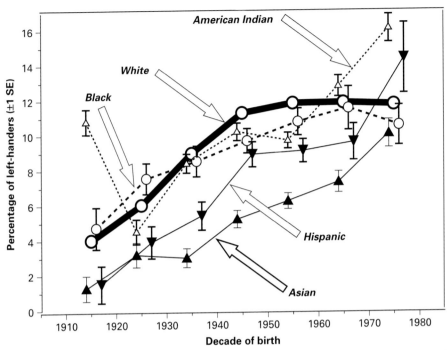

Figure 3.7 Left-handedness rates (± 1 SE) in US respondents from different ethnic groups in the Gilbert and Wysocki study, averaged across sex. Groups are broken down by birth decade (1910–19, 1920–29, etc.) and plotted at the decadal mid-points, with some groups moved slightly to the left or right to prevent standard error bars overlapping. The solid black line with open circles is for White respondents, and standard errors are smaller than the size of the symbol. Ethnic groups are shown as Black (○– – – ○), American Indian (Δ– – – Δ), Hispanic (▼– – – ▼), and Asian (▲– – – ▲). Statistical analysis used hierarchical logistic regression. At the first step, effects of year of birth and sex were entered, the non-linear age trend being taken into account by a quintic polynomial. At the next step, ethnicity showed a highly significant effect (Wald chi-square = 374.7, 4 d.f., $p < 0.001$), with only Asians and Hispanics showing significantly lower rates of handedness from the White reference group ($p < 0.001$ in each case). Ethnicity by sex interactions were tested at the next step, but were not significant (Wald chi-square = 3.508, 4 d.f., $p = 0.477$). Finally, the interaction of linear trend of year of birth by ethnicity was tested, and was highly significant (Wald chi-square = 53.43, 4 d.f., $p < 0.001$), with only the Asian and Hispanic sub-groups showing a significantly lower slope than in the White reference group ($p < 0.001$ in each case).

the US respondents in the Gilbert and Wysocki survey were White, the vast sample size meant there were still sufficient non-White respondents in the USA to allow an analysis by ethnicity and year of birth. Considering only those born from 1910 onwards, numbers being very small before that, there were 8387 respondents describing themselves as Black, 10 080 as Asian (presumably mostly from the Far East), 2513 as American Indian, and 12 049 as Hispanic, numbers that are larger than even most of the largest other studies of handedness.

Figure 3.7 shows the rate of left-handedness in the five ethnic groups in relation to year of birth. The Black and American Indian groups show similar historical changes to the White group, whereas both the Asian and Hispanic groups show lower rates of left-handedness overall, and also a lower rate of increase in the rate of left-handedness than do the other groups. The lower rate of left-handedness in the Asian groups is compatible with other studies suggesting lower rates of left-handedness in China, Japan, and the Indian sub-continent (Iwasaki, 2000; Teng *et al.* 1976), and the lower rate of left-handedness in the Hispanics is similar to that found in the Iberian peninsula in the European data (see Fig. 3.3), and the effects are also similar to those of the large study of Halpern *et al.* (1998), where among US medical school applicants, left-handedness was reported in 13.1% of 92 523 Whites, 10.7% of 11 778 Blacks, 10.5% of 6171 Hispanics, 9.2% of 9055 Indian sub-continent applicants, 6.3% of 3533 Vietnamese, 5.4% of 4087 Koreans, and 5.3% of 7413 Chinese applicants. A striking feature also of Fig. 3.7 is the excess left-handedness in males being similar in all ethnic groups, again suggesting some stable and constant mechanism maintaining sex differences (and hence probably not cultural or social pressures against women, as has sometimes been implied).

Explaining geographical and historical differences in the rate of left-handedness

The analyses of this paper have so far been mainly descriptive, but provide a clear demonstration that rates of left-handedness vary between different countries. Singh and Bryden's (1994) comparisons of India and Canada provide compelling evidence of differences between countries in two different continents, and other studies have shown differences across the continent of Europe and across the states of the USA. There are differences between ethnic groups within the USA, Asians and Hispanics having lower rates of left-handedness, and there are also large historical shifts in the rate of left-handedness across the twentieth century, those historical shifts being paralleled within the separate ethnic groups that comprise the USA. The challenge is to explain the origin of these differences: differences that are present in both space and time.

Explaining geographical differences

Most explanations in biology distinguish nature and nurture, which to a large extent can be conceptualized as genes and environment. When populations differ in their rates of left-handedness then the most important question concerns whether the differences are genetic

or environmental in origin. Distinguishing such explanations were key questions for Phil Bryden during the final years of his life, particularly after he had collected his data showing large and clear differences between Canada and India. However, the obvious theoretical problem is that a low rate of left-handedness in India can result either from social pressure, which results in left-handers being forced, overtly or covertly, to behave as right-handers, or from differences in gene frequency between Canada and India, *and prevalence data alone cannot distinguish between genetic and social causes.* The key insight, however, which Phil Bryden and I developed together in what as it happened were the last months of his life, is that the effects of genes and social pressure can be distinguished if each is modeled separately, and family data are available.

Euchiria, Hipressia, and Lowgenia

In a popular book on handedness (McManus, 2002), I illustrated the separate effects of genes and culture by describing three mythical countries, which I named Euchiria, Hipressia, and Lowgenia. The model is based around the McManus genetic model of handedness (McManus, 1985; McManus & Bryden, 1992), which needs to be briefly described, although it seems likely that any broadly similar genetic model will show similar effects.[1] The model suggests that at a single genetic locus there are two alleles, named *D* (for dextral) and *C* (for chance). One hundred percent of *DD* homozygotes are right-handed, whereas *CC* homozygotes have a 50:50 chance of being right- or left-handed. The alleles are additive in the heterozygote, so that 25% of *DC* individuals are left-handed, and the remaining 75% are right-handed. The model explains not only how handedness runs in families, but also why as a result of the random effects of the *C* allele about one in five monozygotic twin pairs is discordant for handedness. Finally, by assuming that the same alleles determine handedness and language dominance, the

---

[1] An exception may be the Annett model, which as well as a parameters to describe the frequency of the RS-gene, also has a threshold parameter that can be adjusted separately in each population, and which therefore is confounded with rate of handedness.

Table 3.2 Familial patterns of handedness in the mythical countries of Euchiria, Lowgenia, and Hipressia (see text for details). Note that *p(L|DD)* indicates the conditional probability of being left-handed, given that an individual has the *DD* genotype, etc.). L_{par} refers to families in which at least one parent is left-handed.

	Euchiria	Lowgenia	Hipressia
p(C)	0.2	0.1	0.2
p(L|DD)	0	0	0
p(L|DC)	0.25	0.25	0.125
p(L|CC)	0.50	0.50	0.250
p(L)	*0.100*	*0.050*	*0.050*
p(L|R × R)	0.078	0.038	0.045
p(L|L_{par})	0.195	0.160	0.099
Odds ratio	2.87×	4.79×	2.34×

model readily explains why about 5% of right-handers and 35% of left-handers are right hemisphere dominant for language.

Euchiria is a country in which only genes determine handedness, and because the rate of left-handedness, *p(L)*, is set at exactly 10%, the calculations of the McManus model are particularly easy, because the frequency of the *C* allele, *p(C)* is double that of *p(L)*, and hence is 20%. The top of the first column of Table 3.2 shows the frequency of the *C* allele, the probability of each of the three genotypes being left-handed, and the resulting rate of left-handedness, which is 10%. For convenience, and because two left-handed parents is a relatively rare combination, families are divided into those for whom both parents are right-handed (*R × R*) and those in whom at least one parent is left-handed (*L_{par}*). When at least one parent is left-handed, the proportion of left-handers in the offspring, *p(L|L_{par})*, is 19.5%, compared with only 7.8% when both parents are right-handed, *p(L|R × R)*. Calculating a conventional odds ratio, as 19.5 × (100 − 7.8)/(7.8 × (100 − 19.5)), shows a child with at least one left-handed parent is about 2.87 times more likely to be left-handed itself.

Lowgenia is similar in many ways to Euchiria, except that the frequency of the *C* allele is lower, being exactly half that found in Euchiria, so that *p(C)* is 10%, and the

unsurprising consequence is that the rate of left-handedness is also half that found in Euchiria, *p(L)* being 5%. What is rather more counter-intuitive, at least for those not used to genetic calculations, is that the odds ratio for the effect of having at least one left-handed parent is *higher* in Lowgenia than in Euchiria, being 4.79× in Lowgenia, rather than the 2.87× found in Euchiria. A reduction in gene frequency therefore *increases* the odds ratio of the child of a left-handed parent being left-handed.

Hipressia is more complicated, because not only genes but also social pressure affect the rate of left-handedness, both of which need to be modeled. Hipressians do not like left-handers and do their best to make them indistinguishable from right-handers, but human resilience being what it is, they are only successful in half the cases. The gene frequency in Hipressia, *p(C)*, is the same as in Euchiria, but instead of a half of *CC* individuals and a quarter of *DC* individuals becoming left-handed as they would in Euchiria, social pressure against left-handers in Hipressia means that only a quarter of *CC* individuals and an eighth of *DC* individuals become left-handed (or putting it more precisely, a quarter of *CC* individuals and an eighth of *DC* individuals, who would have become left-handed in Euchiria, instead become right-handed in Hipressia because of social pressure, making them what geneticists call "phenocopy right-handers"). The unsurprising result, once again, is that the overall rate of left-handedness in Hipressia is exactly half that found in Euchiria, being 5%. That rate of 5% is exactly the same as the rate found in Lowgenia, showing how two entirely different causal mechanisms result in the same overall rate of left-handedness. However, and it is a key point, the pattern of left-handedness in Hipressian families is very different from that found in Lowgenia, the odds of a Hipressian being left-handed when they have a left-handed parent being 2.34× higher than if both parents are right-handed, compared with 4.79× in Lowgenia. The Hipressian odds ratio is therefore *lower* than in Lowgenia (and indeed is also lower than in Euchiria). The key theoretical conclusion is that gene frequency differences and social pressure can be distinguished by looking at odds ratios in families.

The model that Phil Bryden and I had developed was quickly tested, because Bryden not only had data on the rate of left-handedness in Canada and India, but had already carried out a preliminary analysis of how handedness ran in families in the two countries (Bryden *et al.* 1995). In Canada, where the rate of left-handedness was 9.8%, the odds ratio was 2.09×, whereas in India, where the rate of left-handedness was 5.2%, the odds ratio was 3.07×. The implication was clear: the majority of the difference between Canada and India must be due to differences in gene frequency rather than due to differences in social pressure. Subsequently, Bryden and I collaborated with Taha Amir in the United Arab Emirates (UAE), and Yokahida Ida in Japan, and we also put together larger Western samples (mainly Canada and the UK), and Indian samples. Of 17 850, 14 924, 4485, and 656 offspring in the West, UAE, India, and Japan, for whom $p(L)$ was 11.5%, 7.5%, 5.8%, and 4.0% respectively, the odds ratios for the effect of having a left-handed parent were 2.11×, 2.23×, 3.18× and 3.57× respectively, which is the pattern expected from gene frequency differences. Geographical differences in the modern world seem therefore to be primarily genetic in origin, rather than due to differences in social pressure (or what I will refer to subsequently as "direct social pressure").

Explaining historical differences

If geographical differences in rates of left-handedness can be explained in terms of differences in gene frequency, what about historical differences? "The past is a foreign country", as L. P. Hartley said at the beginning of *The Go-Between* (albeit often being misquoted as "the past is another country"). If so, then the same methods that distinguish the causes of geographical differences should also distinguish the causes of historical differences. Fortunately, a number of family studies of handedness in Western countries have been published over the past century, the earliest being that of Ramaley (1913), who described data collected in a group of undergraduate students (the probands), who therefore would have been born in about 1888. In 1992, Phil Bryden and I (McManus & Bryden, 1992) had already reviewed 25 such studies, and had broken

them down into three groups, those for whom the probands were born between 1880 and 1939, 1940 and 1954, and 1955 and 1979, the rates of left-handedness in the offspring being 7.28%, 10.83%, and 13.25% (whereas, the parents, being born a generation earlier, had rates of left-handedness of 4.44%, 6.11%, and 9.34%). The odds ratios for the effect of having a left-handed parent were 3.29×, 2.08×, and 1.64× in the three groups respectively. Just as with the geographical data, when the rate of left-handedness is lower, so the odds ratio is higher, implying that the historical differences also reflect differences in gene frequency. That suggestion was also strongly supported by a reanalysis of data from the huge study of the German Army by Stier (1911), the conscripts for whom would have been born in about 1890, and of whom 3.87% were left-handed, a lower value than any of the family studies we had analyzed. Stier reported the number of left- and right-handers with left-handed relatives, and by making some reasonable assumptions, one can estimate the odds ratio for the effect of having a left-handed parent as being about 5.2×, a higher value than any of the odds ratios in the other familial studies. Once again, Stier's data suggest that historical differences reflect genetic differences rather than effects of social pressure.

Social pressure can take many forms, and it is useful to distinguish between *direct* and *indirect* social pressure. Direct social pressure involves left-handed individuals being made to write with their right hand, as seems to have happened in some Victorian schools (see, e.g., Ireland, 1880), and has occurred in many other forms around the world to prevent left-handers using their left hands (see McManus, 2002). However, direct social pressure of this sort only alters the phenotype, not the genotype, and the individuals still carry the genes that made them originally left-handed, and if transmitted those genes would allow those individuals' offspring to become left-handed. Indirect social pressure is much more subtle, and does not directly alter the phenotype of the left-hander, but instead acts to make left-handers stigmatized, ostracized, and taboo, so that they find it harder to have offspring. The result is that their genes are less likely to be passed on, and hence the frequency of the genes responsible for left-handedness falls, and left-handedness becomes less common in the next generation. To see how this might happen one must consider the very different social world of relatively small nineteenth-century communities, where most people knew one another, transport was less good, most people married people living less than 30 kilometers away, marriage was relatively early, as also was first childbirth, so that families were large, often with eight or ten children, child-bearing only ceasing at menopause. In such a world, any subtle denigration, mockery, or stigmatization of the left-handed, perhaps for clumsiness or awkwardness at writing or technical skills, or indeed for mere difference itself, might result in marriage and hence childbirth being delayed by five or ten years, so that the number of offspring would be reduced. The consequence would be a fall in the number of C alleles and hence in the rate of left-handedness. Indirect social pressure, although less brutal than direct social pressure, could be of far greater consequence in its eventual effects.

If the theory of indirect social pressure is correct, then there is a clear prediction: left-handers at the end of the nineteenth century should have had fewer children than right-handers. Fortunately that prediction can not only be readily tested, but the data has already been presented in our review of the genetics of handedness (McManus & Bryden, 1992). Family studies typically include all children, and hence if the number of parents is known as well as the number of offspring, then the mean number of offspring can be calculated. Table 3.3 shows that while at the end of the twentieth century, right- and left-handed parents had similar numbers of children, despite parents around the turn of the century in general having more children than modern parents, left-handers had relatively fewer children, two left-handed parents having only 2.32 children, compared with 2.69 children when one parent was left-handed, and 3.10 children when both parents were right-handed. Two right-handed parents therefore had 34% more children than two left-handed parents. It is therefore at least possible that historical shifts in the rate of left-handedness are driven by differences in fertility (and the ultimate test of any evolutionary theories concerns whether groups of individuals differ in the numbers of offspring).

Table 3.3 The average number of offspring in relation to parental handedness, in familial studies of handedness carried out in different periods, classified by the birth year of probands (from McManus & Bryden, 1992).

Birth year of probands	Number of studies	Number of parental pairs	Parental handedness		
			$R \times R$	$R \times L$	$L \times L$
1880–1939	5	4180	3.10	2.69	2.32
1940–54	5	3800	3.17	3.05	3.00
1955–80	6	7323	2.49	2.60	2.57

The consequences of historical and geographical differences in left-handedness

Were the rate of left-handedness to vary, either historically or geographically, and particularly if that variation is due to differences in gene frequency, what consequences does that have for neuropsychology and neuropsychiatry? The answer depends in part on the nature of the genetic system underlying handedness and cerebral dominance, and for obvious reasons I will consider the McManus model, which suggests that 25% of DC individuals and 50% of CC individuals are left-handed. More generally (McManus, 1984; McManus, 1985) the model says that 25% of DC individuals and 50% of CC individuals, but no DD individuals, will have atypically directed lateralization for any character controlled by the gene. A crucial corollary is that the chance processes for each character will be statistically independent.

If there is a probability p_G that any individual modular character will be atypically organized (such as, left-handedness or right-sided language) in a particular genotype, G, and if we consider two modular traits, such as handedness and language, then $(1 - p_G)^2$ will have the typical phenotype (the one described in neuropsychology textbooks, which for handedness and language is right-handedness and left-sided language), $2.p_G.(1 - p_G)$ will have one atypical trait, and p_G^2 will have both traits anomalously organized (in this case, left-handers with right-sided language). For DD, DC, and CC individuals, p_G is 0, 0.25, and 0.5 respectively. However, DD individuals are far more frequent in the population than DC who are more frequent than CC individuals. Combining all the numbers, then it is easy to show that if the rate of left-handedness is 10%, then 7.8% of right-handers and 30.0% of left-handers will have language in the right hemisphere, which corresponds broadly with the data.

There may, however, be multiple modular traits controlled by the D and C alleles, with perhaps several separate modular traits for aspects of spoken and written language, several modular traits for aspects of visuo spatial and facial processing, and so on. If there are n modular traits, then $(1 - p_G)^n$ individuals will have the textbook pattern with no anomalies, and $1 - (1 - p_G)^n$ will have at least one anomaly (such as a right-sided component of language, or a left-sided component of visuo spatial processing). The number of modules is not at present known, but Table 3.4 calculates the percentage of individuals with anomalous organization in relation to the number of modules and the rate of left-handedness in the population. The basic finding is very simple: irrespective of the number of modular traits controlled by the C allele, the proportion of anomalous traits rises approximately linearly with the rate of left-handedness. If it is the case that dyslexia, stuttering, autism, schizophrenia, or other conditions are related to atypical cerebral lateralization, and hence to the presence of a C allele, then the rate of those conditions should change geographically or historically in parallel with the rate of left-handedness.[2] In particular, in the West there may well have been a three- or fourfold increase in the rate of those conditions since Victorian times, and in other cultures the rate might well be rising as left-handedness increases in frequency. That may help to explain how conditions that we now think of as common, were rare and difficult to describe and characterize in the nineteenth century. However, and it is relevant in the context of current speculations about a rising rate of autism, the rate of cerebral dominance related anomalies should be relatively constant for those born in the West after about 1950. Whether or not there are historical and geographical variations in neuropsychiatric conditions remains to be seen; collecting adequate evidence to assess the idea will not be

Table 3.4 The effect of the rate of left-handedness on the percentage of individuals with atypical cerebral organization (e.g., crossed cerebral dominance, "anomalous" dominance).

Rate of left-handedness	Number of modular traits					"Very large"
	1	2	3	5	10	
2.5%	2.5%	4.3%	5.7%	7.5%	9.2%	9.8%
5%	5.0%	8.6%	11.3%	14.7%	18.0%	19.0%
7.5%	7.5%	12.8%	16.7%	21.6%	26.3%	27.8%
10%	10.0%	17.0%	22.0%	28.3%	34.2%	36.0%
12.5%	12.5%	21.1%	27.1%	34.7%	41.6%	43.8%

Note: when the number of modular traits is very large (and is effectively infinite), then all DC and CC individuals will show at least one anomalous trait. If the rate of left-handedness is $p(L)$, then the frequency of the C allele is $2.p(L)$, the frequency of the D allele is $1 - 2.p(L)$, the frequency of DD individuals is $[1 - 2.p(L)]^2$, and hence the combined frequency of DC and CC individuals, which is the proportion of individuals with anomalies, is $1 - [1 - 2.p(L)]^2$.

easy, but the hypotheses relating their rate to handedness and cerebral dominance differences are testable, and have interesting implications for interpreting differences in neuropsychiatric disease prevalence.

ACKNOWLEDGMENTS

I am very grateful to Chuck Wysocki and Avery Gilbert for providing me with raw data from their large study of handedness, and to Michael Peters and Stian Reimers for their collaboration in studying the data from the BBC internet study.

[2] It should also be said that small numbers of anomalies may well be beneficial, while large numbers of anomalies are deleterious. Elsewhere in my "theory of random cerebral variation" (McManus, 2002) I have argued that DC individuals in particular are more likely to have single anomalies that might result in beneficial consequences, perhaps in the form of special talents for particular tasks that involve unusual interactions between modules.

REFERENCES

Aggleton, J. P., Bland, J. M., Kentridge, R. W. & Neave, N. J. (1994). Handedness and longevity: archival study of cricketers. *British Medical Journal*, **309**, 1681–4.

Ambrose, S. H. (2001). Palaeolithic technology and human evolution. *Science*, **291**, 1748–53.

Annett, M. & Annett, J. (1991). Handedness for eating in gorillas. *Cortex*, **27**, 269–75.

Batigne, R. & Bellinger, L. (1953). The significance and technical analysis of ancient textiles as historical documents. *Proceedings of the American Philosophical Society*, **97**, 670–80.

Bertrand, P.-M. (2001). *Histoire des Gauchers*. Paris: Imago.

Brackenridge, C. J. (1981). Secular variation in handedness over ninety years. *Neuropsychologia*, **19**, 459–62.

Bryden, M. P., Ardila, A. & Ardila, O. (1993). Handedness in native Amazonians. *Neuropsychologia*, **31**, 301–8.

Bryden, M. P., Singh, M. & Rogers, T. T. (1995). Heritability for degree and direction of human hand preference. *Society for Neuroscience Abstracts*, **21**, 200.

Burt, C. (1937). *The Backward Child*. London: University of London Press.

Cahen, D., Keeley, L. H. & Van Noten, F. L. (1979). Stone tools, toolkits, and human behavior in prehistory. *Current Anthropology*, **20**, 661–83.

Carrothers, G. E. (1947). Left-handedness among school pupils. *American School Board Journal*, **114**, 17–19.

Cavalli-Sforza, L. L. & Bodmer, W. F. (1971). *The Genetics of Human Populations*. San Francisco: W.H. Freeman.

Cavalli-Sforza, L. L., Menozzi, P. & Piazza, A. (1994). *The History and Geography of Human Genes*. Princeton, NJ: Princeton University Press.

Connolly, K. & Bishop, D. V. M. (1992). The measurement of handedness: a cross-cultural comparison of samples from England and Papua New Guinea. *Neuropsychologia*, **30**, 13–26.

Coren, S. & Halpern, D. F. (1991). Left-handedness: a marker for decreased survival fitness. *Psychological Bulletin*, **109**, 90–106.

Coren, S. & Porac, C. (1977). Fifty centuries of right-handedness: the historical record. *Science*, **198**, 631–2.

Crichton-Browne, J. (1907). Dexterity and the bend sinister. *Proceedings of the Royal Institution of Great Britain*, **18**, 623–52.

Crowfoot, E., Pritchard, F. & Staniland, K. (2001). *Textiles and Clothing c1150–c1450*. Woodbridge: Boydell Press.

de Castro, J. M. B., Bromage, T. G. & Jalvo, Y. F. (1988). Buccal striations on fossil human anterior teeth: evidence of handedness in the middle and early Upper Pleistocene. *Journal of Human Evolution*, **17**, 403–12.

Delacato, C. H. (1963). *The Diagnosis and Treatment of Speech and Reading Problems*. Springfield, IL: C C Thomas.

Ellis, P. J., Marshall, E., Windridge, C., Jones, S. & Ellis, S. J. (1998). Left-handedness and premature death. *Lancet*, **351**, 1634.

Erlenmeyer-Kimling, L., Hans, S., Ingraham, L. *et al.* (2005). Handedness in children of schizophrenic parents: data from three high-risk studies. *Behavior Genetics*, **35**, 351–8.

Faurie, C. & Raymond, M. (2004). Handedness frequency over more than 10,000 years. *Proceedings of the Royal Society of London, Series B*, **271**, S43–S45.

Finger, S. (1994). *Origins of Neuroscience: a History of Explorations into Brain Function*. New York: Oxford University Press.

Finger, S. & Roe, D. (1999). Does Gustave Dax deserve to be forgotten? The temporal lobe theory and other contributions of an overlooked figure in the history of language and cerebral dominance. *Brain and Language*, **69**, 16–30.

Fox, C. L. & Frayer, D. W. (1997). Non-dietary marks in the anterior dentition of the Krapina Neanderthals. *International Journal of Osteoarchaeology*, **7**, 133–49.

Gibbons, B. (1986). The intimate sense of smell. *National Geographic*, **170**, 324–61.

Gilbert, A. N. & Wysocki, C. J. (1987). The Smell Survey results. *National Geographic*, **172**, 514–25.

Gilbert, A. N. & Wysocki, C. J. (1992). Hand preference and age in the United States. *Neuropsychologia*, **30**, 601–8.

Halpern, D. F. & Coren, S. (1988). Do right-handers live longer? *Nature*, **333**, 213.

Halpern, D. F. & Coren, S. (1991). Handedness and life span. *New England Journal of Medicine*, **324**, 998.

Halpern, D. F. & Coren, S. (1993). Left-handedness and life span: a reply to Harris. *Psychological Bulletin*, **114**, 235–41.

Halpern, D. F., Haviland, M. G. & Killian, C. D. (1998). Handedness and sex differences in intelligence: evidence from the Medical College Admission Test. *Brain and Cognition*, **38**, 87–101.

Harris, L. J. (1991). Cerebral control for speech in right-handers and left-handers: an analysis of the views of Paul Broca, his contemporaries, and his successors. *Brain and Language*, **40**, 1–50.

Harris, L. J. (1993a). Broca on cerebral control for speech in right-handers and left-handers: a note on translation and some further comments. *Brain and Language*, **45**, 108–20.

Harris, L. J. (1993b). Do left-handers die sooner than right-handers? Commentary on Coren and Halpern's (1991) "Left-handedness: a marker for decreased survival fitness". *Psychological Bulletin*, **114**, 203–34.

Harris, L. J. (1993c). Reply to Halpern and Coren. *Psychological Bulletin*, **114**, 242–7.

Hopkins, W. D. (2006). Comparative and familial analysis of handedness in great apes. *Psychological Bulletin*, **132**, 538–59.

Hugdahl, K. (1996). Left-handedness and age: comparing writing/drawing and other manual activities. *Laterality*, **1**, 177–83.

Hugdahl, K., Satz, P., Mitrushina, M. & Miller, E. N. (1993). Left-handedness and old age: do left-handers die earlier? *Neuropsychologia*, **31**, 325–33.

Ida, Y. & Bryden, M. P. (1996). A comparison of hand preference in Japan and Canada. *Canadian Journal of Experimental Psychology*, **50**, 234–9.

Ireland, W. W. (1880). Notes on left-handedness. *Brain*, **3**, 207–14.

Iwasaki, S. (2000). Age and generation trends in handedness: an Eastern perspective. In M. K. Mandal, M. B. Bulman-Fleming & G. Tiwari, eds., *Side Bias: A Neuropsychological Perspective*. Dordrecht: Kluwer, pp. 83–100.

Knecht, S., Deppe, M., Dräger, B. *et al.* (2000). Language lateralization in healthy right-handers. *Brain*, **123**, 74–81.

Leask, S. J. & Beaton, A. A. (2007). Handedness in Great Britain. *Laterality*, **12**, 559–72.

Lombroso, C. (1884). Sul mancinismo e destrismo tattile nei sani, nei pazzi, nei ciechi e nei sordomuti. *Archivi di Psichiatria, Neuropsichiatria, antropologia criminale e medicina legale*, vol. **5**.

Marchant, L. F. & McGrew, W. C. (1991). Laterality of function in apes: a meta-analysis of methods. *Journal of Human Evolution*, **21**, 425–38.

Marchant, L. F. & McGrew, W. C. (1996). Laterality of limb function in wild chimpanzees of Gombe National Park: comprehensive study of spontaneous activities. *Journal of Human Evolution*, **30**, 427–43.

Marks, J. S. & Williamson, D. F. (1991). Left-handedness and life expectancy. *New England Journal of Medicine*, **325**, 1042.

McManus, I. C. (1981). Handedness and birth stress. *Psychological Medicine*, **11**, 485–96.

McManus, I. C. (1984). The genetics of handedness in relation to language disorder. In F. C. Rose, ed., *Advances in Neurology, vol 42: Progress in Aphasiology*, New York: Raven Press, pp. 125–38.

McManus, I. C. (1985). *Handedness, Language Dominance and Aphasia: a Genetic Model*. Psychological Medicine, Monograph Supplement No. 8, Cambridge University Press.

McManus, I. C. (1991). The inheritance of left-handedness. In G. R. Bock & J. Marsh, eds., *Biological Asymmetry and Handedness (Ciba Foundation Symposium 162)*, Chichester: Wiley, pp. 251–81.

McManus, I. C. (1999). Handedness, cerebral lateralization and the evolution of language. In M. C. Corballis & S. E. G. Lea, eds., *The Descent of Mind: Psychological Perspectives on Hominid Evolution*. Oxford: Oxford University Press, pp. 194–217.

McManus, I. C. (2002). *Right Hand, Left Hand: The Origins of Asymmetry in Brains, Bodies, Atoms and Cultures*. London, UK/Cambridge, MA: Weidenfeld and Nicolson/Harvard University Press.

McManus, I. C. (2004). Grappling with the hydra: review of *Handedness and Brain Asymmetry*, by Marian Annett. *Cortex*, **40**, 139–41.

McManus, I. C. & Bryden, M. P. (1992). The genetics of handedness, cerebral dominance and lateralization. In I. Rapin & S. J. Segalowitz, eds., *Handbook of Neuropsychology*, Volume 6, Section 10: Child neuropsychology (Part 1), Amsterdam: Elsevier, pp. 115–44.

McManus, I. C. & Bryden, M. P. (1993). Handedness on Tristan da Cunha: the genetic consequences of social isolation. *International Journal of Psychology*, **28**, 831–43.

McManus, I. C. & Hartigan, A. (2007). Declining left-handedness in Victorian England seen in the films of Mitchell and Kenyon. *Current Biology*, **17**, R793–4.

McManus, I. C., Moore, J., Freegard, M. & Rawles, R. (in press a). Science in the making: right hand, left hand: III: the incidence of left-handedness. *Laterality*.

McManus, I. C. & Peters, M. (in press). Handedness in Europe: analysis of data from the BBC internet study.

McManus, I. C., Rawles, R., Moore, J. & Freegard, M. (in press b). Science in the making: Right Hand, Left Hand: I: a BBC television programme broadcast in 1953. *Laterality*.

McManus, I. C., Richards, P. & Maitlis, S. L. (1989). Prospective study of the disadvantage of people from ethnic minority groups applying to medical schools in the United Kingdom. *British Medical Journal*, **298**, 723–6.

McManus, I. C., Richards, P., Winder, B. C., Sproston, K. A. & Styles, V. (1995). Medical school applicants from ethnic minorities: identifying if and when they are disadvantaged. *British Medical Journal*, **310**, 496–500.

McManus, I. C. & Wysocki, C. J. (in press). Variation in handedness across the United States.

Medland, S. E., Perelle, I. B., De Monte, V. & Ehrman, L. (2004). Effects of culture, sex, and age on the distribution of handedness: an evaluation of the sensitivity of three measures of handedness. *Laterality*, **9**, 287–97.

Minar, C. J. (2001). Motor skills and the learning process: the conservation of cordage final twist direction in communities of practice. *Journal of Anthropological Research*, **57**, 381–405.

Ogle, W. (1871). On dextral pre-eminence. *Medical – Chirurgical Transactions (Transactions of the Royal Medical and Chirurgical Society of London)*, **54**, 279–301.

Olivier, G. (1978). Anthropometric data on left-handed. *Biométrie Humaine*, **13**, 13–22.

Parson, B. S. (1924). *Lefthandedness: a New Interpretation*. New York: Macmillan.

Perelle, I. B. & Ehrman, L. (1994). An international study of human handedness: the data. *Behavior Genetics*, **24**, 217–27.

Peters, M., Reimers, S. & Manning, J. T. (2006). Hand preference for writing and associations with selected demographic and behavioral variables in 255,100 subjects: the BBC internet study. *Brain and Cognition*, **62**, 177–89.

Phillipson, L. (1997). Edge modification as an indicator of function and handedness of Acheulian handaxes from Kariandusi, Kenya. *Lithic Technology*, **22**, 171–83.

Pujol, J., Deus, J., Losilla, J. M. & Capdevila, A. (1999). Cerebral lateralization of language in normal left-handed people studied by functional MRI. *Neurology*, **52**, 1038–43.

Pye-Smith, P. H. (1871). On left-handedness. *Guy's Hospital Reports*, **16**, 141–6.

Ramaley, F. (1913). Inheritance of left-handedness. *American Naturalist*, **47**, 730–9.

Raymond, M. & Pontier, D. (2004). Is there geographical variation in human handedness? *Laterality*, **9**, 35–51.

Reimers, S. (2007). The BBC Internet Study: general methodology. *Archives of Sexual Behaviour*, **36**, 147–61.

Roberts, M. B. & Parfitt, S. A. (1999). *Boxgrove: A Middle Pleistocene Hominid Site at Eartham Quarry, Boxgrove, West Sussex*. London: English Heritage.

Ross, G., Lipper, E. & Auld, P. A. M. (1992). Hand preference, prematurity and developmental outcome at school age. *Neuropsychologia*, **30**, 483–94.

Sadler, N. (1997). A sinister way of life: a search for left-handed material culture. In S. M. Pearce, ed., *Experiencing Material Culture in the Western World*. London: Leicester University Press, pp. 140–53.

Salmaso, D. & Longoni, A. M. (1983). Hand preference in an Italian sample. *Perceptual and Motor Skills*, **57**, 1039–42.

Schäfer, M. (1911). Die Linkshänder in den Berliner Gemeindeschulen. *Berliner klinische Wochenschrift*, **48**, 295.

Singh, M. & Bryden, M. P. (1994). The factor structure of handedness in India. *International Journal of Neuroscience*, **74**, 33–43.

Singh, M., Manjary, M. & Dellatolas, G. (2001). Lateral preferences among Indian school children. *Cortex*, **37**, 231–41.

Spenneman, D. R. (1984). Handedness data on the European Neolithic. *Neuropsychologia*, **22**, 613–15.

Spindler, K. (1994). *The Man in the Ice*. London: Weidenfeld and Nicolson.

Steele, J. (2000). Handedness in past human populations: skeletal markers. *Laterality*, **5**, 193–220.

Steele, J. & Mays, S. (1995). Handedness and directional asymmetry in the long bones of the human upper limb. *International Journal of Osteoarchaeology*, **5**, 39–49.

Steele, J. & Uomini, N. (2005). Humans, tools and handedness. In V. Roux & B. Bril, eds., *Stone Knapping: the Necessary Conditions for a Uniquely Hominin Behaviour*. Cambridge: McDonald Institute, pp. 217–39.

Stephens, W. B. (1990). Literacy in Scotland, England and Wales, 1500–1900. *History of Education Quarterly*, **30**, 545–71.

Stier, E. (1911). *Untersuchungen über Linkshändigkeit und die funktionellen Differenzen der Hirnhälften. Nebst einem Anhang, "Über Linkshändigkeit in der deutschen Armee"*. Jena: Gustav Fischer.

Stone, L. (1969). Literacy and education in England 1640–1900. *Past and Present*, **42**, 69–139.

Teng, E. L., Lee, P. & Chang, P. C. (1976). Handedness in a Chinese population: biological, social and pathological factors. *Science*, **193**, 1148–50.

Toth, N. (1985). Archaeological evidence for preferential right handedness in the lower and middle Pleistocene and its possible implications. *Journal of Human Evolution*, **14**, 607–14.

Viggiano, M. P., Borelli, P., Vannucci, M. & Rocchetti, G. (2001). Hand preference in Italian students. *Laterality*, **6**, 283–6.

Watson, T. (1836). An account of some cases of transposition observed in the human body. *London Medical Gazette*, **18**, 393–403.

West, E. G. (1978). Literacy and the Industrial Revolution. *Economic History Review*, **31**, pp. 369–83.

Wolf, P. A., D'Agostino, R. B. & Cobb, J. (1991). Left-handedness and life expectancy. *New England Journal of Medicine*, **325**, 1042.

Wysocki, C. J. & Gilbert, A. N. (1989). National Geographic Smell Survey: effects of age are heterogenous. In C. Murphy, W. S. Cain & D. M. Hegsted, eds., *Nutrition and the Chemical Senses in Aging: Recent Advances and Current Research Needs*. New York: New York Academy of Sciences, pp. 12–28.

Wysocki, C. J., Pierce, J. D. & Gilbert, A. N. (1991). Geographic, cross-cultural, and individual variation in human olfaction. In T. V. Getchell *et al.*, eds., *Smell and Taste in Health and Disease*, New York: Raven Press, pp. 287–314.

4

The association between hand preference and language lateralization

Bianca Stubbe-Dräger and Stefan Knecht

Summary

Specialization of the left hemisphere for language has been generally accepted for more than a century. But across individuals, hemispheric specialization is a variable trait – not only with respect to the side but also with respect to the degree. Thus, the neural correlates of language are also found in the right side, and in some individuals in both hemispheres. The degrees of hand and language lateralization in humans are correlated, although right-handedness is not a precondition for left-hemispheric language lateralization. The mechanisms underlying hemispheric lateralization in humans are still unclear. Because a selective advantage for either brain organization is missing, the freedom with which the brain can instantiate language, invites speculation about the underlying neural causes for language lateralization. Present evidence suggests that language builds on a bilateral symmetric sensorimotor neural architecture dedicated to action, which supports dexterity as well as motor observation, imitation, learning, and understanding.

This chapter summarizes literature on handedness, language, and cerebral asymmetry as evidenced by lesion and neuroimaging studies. It will comment on the possible origin of dexterity and language lateralization, the individual differences in laterality, as well as the distribution of laterality at the population level.

The beginnings

In 1836, the medical practitioner Mark Dax gave a lecture for the medical association in Montpellier on patients suffering from speech loss after brain lesion. This observation was not new. The old Greeks had already described aphasias. However, Mark Dax was the first to realize that all of his aphasic patients had a lesion of the left hemisphere – and none showed damage of the right (Harris, 1991). Nevertheless, because no one was really interested in this observation, the lecture remained his only documented one. Mark Dax died about one year later without knowing that he had been a pioneer of one of the most fascinating research fields of the twentieth century.

Paul Broca was the one who revolutionized general conceptions of the brain in 1861. He had a patient named "Tan", this being the only syllable the patient could speak. Tan had a lesion of the left hemisphere, which had induced his speech loss. By contrast, none of Broca's patients with a lesion of the right hemisphere had aphasia. The observation that a palsy of the right half of the body is often accompanied by speech loss, whereas a palsy of the left half is not, established the relationship between the left hemisphere and language functions. After this description, it was speculated that the reverse, i.e., right-hemispheric language dominance, should be true for left-handers. This claim has been widely accepted as the "Broca rule" although Broca never explicitly postulated such a rule (Harris, 1991). Interestingly, Broca invoked the idea that early brain damage could change language dominance (Broca, 1863; 1865).

Luria was among the first to point out that the proposed tight relation between left-handedness and right-hemispheric language dominance could not be true. A sizable number of left-handers, following a stroke to their left hemisphere, displayed severe language impairment and thus had to be left-hemisphere dominant for language (Luria, 1970).

Language Lateralization and Psychosis, ed. Iris E. C. Sommer and René S. Kahn. Published by Cambridge University Press.
© Cambridge University Press 2009.

If the brain was believed to be a uniform structure up to Broca's time, it was now recognized that anatomically identical hemispheres differ functionally.

Handedness, language, and cerebral asymmetry

Today's knowledge of the variability of language lateralization in the healthy population is derived from studies of aphasias resulting from stroke. From these studies it was concluded that right-hemispheric language dominance should be rare and only found in left-handers. Further insights were obtained with functional imaging techniques. The use of these techniques arose from the need to determine higher cognitive functions in patients prior to neurosurgical interventions. In the meantime, the development of non-invasive techniques has allowed us to determine functional brain asymmetries even in healthy subjects.

Evidence from patients with aphasia

Aphasia occurs frequently after left-sided brain damage, but can also be found after right-sided lesions. Studies on the occurrence of aphasia after stroke in relation to handedness have provided widely diverging results. Aphasia following a right-hemisphere lesion ("crossed aphasia") in right-handed individuals is rare, most studies show a prevalence of less than 3% (Borod et al., 1985; Carr et al., 1981; Gloning, 1977; Zangwill, 1979). Two groups reported an increased incidence of about 20% to 25% for language deficits in left- or non-right-handers after right-hemispheric stroke (Basso et al., 1990; Gloning, 1977). Another group found no such increase and suggested a negligible role of the right-hemisphere in speech function in most left-handers without a history of early left-hemisphere damage (Kimura, 1983). A study with nearly three hundred patients demonstrated that variability of language lateralization occurs more frequently in left- than in right-handers (Hecaen et al., 1971; Hecaen & Sauguet, 1971).

Only 38% of hemispheric lesions in the language dominant hemisphere will result in transient, and 18% in permanent aphasia (Pedersen et al., 1995). Difficulties in the assessment of language performance due to physical exhaustion and deficits in attention in the early stages after stroke and restitution in the later stages may have led to an underdiagnosis of aphasia in right-hemispheric stroke patients. Another shortcoming of studies on differences in aphasia incidences in left- and right-handers is the small number of left-handers with right-hemispheric stroke and aphasia. Additionally, patients with language disturbances after cerebral infarction do not infrequently have pre-existing lesions in the other hemisphere rendering conjectures on the original hemispheric language dominance ambiguous (Pedersen et al., 1995). In addition, patients with crossed aphasia often have subcortical lesions instead of lesions of classical language areas (Alexander et al., 1989).

Because single case studies suggested that brain-damaged left-handers become aphasic more frequently than right-handers but recover quicker and better (Bakan et al., 1973; Bakan, 1977; Gloning, 1977; Luria, 1970), the degree of language lateralization has often been considered important for the likelihood of aphasia and recovery after unilateral brain damage. Lower degrees of lateralization have been related to a better recovery from aphasia. Left-handedness and right-hemispheric language lateralization are discussed as factors that may result in a more bilateral language representation. Data, however, are very diverging (Bakan et al., 1973; Gloning, 1977; Luria, 1970). Retrospective analysis of aphasia profiles suggests that the differences in the side of lesion as well as the differences between left-handers and right-handers have been overemphasized (Basso et al., 1990; Pedersen et al., 1995). Also, a thorough analysis of published crossed aphasia cases shows that these patients are comparable to subjects with aphasia after left-hemispheric lesions in terms of age, gender distribution, and aphasia type distribution (Coppens et al., 2002). Taken together, aphasia profiles induced by left- or right-hemispheric lesions and, in consequence, aphasia profiles of right- and left-handers seem to differ only in frequency.

Evidence from the intracarotid sodium amobarbital procedure (Wada test)

For a long time this test was the gold standard to determine hemispheric specialization. Due to its invasiveness it is used in pre-surgical patients only. Taken together, studies that make use of the Wada test[1] confirm that right-hemispheric language dominance is more frequent in left- than in right-handers (Benbadis *et al.*, 1995a; Loring *et al.*, 1990; Rasmussen & Milner, 1977; Risse *et al.*, 1997; Strauss & Wada, 1983; Wyllie *et al.*, 1990). However, the number of right-handers with right-hemisphere language dominance was 4% in a large series and rose to 12% when a left-hemisphere lesion was defined (Rasmussen & Milner, 1977). The Wada test is only performed in patients with brain lesions, which are often associated with a secondary transfer of cortical functions from the damaged to the intact hemisphere (Helmstaedter *et al.*, 1994). Thus, the knowledge concerning the variability of language dominance is heavily biased by pathological states in which there is, among other problems, a high likelihood of functional hemispheric reorganization with a shift of handedness and language dominance to the right hemisphere after left-hemispheric lesion (Helmstaedter *et al.*, 1997; Isaacs *et al.*, 1996; Jokeit *et al.*, 1996).

Lesion studies have also led to conjectures on a neural implementation of language and suggested a higher proportion of ambilateral patterns in left-handers. However, in the literature based on the intracarotid amobarbital procedure the definition of bilaterality of language varies considerably. Rasmussen and Milner reported 19% and Risse *et al.* 20% of non-right-handed patients with bilateral speech representation (Rasmussen & Milner, 1977; Risse *et al.*, 1997). Benbadis *et al.* reported evidence for speech in both hemispheres in 12% of patients (Benbadis *et al.*, 1995a). In about half of these patients they found return of speech soon after injection of amobarbital into either side of the brain, suggesting that in these subjects each hemisphere was capable of supporting language independently of the other. In the other patients speech impairment occurred after injection of either side. This shows that even if the technique of the Wada test seems to be relatively consistent, the interpretation of its results is subjective. Additionally, the procedure varies between centers (Dodrill, 1993; Benbadis *et al.*, 1995b; Loring *et al.*, 1990).

As a result of functional reorganization in brain-lesioned patients the relationship between handedness and language dominance is weak. If the lesion has occurred early in life, both language and handedness are shifted to the other hemisphere; after lesions later in life it is likely that only language shifts (Satz *et al.*, 1988). However, for every single patient it is unclear how the brain was organized before the brain injury. Therefore, predictions about brain organization based on studies with brain-injured patients are difficult.

Evidence from functional imaging

Due to non-invasive technology it is possible to directly assess language lateralization in the healthy population. Using fMRI,[2] Frost *et al.* studied 100 right-handers: none of them was right dominant for language, 94% were strongly left lateralized (Frost *et al.*, 1999). Pujol *et al.* addressed the question of language dominance in the healthy population by studying 50 left- and 50 right-handers with fMRI. They found a high prevalence of left-hemispheric specialization in right-handers and more frequent atypical ambilateral and rightward lateralization patterns in left-handers, but

---

[1] In most epilepsy surgery programs, hemispheric dominance for language is assessed by intra-arterial administration of amobarbital via a transfemoral catheter placed in an internal carotid artery (Wada 1949). The injection of amobarbital in the left or right internal carotid artery causes a function loss of the ipsilateral hemisphere with hemianopia and hemiplegia for some minutes. This enables the study of the functions of each hemisphere separately (Meador and Loring 1999; Loring 1997).

[2] Functional magnetic resonance imaging (fMRI) measures the hemodynamic response related to neural activity in the brain. Nerve cells consume oxygen for neural activation. The local response to this oxygen use is an increase in blood flow to regions of increased neural activity. After deoxygenation, hemoglobin causes a slightly different signal of the blood, which can be detected using an MR pulse sequence as blood-oxygen-level-dependent (BOLD) contrast. Therefore, fMRI can be used to map changes in brain hemodynamics that correspond to mental operations. Due to the good spatial resolution it extends traditional anatomical imaging to include maps of human brain function. There are various approaches to describe hemispheric language dominance (Turner *et al.*, 1998; Jansen *et al.*, 2006).

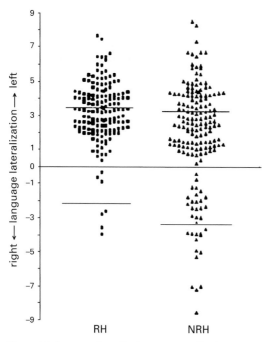

Figure 4.1 Language lateralization as assessed by fTCD in 326 healthy subjects.

RH = right-handers; NRH = non-right-handers; – = mean.

most of the left-handers still presented left-hemispheric specialization (Pujol *et al.*, 1999).

Using fTCD,[3] we studied 326 healthy subjects of whom over 100 were left-handers. We showed that 1 in 20 right-handers is right-hemisphere language lateralized, as well as every fourth left-hander (Knecht *et al.*, 2000b). (See Fig. 4.1.)

---

[3] Functional transcranial Doppler ultrasonography (fTCD) is a non-invasive method to establish cerebral lateralization. It can assess event-related changes in cerebral blood flow velocities and, by comparison between sides, can provide a measure of lateralization of hemispheric perfusion. The changes in cerebral perfusion during cognitive tasks result in corresponding alterations of blood flow velocities in the feeding basal arteries. These task-related alterations can be non-invasively and conveniently assessed by fTCD. A cued word generation task was established to determinate language lateralization in single subjects. The technique provides a highly reliable language laterality index, which is proportional to the Wada and fMRI index (Deppe *et al.*, 2004; Stroobant & Vingerhoets, 2000).

We also found that handedness or the dominant hemisphere as a single determinant does not influence differences in the degree of language lateralization. Rather the degree of language lateralization is related to an interaction of hand preference and side of the dominant hemisphere. Subjects with control for language and handedness lateralized to the same hemisphere have a stronger lateralization for language than subjects with control for language and handedness lateralized to different hemispheres (Drager *et al.*, 2000; Knecht *et al.*, 2001).

The distribution of hemispheric language dominance was found to vary with the degree of handedness. The more right-handed the subjects were, the lower was the relative incidence of right-hemispheric language dominance and vice versa. Overall, strong left-handers demonstrated a nearly sixfold higher incidence of right dominance than strong right-handers: extreme left-handers had a 27%, and extreme right-handers a 4% incidence of right-hemispheric language dominance. The intermediate groups showed a 27%, 22%, 11%, 10%, and 6% incidence, respectively. The rate of right-hemispheric language dominance can be approximated by the formula: *likelihood of right-hemispheric language dominance (%) = 15% – handedness by the Edinburgh inventory (%)/10* (Knecht *et al.*, 2000b).

An fMRI study focusing on the Broca region corroborated this finding by reporting "bilateral" activation in 14% of 100 healthy subjects during word generation (Pujol *et al.*, 1999).

From studies with the Wada test we know that there are subjects with bilateral language lateralization whose hemispheres are capable of supporting language independently of the other, because after injection of amobarbital into either side of the brain no speech loss was found. On the other hand, there were other subjects in whom speech impairment occurred after injection of either side (Benbadis *et al.*, 1995b). Studies of brain lateralization as assessed by functional activation, which underlies both fTCD and fMRI, can not provide information about the functional relevance of task-related activation. Therefore, we used TMS to disturb language functions of healthy subjects with known language lateralization from strong left over bilateral to strong right-hemispheric lateralization as assessed by fTCD.[4] Both, side and degree of language lateralization, correlated with a person's susceptibility to language disruption after neural deactivation with TMS. Subjects with weak lateralization (more bilaterality) were less affected by either left- or right-sided TMS than were subjects with strong lateralization to one hemisphere (Knecht *et al.*, 2002).

Accordingly, the degree and not the side of language lateralization seems to be important for the susceptibility of suffering aphasia after unilateral brain lesions. In line with this view, an fMRI study showed no differences in the pattern of brain activation between subjects with right- and left-language lateralization. Subjects with right-hemispheric language lateralization showed patterns of brain activation that were just the mirror reverse of the patterns of subjects with left-hemispheric language lateralization (Knecht *et al.*, 2003). (See Fig. 4.2.)

Functional imaging is also conducted in patients following stroke and has led to new insights into changes in brain activation associated with neural reorganization. Following the old idea that the homologous regions of the right hemisphere play a crucial role in recovery from aphasia, it has been assumed that the observed activation of the unaffected hemisphere in stroke patients is due to language recovery (Weiller *et al.*, 1995; Silvestrini *et al.*, 1995). Some patients show recruitment of areas of the language-dominant hemisphere (Karbe *et al.*, 1998b), whereas others recruit homologous areas of the language-subdominant hemisphere (Thulborn *et al.*, 1999; Musso *et al.*, 1999). Whether the activation is language relevant is unclear. Critics interpret the activation of contralateral homologous areas as effort of the subject to overcome his or her deficit (Heiss *et al.*, 1997). However, in healthy subjects an increase in difficulty of word

retrieval does not lead to an increased activation of the dominant or of the subdominant hemisphere. These findings lend support to the view that in aphasics activation of the unaffected hemisphere should not be interpreted as unspecific effect but reflects activation specific to language (Drager & Knecht, 2002; Drager *et al.*, 2004).

Therefore, activation studies of aphasics may reflect different pre-lesioned brain organizations between patients. This does not mean that every right-hemispheric activation is due to recovery. In some cases right-hemispheric activation could simply be due to a premorbid "bilateral" language network of the patient and may not reflect functional reorganization. But studies with partially recovered aphasics suggest that right-brain activation is functionally relevant (Weiller *et al.*, 1995; Silvestrini *et al.*, 1995). As a whole, studies of aphasic patients show that the functional dominance of the left hemisphere varies between individuals, and that language recovery after stroke depends on the restitution of the speech-relevant network in both brain hemispheres.

Evidence from anatomical imaging

Anatomical studies measuring the planum temporale in healthy subjects showed that left-handers as a whole are more likely to present symmetry (Foundas *et al.*, 2002; Steinmetz *et al.*, 1991). With regards to Broca's area, data are contradictory. Some authors found a weaker asymmetry for left-handers (Foundas *et al.*, 1998) while others found no asymmetry between the hemispheres for any group (Watkins *et al.*, 2001; Tomaiuolo *et al.*, 1999).

Whether a relationship between anatomical structures and functional asymmetry exists is still unclear. Using magnetic resonance imaging (MRI) in patients who underwent the Wada test, Foundas *et al.* found that the left hemisphere was dominant for language in patients with leftward asymmetry of both the planum temporale and the pars triangularis, which is part of Broca's area. A patient who had a rightward asymmetry of both the planum temporale and the pars triangularis presented right-hemisphere dominance for language. However, one patient had a leftward asymmetry of the

---

[4] Transcranial magnetic stimulation (TMS) allows the induction of an electrical current in neurons via non-invasive excitation. In contrast to most other techniques, which give evidence about brain regions that are active during a task without differentiating if this activation is necessary for the task, TMS can induce virtual lesions and therefore give evidence about activation of brain regions that are necessary for performing a specific task (Pascual-Leone *et al.*, 2002).

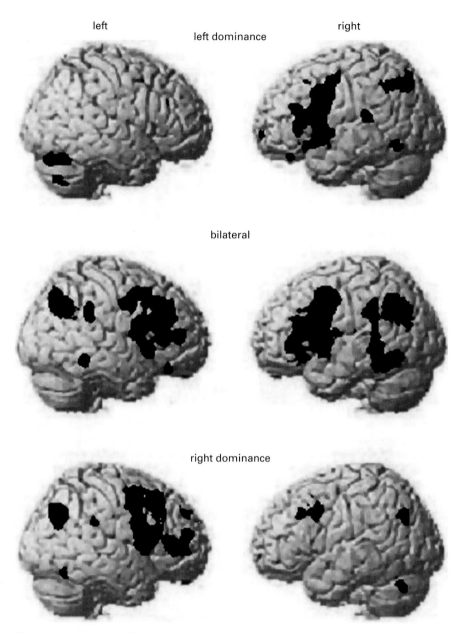

Figure 4.2 Language lateralization as assessed by fMRI.

planum temporale, a rightward asymmetry of the pars triangularis, and a left-hemisphere specialization for language (Foundas *et al.*, 1994; Foundas *et al.*, 1996). Other authors assumed a relationship of the planum temporale and handedness (Annett, 1992; Beaton, 1997). A combined anatomical MRI and PET study during story listening did not detect a relationship between the anatomical asymmetry of the planum temporale and the functional asymmetry of the temporal lobe related to language (Tzourio *et al.*, 1998).[5] But this study evidenced a relationship between the surface of the left planum temporale and left activations: subjects with the largest left planum temporale were also those who activated their left temporal regions the most. This result was confirmed by a further study that showed this relationship also for parts of the inferior parietal lobule and the rolandic operculum (Josse *et al.*, 2003).

A volumetric resonance imaging study (VBM) suggested a high occurrence of leftward asymmetry for relative white matter content in language-related regions (Pujol *et al.*, 2002).[6] Using tractography,[7] Nucifora *et al.* reported a strong asymmetry in the relative fiber density of the arcuate fasciculus, a white-matter pathway associated with language that connects the frontal, temporal, and parietal lobes (Nucifora *et al.*, 2005). A recent combined tractography and fMRI study showed that tract volumes and mean fractional anisotropy were significantly greater on the left than the right and demonstrated a correlation between measures of structure and function, in which subjects with more lateralized fMRI activation had a more highly lateralized mean

fractional anisotropy of their connections (Powell *et al.*, 2006). Comparing the brain morphology of healthy subjects with known left- and right-hemisphere language dominance these findings could be corroborated by our group. Additionally, the asymmetries of the planum temporale showed no functional relevance for language lateralization, but interestingly, we found structural differences between the language dominance groups in the hippocampus. Subjects with right-hemisphere language dominance had larger gray matter volume in the right hippocampus than subjects with left-hemisphere language dominance. This is in line with the view that the hippocampus might even be the driving force for the development of language lateralization, and with the role of the hippocampus for learning semantic information (Breitenstein *et al.*, 2005; Knecht, 2004). Therefore, the study underlines the role of the hippocampus for the language network (Jansen *et al.*, 2008; Mohammadi *et al.*, 2006).

Taken together, several functional studies confirmed the high degree of freedom with which the brain can instantiate language. Language lateralization in humans follows a bimodal distribution. The majority of individuals are lateralized to the left and a minority of individuals are lateralized to the right side of the brain (Knecht *et al.*, 2000a; 2000b; 2001; Pujol *et al.*, 1999). But across individuals, hemispheric specialization is a variable trait – not only with respect to the side but also with respect to the degree.

Even under natural conditions the association between handedness and language dominance is not an absolute one. The phenotypic association of handedness and language lateralization in healthy subjects demonstrates that left-handedness is neither a precondition nor a necessary consequence of right-hemispheric language dominance. It remains the question: what is the missing link between handedness and language lateralization?

Origins of language: from gesture to speech?

The relation between handedness and language lateralization invites speculation on the underlying neural causes.

---

[5] Positron emission tomography (PET) measures emissions from radioactively labeled metabolically active chemicals that have been injected into the bloodstream. Via sensors in the PET scanner, the radioactivity can be detected as the compound accumulates in various regions of the brain. Areas of high radioactivity are associated with brain activity. With PET cognitive processes can be made visible even in the working brain (Heiss & Herholz, 2006).

[6] Voxel based morphometry (VBM) is an MRI technique that allows statistical parametric mapping of focal differences in brain volume. Every brain is registered to a brain template that compensates for anatomical differences among subjects. After this procedure the images are smoothed. As a result, every voxel represents the average of itself and its neighbor. This allows the identification of differences in the local gray matter volume between groups (Ashburner & Friston, 2000).

[7] Tractography is a diffusion tensor imaging (DTI) technique using MRI that enables the measurement of restricted diffusion of water in tissue. With DTI, information about anatomical connectivity between different brain areas can be won. White matter bundles carry functional information between brain regions. The diffusion of water molecules is hindered across the axes of these bundles, such that measurements of water diffusion can reveal information about the location of large white-matter pathways (Lee *et al.*, 2005; Mori & Zhang, 2006; Sundgren *et al.*, 2004).

The motor theory of speech

During early development there is a co-emergence of gesture and language. At the age of 6 months, children begin canonical babbling and rhythmic hand movements; the beginning of word comprehension at the age of eight months correlates with deictic gesture and first tool use; three months later a child starts to produce words and uses recognitory gestures at the same time. When the child begins to combine words at the age of eighteen months, it combines gestures and words as well as gestures and gestures. Between two and two-and-a-half years of age the onset and growth of grammar is linked with the child's ability to remember and imitate arbitrary sequences of manual action (for a review see Bates & Dick, 2002).

The link between gesture and language is also traceable in adults. Subjects make faster semantic sensibility judgments of phrases describing meaningful and nonsensical physical acts (e.g., aim a dart or close a nail) when they perform appropriate physical hand motions (e.g., pinching or clenching) (Klatzky et al., 1989). Conversely, automatic word reading influences processes of visuo-motor transformation. Subjects are slower at grasping an object if a word that is incompatible with the target object is printed on the object (e.g., the word "high" on a low object) (Gentilucci et al., 2000). In view of such findings, it has been suggested that the phylogenetic evolution of language may have resembled the ontogenetic development of language in children.

Maybe the capability for skilled action and tool use did provide the basis for computing a broad variety of action-object frames, which then could also be used for gestures in the absence of concrete objects. Facial and vocal elements may gradually have been introduced, and evolved to the point that vocalization predominated (Arbib, 2005; Gentilucci & Corballis, 2006). Indeed, research has shown that modern apes use the same brain areas to interpret hand signals as humans do to process spoken language (Pollick & de Waal, 2007).

Further support for a gesture–language connection was provided by the detection of the mirror-neuron system in the F5 – among other – regions in the monkey brain (Gallese et al., 1996; Rizzolatti et al., 1996a;

1996b). A mirror neuron fires both when someone performs an action and when someone observes the same action performed by another. Studying monkeys, Fogassi et al. showed that during observation of a specific act, motor neurons of the inferior parietal lobe coding for the specific act show markedly different activations for acts that are part of different activities (e.g., simple grasping versus eating). The neurons discriminate the very same act (e.g., grasping) according to the context in which the act is embedded (e.g., grasping a tool or grasping food). These neurons are an example of how action and cognition are linked with one another and how the augmentation of motor neurons during evolution may have provided the basis for developing complex cognitive functions (Fogassi et al., 2005). Mirror neurons allow the observing individual to understand the goal of the observed motor act. Even in humans observing, imagining, preparing, or in any way representing an action, stimulates the motor program used to execute the same action (Buccino et al., 2001; Rizzolatti et al., 1996; Nishitani & Hari, 2000).

But what is the link between the mirror neuron system and language? Human brain imaging studies frequently show coactivation of Broca's area, the human homolog of the F5 region in monkeys, during observation of hand action (Buccino et al., 2001; Rizzolatti et al., 1996; Nishitani & Hari, 2000); the neural architecture for imitation of finger movements overlaps with language areas in the human brain (Aziz-Zadeh et al., 2006). Additionally, the hand motor system has been shown to be activated by linguistic tasks, most notably by pure linguistic perception, but not by auditory or visuospatial processing in humans (Tokimura et al., 1996; Floel et al., 2003; Pulvermuller et al., 2001; Rogalewski et al., 2004).

Human brain imaging studies indicate that Broca's area, which is located in the pars opercularis of the inferior frontal gyrus, may be part of the human mirror neuron system as well as the superior temporal sulcus and the inferior parietal lobule. The pars opercularis may serve as a core neural network for action understanding (Carr et al., 2003; Iacoboni et al., 2005; Mazziotta et al., 2001).

The dual use of classical language areas in humans suggests an evolutionary continuity between action perception, simulation, execution, and language. Because the mirror neuron system may be the neural basis for using own experience for interacting with the world, it is suggested that it plays an important role in imitation, observational learning, and social skills in humans. As such, language can be viewed as symbolic mirror function. As someone is able to understand the goal of an action irrespective of performing the action himself or observing the action by another, he or she is also able to understand the meaning of spoken language, irrespective of being the speaker or the hearer. Language may be the culmination of symbolic goal-directed action.

Brain asymmetry at the individual level

In most individuals handedness and language are lateralized brain functions. But why?

First of all: why not? There is no need for brain functions such as handedness and language to be organized bilaterally. Functions related to locomotion are organized symmetrically because bisymmetric organisms can move faster in fight and flight than can radial-symmetric organisms (Kinsbourne, 1978). For neural function unrelated to locomotion, such as action perception, action simulation, and goal-directed actions, and therefore handedness and language, a strictly symmetrical bilateral implementation in the neuronal structure of the brain is not mandatory.

It was further postulated that in the case of a bilateral organization of language functions, transfer of language information within only one hemisphere would be more efficient than across hemispheres. Repeated transcallosal transitions of neural impulses between hemispheres during complex linguistic operations were believed to decrease processing speed and efficacy (Ringo et al., 1994). Lateralization of language functions should aid the processing demands required for a full exhaustion of linguistic capacities (Geschwind & Galaburda, 1985; Luria, 1973).

The mechanisms underlying hemispheric lateralization in humans are still unclear. Until now, there is no evidence that the motor mirror neuron system itself is lateralized in humans (Aziz-Zadeh et al., 2006). But there is evidence that the auditory mirror neuron system (Kohler et al., 2002) may be lateralized (Aziz-Zadeh et al., 2004; Gazzola et al., 2005; 2006). The progression toward left lateralization of language functions may have been facilitated by the influence of a left-lateralized auditory component of a multimodal mirror neuron system.

It is also possible that factors independent from the mirror neuron system play a role in the development of brain asymmetries. For the motor system, transcallosal inhibition presents an important mechanism to optimize performance. It serves to solve incompatibilities between sensorimotor functions of homologous hemispheric regions during limb movements and may be a mechanism underlying the development of handedness (Karbe et al., 1998a; Meyer et al., 1998). Overall, the language-dominant hemisphere seems to exert more inhibition of the non-language-dominant hemisphere than vice versa (Netz et al., 1995). Transcallosal inhibition is not fully developed before the age of five years (Heinen et al., 1998). This correlates with the time window for transhemispheric shift of language functions after brain lesions in children, and may determine the freedom of the brain to instantiate language functions during childhood (Vargha-Khadem et al., 1985).

Brain asymmetry at the population level

The right–left ratio of handedness is 50:50 in chimpanzees and 90:10 in humans (Marchant & Mcgrew, 1996). There is no human culture in which right-handedness and left-handedness occur in equal parts (Provins, 1997). A survey of more than 5000 years of art-work, encompassing 1180 instances of unimanual tool or weapon usage, revealed no systematic trends in hand usage. The right hand was used on an average of 93% of the cases, regardless of which historical era or geographic region was assessed (Coren & Porac, 1977). A large adoption study demonstrated that handedness has a genetic component (Carter-Saltzman, 1980). Moreover, the first quantitative trait loci related to handedness have been identified (Francks et al., 2002; 2003a; 2003b).

The frequency distribution of language lateralization is similar to that of handedness, with approximately 90% of humans being left-hemisphere language dominant (Knecht *et al.*, 2000b). Despite the epidemiological dominance of left-hemispheric specialization for dexterity and language, no clear behavioral disadvantages for inverse or mixed patterns of hemispheric specialization have emerged so far (Knecht *et al.*, 2001).

However, it is conceivable that an adaptive advantage of lateralized neural processing during brain evolution may have biased our brain toward lateralization of language and handedness. This advantage may have been so small that it is not detectable at the individual level today.

Handedness and language lateralization: what does it tell us?

Present evidence suggests that language builds on a bilateral symmetric sensorimotor neural architecture dedicated to action, which supports dexterity as well as motor observation, imitation, learning, and understanding. Independence from locomotion requirements for symmetry allowed this architecture to become lateralized to some degree.

On the population level there is a strong tendency for left-hemispheric lateralization of language and handedness. But across individuals, hemispheric specialization is a variable trait with no apparent behavioral costs of any brain organization. However, as evidenced by severe language impairment in adults after unilateral brain lesions, once developed, lateralized brain systems become dedicated and homologous brain regions are hard to recruit.

REFERENCES

Alexander, M. P., Fischette, M. R. & Fischer, R. S. (1989). Crossed aphasias can be mirror image or anomalous. Case reports, review and hypothesis? *Brain*, **112**(4), 953–73.

Annett, M. (1992). Parallels between asymmetries of planum-temporal and of hand skill. *Neuropsychologia*, **30**(11), 951–62.

Arbib, M. A. (2005). From monkey-like action recognition to human language: an evolutionary framework for neurolinguistics. *Behavioral and Brain Sciences*, **28**(2), 105–11.

Ashburner, J. & Friston, K. J. (2000). Voxel-based morphometry – the methods. *Neuroimage*, **11**(6 Pt 1), 805–21.

Aziz-Zadeh, L. *et al.* (2004). Left hemisphere motor facilitation in response to manual action sounds. *European Journal of Neuroscience*, **19**(9), 2609–12.

Aziz-Zadeh, L. *et al.* (2006). Lateralization of the human mirror neuron system. *Journal of Neuroscience*, **26**(11), 2964–70.

Bakan, P. (1977). Left handedness and birth order revisited. *Neuropsychologia*, **15**(6), 837–9.

Bakan, P., Dibb, G. & Reed, P. (1973). Handedness and birth stress. *Neuropsychologia*, **11**(3), 363–6.

Basso, A. *et al.* (1990). Aphasia in left-handers. Comparison of aphasia profiles and language recovery in non-right-handed and matched right-handed patients. *Brain and Language*, **38**(2), 233–52.

Bates, E. & Dick, F. (2002). Language, gesture, and the developing brain. *Developmental Psychobiology*, **40**, 293–310.

Beaton, A. A. (1997). The relation of planum temporale asymmetry and morphology of the corpus callosum to handedness, gender, and dyslexia: a review of the evidence. *Brain and Language*, **60**(2), 255–322.

Benbadis, S. *et al.* (1995a). Autonomous versus dependent: a classification of bilateral language representation by intracarotid amobarbital procedure. *Journal of Epilepsy*, **8**, 255–66.

Benbadis, S. R. *et al.* (1995b). Objective criteria for reporting language dominance by intracarotid amobarbital procedure. *Journal of Clinical and Experimental Neuropsychology*, **17**(5), 682–690.

Borod, J. C. *et al.* (1985). Left-handed and right-handed aphasics with left hemisphere lesions compared on nonverbal performance measures. *Cortex*, **21**(1), 81–90.

Breitenstein, C. *et al.* (2005). Hippocampus activity differentiates good from poor learners of a novel lexicon. *Neuroimage*, **25**(3), 958–68.

Broca, P. (1863). Remarques sur le siège, le diagnostic et la nature de l'aphemie. *Bullitin of Comparative Anatomy*, **38**, 379–85.

Broca, P. (1865). Sur le siege de la faculté du langage articlé. *Bulletin de la Société d'Anthropologie de Paris*, **6**, 377–93.

Buccino, G. *et al.* (2001). Action observation activates premotor and parietal areas in a somatotopic manner: an fMRI study. *European Journal of Neuroscience*, **13**(2), 400–4.

Carr, L. *et al.* (2003). Neural mechanisms of empathy in humans: a relay from neural systems for imitation to limbic areas. *Proceedings of the National Academy of Sciences of the United States of America*, **100**(9), 5497–502.

Carr, M. S., Jacobson, T. & Boller, F. (1981). Crossed aphasia: analysis of four cases. *Brain and Language*, **14**(1), 190–202.

Carter-Saltzman, L. (1980). Biological and sociocultural effects on handedness: comparison between biological and adoptive families. *Science*, **209**(4462), 1263–5.

Coppens, P. *et al.* (2002). Crossed aphasia: an analysis of the symptoms, their frequency, and a comparison with left-hemisphere aphasia symptomatology. *Brain and Language*, **83**(3), 425–63.

Coren, S. & Porac, C. (1977). 50 centuries of right-handedness – historical record. *Science*, **198**(4317), 631–2.

Deppe, M., Ringelstein, E. B. & Knecht, S. (2004). The investigation of functional brain lateralization by transcranial Doppler sonography. *Neuroimage*, **21**(3), 1124–46.

Dodrill, C. B. (1993). Preoperative criteria for identifying eloquent brain. Intracarotid amytal for language and memory testing. *Neurosurg Clinics of North America*, **4**(2), 211–16.

Drager, B. *et al.* (2000). Association and dissociation of language dominance and handedness – possible impact on recovery from aphasia. *Journal of Neurolinguistics*, **13**(4), 279–82.

Drager, B. *et al.* (2004). How does the brain accommodate to increased task difficulty in word finding? A functional MRI study. *Neuroimage*, **23**(3), 1152–60.

Drager, B. & Knecht, S. (2002). When finding words becomes difficult: is there activation of the subdominant hemisphere? *Neuroimage*, **16**(3), 794–800.

Floel, A. *et al.* (2003). Language perception activates the hand motor cortex: implications for motor theories of speech perception. *European Journal of Neuroscience*, **18**(3), 704–8.

Fogassi, L. *et al.* (2005). Parietal lobe: from action organization to intention understanding. *Science*, **308**(5722), 662–7.

Foundas, A. L. *et al.* (1998). MRI asymmetries of Broca's area: the pars triangularis and pars opercularis. *Brain and Language*, **64**(3), 282–96.

Foundas, A. L. *et al.* (1994). Planum temporale asymmetry and language dominance. *Neuropsychologia*, **32**(10), 1225–31.

Foundas, A. L. *et al.* (1996). Pars triangularis asymmetry and language dominance. *Proceedings of the National Academy of Sciences of the United States of America*, **93**(2), 719–22.

Foundas, A. L., Leonard, C. M. & Hanna-Pladdy, B. (2002). Variability in the anatomy of the planum temporale and posterior ascending ramus: do right- and left-handers differ? *Brain and Language*, **83**(3), 403–24.

Francks, C. *et al.* (2003a). Parent-of-origin effects on handedness and schizophrenia susceptibility on chromosome 2p12-q11. *Human Molecular Genetics*, **12**(24), 3225–30.

Francks, C. *et al.* (2002). A genome-wide linkage screen for relative hand skill in sibling pairs. *American Journal Human Genetics*, **70**(3), 800–5.

Francks, C. *et al.* (2003b). Familial and genetic effects on motor coordination, laterality, and reading-related cognition. *American Journal of Psychiatry*, **160**(11), 1970–7.

Frost, J. A. *et al.* (1999). Language processing is strongly left lateralized in both sexes – evidence from functional MRI. *Brain*, **122**, 199–208.

Gallese, V. *et al.* (1996). Action recognition in the premotor cortex. *Brain*, **119**, 593–609.

Gazzola, V., Aziz-Zadeh, L. & Keysers, C. (2005). I hear what you are doing: an fMRI study of the auditory mirror system in humans. In: *Cognitive Neuroscience Society Abstracts*. New York: Cognitive Neuroscience Society.

Gazzola, V., Aziz-Zadeh, L. & Keysers, C. (2006). Empathy and the somatotopic auditory mirror system in humans. *Current Biology*, **16**(18), 1824–9.

Gentilucci, M. *et al.* (2000). Language and motor control. *Experimental Brain Research*, **133**(4), 468–90.

Gentilucci, M. & Corballis, M. C. (2006). From manual gesture to speech: a gradual transition. *Neuroscience and Biobehavioral Reviews*, **30**(7), 949–60.

Geschwind, N. & Galaburda, A. M. (1985). Cerebral lateralization. Biological mechanisms, associations, and pathology: III. A hypothesis and a program for research. *Archives of Neurology*, **42**(7), 634–54.

Gloning, K. (1977). Handedness and aphasia. *Neuropsychologia*, **15**(2), 355–8.

Harris, L. J. (1991). Cerebral control for speech in right-handers and left-handers: an analysis of the views of Paul Broca, his contemporaries, and his successors. *Brain and Language*, **40**(1), 1–50.

Hecaen, H. *et al.* (1971). Crossed aphasia in a right-handed bilingual (Vietnamese–French) subject. *Review of Neurology*, **124**(4), 319–23.

Hecaen, H. & Sauguet, J. (1971). Cerebral dominance in left-handed subjects. *Cortex*, **7**(1), 19–48.

Heinen, F. *et al.* (1998). Absence of transcallosal inhibition following focal magnetic stimulation in preschool children. *Annals of Neurology*, **43**(5), 608–12.

Heiss, W. D. & Herholz, K. (2006). Brain receptor imaging. *Journal of Nuclear Medicine*, **47**(2), 302–12.

Heiss, W. D. *et al.* (1997). Speech-induced cerebral metabolic activation reflects recovery from aphasia. *Journal of Neurological Sciences*, **145**(2), 213–17.

Helmstaedter, C. *et al.* (1994). Right hemisphere restitution of language and memory functions in right hemisphere language-dominant patients with left temporal lobe epilepsy. *Brain*, **117**(4), 729–37.

Helmstaedter, C. *et al.* (1997). Natural atypical language dominance and language shifts from the right to the left hemisphere in right hemisphere pathology. *Naturwissenschaften*, **84**(6), 250–2.

Iacoboni, M. *et al.* (2005). Grasping the intentions of others with one's own mirror neuron system. *PLoS Biology*, **3**(3), 529–35.

Isaacs, E. *et al.* (1996). Effects of hemispheric side of injury, age at injury, and presence of seizure disorder on functional ear and hand asymmetries in hemiplegic children. *Neuropsychologia*, **34**(2), 127–37.

Jansen, A. *et al.* (2006). The assessment of hemispheric lateralization in functional MRI – robustness and reproducibility. *Neuroimage*, **33**(1), 204–17.

Jansen, A., Luzzi, J., Deppe, M. *et al.* (2008). Structural correlates of functional language dominance – a voxel based morphometry study. *Journal of Neuroimaging*.

Jokeit, H. *et al.* (1996). Reorganization of memory functions after human temporal lobe damage. *NeuroReport*, **7**(10), 1627–30.

Josse, G. *et al.* (2003). Left planum temporale: an anatomical marker of left hemispheric specialization for language comprehension. *Cognitive Brain Research*, **18**(1), 1–14.

Karbe, H. *et al.* (1998a). Collateral inhibition of transcallosal activity facilitates functional brain asymmetry. *Journal of Cerebral Blood Flow and Metabolism*, **18**(10), 1157–61.

Karbe, H. *et al.* (1998b). Brain plasticity in poststroke aphasia: what is the contribution of the right hemisphere? *Brain and Language*, **64**(2), 215–30.

Kimura, D. (1983). Sex differences in cerebral organization for speech and praxic functions. *Canadian Journal of Psychology*, **37**(1), 19–35.

Kinsbourne, M. (1978). Evolution of language in relation to lateral action. In: Kinsbourne, M. (ed.) *Asymmetrical Function of the Brain*. Cambridge: Cambridge University Press, pp. 553–66.

Klatzky, R. L. *et al.* (1989). Can you squeeze a tomato – the role of motor representations in semantic sensibility judgments. *Journal of Memory and Language*, **28**(1), 56–77.

Knecht, S. (2004). Does language lateralization depend on the hippocampus? *Brain*, **127**, 1217–18.

Knecht, S. *et al.* (2000a). Language lateralization in healthy right-handers. *Brain*, **123**, 74–81.

Knecht, S. *et al.* (2000b). Handedness and hemispheric language dominance in healthy humans. *Brain*, **123**, 2512–18.

Knecht, S. *et al.* (2001). Behavioural relevance of atypical language lateralization in healthy subjects. *Brain*, **124**, 1657–65.

Knecht, S. *et al.* (2002). Degree of language lateralization determines susceptibility to unilateral brain lesions. *Nature Neuroscience*, **5**(7), 695–9.

Knecht, S. *et al.* (2003). How atypical is atypical language dominance? *Neuroimage*, **18**(4), 917–27.

Kohler, E. *et al.* (2002). Hearing sounds, understanding actions: action representation in mirror neurons. *Science*, **297**(5582), 846–8.

Lee, G. P. *et al.* (2005). Prediction of verbal memory decline after epilepsy surgery in children: effectiveness of Wada memory asymmetries. *Epilepsia*, **46**(1), 97–103.

Loring, D. W. (1997). Neuropsychological evaluation in epilepsy surgery. *Epilepsia*, **38**(4), S18–23.

Loring, D. W. *et al.* (1990). Cerebral language lateralization: evidence from intracarotid amobarbital testing. *Neuropsychologia*, **28**(8), 831–8.

Luria, A. (1970). *Traumatic Aphasia*. The Hague: Mouton.

Luria, A. (1973). *The Working Brain*. New York: Basic Books.

Marchant, L. F. & Mcgrew, W. C. (1996). Laterality of limb function in wild chimpanzees of Gombe National Park: comprehensive study of spontaneous activities. *Journal of Human Evolution*, **30**(5), 427–43.

Mazziotta, J. *et al.* (2001). A probabilistic atlas and reference system for the human brain: International Consortium for Brain Mapping (ICBM). *Philosophical Transactions of the Royal Society of London Series B – Biological Sciences*, **356** (1412), 1293–1322.

Meador, K. J. & Loring, D. W. (1999). The Wada test: controversies, concerns, and insights. *Neurology*, **52**(8), 1535–6.

Meyer, B. U., Roricht, S. & Woiciechowsky, C. (1998). Topography of fibers in the human corpus callosum mediating interhemispheric inhibition between the motor cortices. *Annals of Neurology*, **43**(3), 360–9.

Mohammadi, S., Jansen, A., Schwindt, W., Knecht, S. & Deppe, M. (2006). *Anatomisches Korrelat rechtshemisphärischer Sprachlateralisation: eine DTI Studie*. Wissenschaftszentrum NRW Netzwerk Neuro NRW, Neurovisionen, Duisburg, Deutschlang.

Mori, S. & Zhang, J. (2006). Principles of diffusion tensor imaging and its applications to basic neuroscience research. *Neuron*, **51**(5), 527–39.

Musso, M. *et al.* (1999). Training-induced brain plasticity in aphasia. *Brain*, **122**(9), 1781–90.

Netz, J., Ziemann, U. & Homberg, V. (1995). Hemispheric-asymmetry of transcallosal inhibition in man. *Experimental Brain Research*, **104**(3), 527–33.

Nishitani, N. & Hari, R. (2000). Temporal dynamics of cortical representation for action. *Proceedings of the National Academy of Sciences of the United States of America*, **97**(2), 913–18.

Nucifora, P. G. P. *et al.* (2005). Leftward asymmetry in relative fiber density of the arcuate fasciculus. *NeuroReport*, **16**(8), 791–4.

Pascual-Leone, A. *et al.* (eds.) (2002). *Handbook of Transcranial Magnetic Stimulation*. New York: Oxford University Press.

Pedersen, P. M. *et al.* (1995). Aphasia in acute stroke: incidence, determinants, and recovery. *Annals of Neurology*, **38**(4), 659–66.

Pollick, A. S. & de Waal, F. B. (2007). Ape gestures and language evolution. *Proceedings of the National Academy of Sciences of the United States of America*, **104**(19), 8184–9.

Powell, H. W. R. *et al.* (2006). Hemispheric asymmetries in language-related pathways: a combined functional MPI and tractography study. *Neuroimage*, **32**(1), 388–99.

Provins, K. A. (1997). Handedness and speech: a critical reappraisal of the role of genetic and environmental factors in the cerebral lateralization of function. *Psychological Review*, **104**(3), 554–71.

Pujol, J. *et al.* (1999). Cerebral lateralization of language in normal left-handed people studied by functional MRI. *Neurology*, **52**(5), 1038–43.

Pujol, J. *et al.* (2002). The lateral asymmetry of the human brain studied by volumetric magnetic resonance imaging. *Neuroimage*, **17**(2), 670–9.

Pulvermuller, F. *et al.* (2001). Constraint-induced therapy of chronic aphasia after stroke. *Stroke*, **32**(7), 1621–6.

Rasmussen, T. & Milner, B. (1977). The role of early left-brain injury in determining lateralization of cerebral speech functions. *Annals of the New York Academy of Sciences*, **299**, 355–69.

Ringo, J. L. *et al.* (1994). Time is of the essence: a conjecture that hemispheric specialization arises from interhemispheric conduction delay. *Cerebral Cortex*, **4**(4), 331–43.

Risse, G. L., Gates, J. R. & Fangman, M. C. (1997). A reconsideration of bilateral language representation based on the intracarotid amobarbital procedure. *Brain and Cognition*, **33**(1), 118–32.

Rizzolatti, G. *et al.* (1996a). Premotor cortex and the recognition of motor actions. *Cognitive Brain Research*, **3**(2), 131–41.

Rizzolatti, G., Luppino, G. & Matelli, M. (1996b). The classic supplementary motor area is formed by two independent areas. *Supplementary Sensorimotor Area*, **70**, 45–56.

Rogalewski, A. *et al.* (2004). Prosody as an intermediary evolutionary stage between a manual communication system and a fully developed language faculty. *Behavioral and Brain Sciences*, **27**(4), 521–2.

Satz, P. *et al.* (1988). Some correlates of intra- and inter-hemispheric speech organization after left focal brain injury. *Neuropsychologia*, **26**(2), 345–50.

Silvestrini, M. *et al.* (1995). Involvement of the healthy hemisphere in recovery from aphasia and motor deficit in patients with cortical ischemic infarction: a transcranial Doppler study. *Neurology*, **45**(10), 1815–20.

Steinmetz, H. *et al.* (1991). Anatomical left–right asymmetry of language-related temporal cortex is different in left-handers and right-handers. *Annals of Neurology*, **29**(3), 315–19.

Strauss, E. & Wada, J. (1983). Lateral preferences and cerebral speech dominance. *Cortex*, **19**(2), 165–77.

Stroobant, N. & Vingerhoets, G. (2000). Transcranial Doppler ultrasonography monitoring of cerebral hemodynamics during performance of cognitive tasks: a review. *Neuropsychological Review*, **10**(4), 213–231.

Sundgren, P. C. *et al.* (2004). Diffusion tensor imaging of the brain: review of clinical applications. *Neuroradiology*, **46**(5), 339–50.

Thulborn, K. R., Carpenter, P. A. & Just, M. A. (1999). Plasticity of language-related brain function during recovery from stroke. *Stroke*, **30**(4), 749–54.

Tokimura, H. *et al.* (1996). Speech-induced changes in corticospinal excitability. *Annals of Neurology*, **40**(4), 628–34.

Tomaiuolo, F. *et al.* (1999). Morphology, morphometry and probability mapping of the pars opercularis of the inferior frontal gyrus: an in vivo MRI analysis. *European Journal of Neuroscience*, **11**(9), 3033–46.

Turner, R. *et al.* (1998). Functional magnetic resonance imaging of the human brain: data acquisition and analysis. *Experimental Brain Research*, **123**(1–2), 5–12.

Tzourio, N., Nkanga-Ngila, B. & Mazoyer, B. (1998). Left planum temporale surface correlates with functional dominance during story listening. *NeuroReport*, **9**(5), 829–33.

Vargha-Khadem, F., O'Gorman, A. M. & Watters, G. V. (1985). Aphasia and handedness in relation to hemispheric side, age at injury and severity of cerebral lesion during childhood. *Brain*, **108**(3), 677–96.

Wada, J. (1949). A new method for determination of the side of cerebral speech dominance: a preliminary report on the intracarotid injection of sodium amytal in man. *Igaku Seibutsugaku*, **4**, 221–2.

Watkins, K. E. *et al.* (2001). Structural asymmetries in the human brain: a voxel-based statistical analysis of 142 MRI scans. *Cerebral Cortex*, **11**(9), 868–77.

Weiller, C. *et al.* (1995). Recovery from Wernicke's aphasia: a positron emission tomographic study. *Annals of Neurology*, **37**(6), 723–32.

Wyllie, E. *et al.* (1990). Intracarotid amobarbital (Wada) test for language dominance: correlation with results of cortical stimulation. *Epilepsia*, **31**(2), 156–61.

Zangwill, O. L. (1979). Two cases of crossed aphasia in dextrals. *Neuropsychologia*, **17**(2), 167–72.

5

The genetic basis of lateralization

Marian Annett

Summary

Modern theories of genetic influence on lateralization suggest that random or fluctuating asymmetry has an important role. Theories of directional asymmetry *or* chance can be distinguished from the right shift (RS) theory that accidental asymmetries are universal for bilaterally symmetrical organisms, but that in most humans left hemisphere advantage gives an incidental bias of the random distribution toward the right hand. Whereas many assume there is a true incidence of left-handedness, the RS theory suggests that degrees of hand preference map onto a continuous baseline of asymmetry that can be cut at any point to represent observed incidences of left-handedness. The parameters of the RS genetic model were derived from findings for speech lateralization in aphasics, supporting the argument that the relevant genetic locus is "for" cerebral dominance, not handedness. Genetic predictions are given for two levels of parental left-handedness (10% and 20%). Studies of family handedness distinguishing for sex in both generations gave generally good fits where handedness was assessed by self-report, but more variable fits for indirect report of relatives' handedness. The tendency to find a higher proportion of left-handed children born to left-handed mothers than left-handed fathers is not likely due to X-linked inheritance, but rather to slightly stronger expression of the *RS+* gene in females than males, and also under-reporting of left-handedness in mothers by right-handed children.

Monozygotic (MZ) twins discordant for handedness have led to doubts about genetic influence but these doubts are misplaced if random asymmetry affects every individual, twin and singleborn. The similarity of handedness distributions in MZ and dizygotic (DZ) twin pairs suggests that similar mechanisms are at work in both types of pair. Twins are more likely to be left-handed than the singleborn, by some 3% to 4%. There is greater concordance in MZ than DZ pairs, but this is difficult to detect because variability due to accidental asymmetries is large in comparison with the small genetic variability (due to the high prevalence of dextral genetic bias).

The inheritance of brain asymmetries is difficult to research but findings are consistent with models developed for handedness. There is a continuous normal distribution of asymmetry, biased in a typical direction with negative skew. A study of strength of language lateralization in families suggests genetic influence. Studies of asymmetries of cerebral anatomy and function in twins support theories of bias in a typical direction, which is reduced in the presence of left-handers. The theory that asymmetries occur at random in the absence of the typical pattern is consistent with findings for language and visuospatial functions. The suggestion that the *RS+* gene might lose directional coding and cause random impairment of the cerebral hemispheres offers a possible explanation for disorders of language and loss of cerebral asymmetry in psychosis.

Introduction

The search for genetic bases for handedness began almost a hundred years ago. There is strong evidence for a gene for normal lateralization of the viscera. There is evidence for genetic influence on hand preference but some reject genetic arguments in favor of explanations in terms of pathology, culture, or learning. The handedness of twins poses particular problems because conventional expectations about concordance in MZ versus DZ twin pairs appear not to be fulfilled. Whether there is a genetic basis for lateralization of the brain is difficult to research. However, the correlation between right-handedness and left hemisphere speech suggests that theory and research on handedness might offer clues to the inheritance of cerebral asymmetries.

Language Lateralization and Psychosis, ed. Iris E. C. Sommer and René S. Kahn. Published by Cambridge University Press.
© Cambridge University Press 2009.

Jordan (1911) suggested that left-handedness might be due to the recessive allele of a classic Mendelian locus. Studies of the families of students disproved this model because two left-handed parents (L × L families) had many right-handed children (Chamberlain, 1928; Ramaley, 1913; Rife, 1940). Trankell (1955) showed that although these three studies differed in incidences of left-handedness, they gave consistent estimates for a recessive allele with imperfect penetrance (frequency about 0.40–0.43). Current theories propose a recessive allele with imperfect penetrance in the sense that it is neutral for directional asymmetry and leads to a right- or left-handed phenotype by chance (Annett, 1972; Klar, 1996; McManus, 1985). There must be many ways in which genetic and non-genetic influences combine to determine asymmetries of early growth (Rutter *et al.*, 2006). The task of this chapter is to try to discern the recipe.

Theories of directional *or* chance asymmetry

Layton (1976) studied a mutant strain of mice with a high frequency of *situs inversus*. He hypothesized that a gene for typical situs was lost and that a mutant *iv* gene gave random bias to either side. Some twenty years later it was discovered that left–right orientation in early embryos depends on the directional beating of cilia, which direct the flow of essential substances to one side (Nonaka *et al.*, 1998). *Situs inversus* is associated with abnormal flow (Okada *et al.*, 1999). In humans, *situs inversus* is associated with loss of ciliary motion (primary ciliary dyskinesia, PCD) and occurs in 50% of affected cases, as in mutant mice.

Are the same genes involved in visceral and cerebral lateralization in humans? There is no increase in left-handedness in people with PCD (McManus *et al.*, 2004). Tanaka *et al.* (1999) gave a dichotic listening test to nine subjects with *situs inversus* and found eight had typical right-ear advantage. Kennedy *et al.* (1999) examined three individuals with *situs inversus* and found them strongly right-handed, with left hemisphere language by fMRI. Therefore, although similar models of directional asymmetry or chance have been proposed for asymmetries of gut and brain, the same genes are not likely to be involved.

McManus (1985) suggested a model for handedness like that of Layton (1976), a single locus with alleles coding for directional asymmetry (*D*, dextrality) *or* random asymmetry (*C*, chance). The model assumed heterozygote variability, with *C* expressed in 50% of *DC* genotypes and 25% becoming left-handed. In *CC* genotypes there is 50% left-handedness while in *DD* genotypes there is 100% right-handedness. McManus suggested a "true" incidence (7.75%) of left-handedness in the population. In actual data many different incidences occur and discrepancies from the true value were treated as error. In tests of the model, right- and left-handers were moved between genotypes to match observed incidences. The model cannot fail, therefore, unless observed incidences are very different from the supposed true incidence. With regard to cerebral dominance, *D* is expected to give left hemisphere speech, while *C* gives random specialization. The *C* allele is expressed in 50% of heterozygotes but independently of handedness. This implies that a large proportion of atypical speakers should carry the *D* allele.

Klar (1996) proposed a version of the dextrality *or* chance model resembling that of the *iv* gene most directly, a dominant allele for dextrality (*R*) and a recessive allele (*r*) for chance asymmetry. *RR* and *Rr* genotypes are right-handed and *rr* genotypes are right- or left-handed by chance. All left-handers are of *rr* genotype so that in L × L families 50% of children should be left-handed. Klar supported his theory by citing Rife (1940) where 6 out of 11 children in L × L families were left-handed. However, this high proportion is unusual (McManus & Bryden, 1992). In three new samples there were 94 children in L × L families, of whom 37.2% were left-handed, significantly fewer than the 50% predicted by Klar (Annett, 2008).

Klar argued that Rife's (1940) data give the "true" incidence of left-handedness in the population because the criterion was use of the left hand for any of several actions. More recent studies using the same criterion find higher incidences (below). In Rife's sample incidences differed for fathers, mothers, sons, and daughters. Klar estimated gene frequencies from the proportion of left-handed sons, about 9%, thus giving 18% in the population with *rr* genotype and gene frequency of about 0.43. The parallel with the estimates of Trankell (above) and Annett (below) is striking, but the reasoning behind the estimate does not withstand scrutiny. Klar has not attempted to fit his model to other studies in the literature.

A basic problem is that frequencies of left-handedness vary widely. If preference is treated as a discrete variable, then incidences are unstable and theories are restricted in the range of incidences to which they apply.

The right shift theory: chance asymmetry for all plus directional asymmetry for most but not all

The RS theory (Annett, 1972) developed through a series of stages of empirical research and theoretical analysis (Annett, 2002). The chief conclusion of the RS analysis was that the genetic agent is for cerebral dominance, not handedness.

Briefly, the theory suggests that degrees of hand preference map onto a non-genetic normal distribution of asymmetry for hand skill, a continuum of right minus left (R – L) skill. Accidental differences in the early growth of the body give differences between the sides, different for every individual and for every individual twin. An agent of left cerebral advantage (RS+ gene) displaces the accidental distribution of handedness in a dextral direction. The relative advantage to the left hemisphere probably depends on a *disadvantage* to the right hemisphere (Kilshaw & Annett, 1983). All gene carriers are expected to develop left hemisphere speech but the mechanisms involved probably have additive effects (below). RS–– genotypes are hypothesized to develop right or left hemisphere speech at random, and independently of handedness. There is no intrinsic link between cerebral lateralization and handedness, except as mediated by the RS+ gene. RS–– genotypes are distributed for handedness about R – L = 0, but many are evenly balanced between the sides and easily persuaded, therefore, to use the right hand for socially significant actions such as writing and eating. An important element of the model is the threshold, or cut-point along the continuum of asymmetry, which divides right- from left-handers. When 10% of the population is classified as left-handed, the threshold is to the left of zero (of the R – L distribution) and some 35% of RS–– genotypes will be left-handed. When 16% of the population is left-handed, the threshold is near zero and about 50% should be left-handed. For critical reviews of Annett (2002) see Corballis (2004), Crow (2004), Elias (2004), McManus (2004), and author's reply (Annett, 2004).

It is important to emphasize that the RS genetic model was not developed by fitting parameters to studies of family handedness. Rather, it was discovered that parameters derived from studies of aphasics representative of the general population (Annett, 1975) could be applied to family data, using straightforward Mendelian laws of segregation. The RS model explains relations between handedness and cerebral speech laterality (Alexander & Annett, 1996: Annett & Alexander, 1996). The theory suggests that right hemisphere speakers (9.27%, see also Pederson *et al.*, 1995) represent 50% of RS–– genotypes (18.54%) and the square root of this value gives the frequency of the RS– gene (0.43) and the RS+ gene (0.57). The extent of shift was estimated from the percentages of left-handers with right versus left hemisphere speech. This approach required an assumption of dominance for cerebral speech and also handedness, and did not distinguish for sex. Predictions for handedness in families were good for all studies available at that time (Annett, 1978) except Ramaley (1913). Fits were good for strict criteria (left-writing) and also generous criteria (non-right-handedness). The original dominant model remains more powerful that rival models (Annett, 1996). A worked example of the calculations was given (Annett, 2002, Appendix VIII).

Further studies led to elaborations in terms of additive effects and sex differences. The genotype frequencies that follow from the above estimates of gene frequency (RS++ 0.3242, RS+– 0.4904, RS–– 0.1854) have the interesting property that the heterozygote is the most frequent, and about as high as possible for a pair of alleles at a single locus. This suggests a genetic balanced polymorphism with heterozygote advantage. Evidence has been sought for advantages associated with the RS+ gene for speech and language-related abilities and perhaps costs for non-verbal abilities

Table 5.1 Data of Ashton (1982): predicted and observed percentages of left-handers in family types for sons and daughters. (Sum chi squares for right-handers)

Father × Mother	Sons				Daughters			
	N	Exp. %	Obs. %	Chi square	N	Exp. %	Obs. %	Chi square
R × R	1210	15.1	15.8	0.34	1220	12.8	13.2	0.14
R × L	88	24.7	19.3	1.04	118	22.4	24.6	0.24
L × R	128	23.6	21.1	0.34	143	21.3	14.7	2.94
L × L	9	37.1	44.4	0.13	10	36.1	30.0	0.10
			Sum	1.86				3.42
				(0.59)				(0.95)
		Total	d.f. 3	2.45				4.37

(review Annett, 2002; Smythe & Annett, 2006). Research into a balanced polymorphism is beyond the scope of this chapter, except for possible relevance to psychosis, considered below. The important point here is that heterozygote advantage implies that for at least some purposes the expression of the *RS+* gene must be greater in double than in single dose.

There are small differences in incidence between the sexes, which suggest that the *RS+* gene is expressed a little more strongly in females than males. Family data showed good fits to predictions if shift values were as follows (shifts of 0.0z, 1.0z, 2.0z for males and 0.0z, 1.2z, and 2.4z for females, for the *RS−−*, *RS+−*, and *RS++* genotypes respectively). Annett (1999a) showed that when family data were collected by self-report (parents and children describing their own handedness) these shift parameters gave matching values for corresponding thresholds of males and females (fathers and mothers or sons and daughters in the same sample).

Tests of the RS genetic theory on family data

Annett (1999a) tested the additive model against 14 sets of family data in which sex was distinguished for parents and children. Annett (2008) tested three further samples. The calculations depend on Mendelian laws, as stated above, but the genotype frequencies must be matched to thresholds that are defined by incidences (Annett, 2002, Appendix III). The genotype proportions predicted for children must be matched to the frequency of

left-handedness observed for children. Appendix I gives two examples of the percentages of left-handed sons and daughters expected in family types (R × R, R × L, etc. father × mother), when parental incidences are 10% and 20% and incidences for children range from 5% to 40%. (Further predictions across a range of incidences are given by Annett, 2008). Graphical plots of the percentages would allow intermediate values to be interpolated.

Table 5.1 gives the predicted and observed percentages of left-handed children for the data of Ashton (1982). This was a large sample of individually questioned parents and children in Hawaii. There were differences between ethnic groups for the writing hand but not for the question "any use of the left hand?" (The data in Table 5.1 combine "left" and "ambidextrous" responses in Ashton's Table 3.) Incidences for children (sons 16.6%, daughters 14.3%) were higher than for parents (fathers 9.0%, mothers 7.6%) as in all family studies. The expected proportions for family types are close to those given in Appendix Ia (10% for parents), for filial incidences at about 15%. Exact predictions are given in Table 5.1. Chi square values were low, showing good fit. (For d.f. = 3, chi square at the 5% level of confidence is 7.81, the minimum value needed to show significantly poor fit.)

Table 5.2 makes a similar analysis for McGee and Cozad (1980). Parents and children completed a questionnaire and were classified as left-handed if they performed any of ten actions with the left hand. This resembled the criterion of Rife (1940) but incidences here were very different (fathers 19.6%, mothers 16.7%,

Table 5.2 Data of McGee and Cozad (1980): predicted and observed percentages of left-handers in family types for sons and daughters. (Sum chi squares for right-handers)

Father × Mother	Sons				Daughters			
	N	Exp. %	Obs. %	Chi square	N	Exp. %	Obs. %	Chi square
R × R	489	23.2	22.9	0.02	570	17.5	17.4	0.00
R × L	91	35.0	41.8	1.19	123	28.8	28.4	0.00
L × R	130	33.5	30.0	0.47	131	27.3	29.0	0.13
L × L	27	47.9	44.4	0.07	25	42.9	40.0	0.05
			Sum	1.74				0.19
				(0.94)				(0.09)
		Total	d.f. 3	2.68				0.28

sons 27.3%, and daughters 21.4%). The percentages expected in family types were now close to those listed in Appendix Ib (20% for parents), and around 25% for children. Exact predictions and tests against observed percentages are given in Table 5.2. There were good fits for both sexes.

Annett (1999a) found good fits to predictions for these studies and four others where data were collected by self-report except for one marginally poor fit for sons. In eight studies where parent and sibling data depended on student report, fits were more variable. Children tend to underestimate left-handedness in parents (Porac & Coren, 1979) and right-handers are more likely than left-handers to be inaccurate (Kang & Harris, 1996; McGuire & McGuire, 1980). Annett (2008) found good fit to predictions for a relatively small self-report sample but poorer fits for two indirect report samples. One of the latter (McKeever, 2000) was not representative of students but inflated by the recruitment of left-handers for psychology experiments, giving an incidence of about 17.5%. The parental incidence, reported by the students, was about 10%. Of the eight family analyses available for the McKeever sample (four family types × two sexes), only one was markedly discrepant with RS predictions, a shortfall of left-handed sons in L × R families. McKeever (2004) interpreted these findings as showing an excess of left-handed sons in R × L families, but the fit for the latter to RS predictions was particularly good.

These analyses show that fits to the RS model were generally good in self-report samples. Discrepancies occurred in indirect report samples but varied between studies. Poor fits were probably due to sampling variations and inaccurate report of parental handedness, as considered further below.

Is there an X-linked gene for handedness?

There is a small trend to higher frequencies of left-handedness in males than females but rarely statistically significant in individual studies. There is also a tendency to find more left-handed children in the families of left-handed mothers than fathers. McManus and Bryden (1992) suggested an elaboration of the McManus (1985) model, a rare X-linked recessive modifier gene, which suppressed the expression of the D allele and thereby raised the proportion of left-handers. These proposals were not submitted to tests against findings for handedness in families, either for specific studies or combined data. Corballis (1997) asked whether there are genes for handedness located in the homologous regions of the X and Y chromosomes but considered this implausible. Jones and Martin (2000) showed that it was possible to model sex differences, either for additive genes located in the homologous regions, or for a recessive model of X-linked inheritance. It is possible to model any set of data, of course, with appropriate choice of parameters, but those used by Jones and Martin were not plausible theoretically, nor did the model fit the data well (Corballis, 2001; rejoinder Jones & Martin, 2001).

McKeever (2004) suggested a model with three alleles on the sex chromosomes to fit his own data. None of these attempts to model X-linked inheritance was tested against specific studies in the literature.

The RS analysis suggests that the observation of more left-handed children in R × L than L × R families could be due to a Carter (1961) effect. That is, traits that are expressed less often in females than males tend to be observed more often in the relatives of affected females than affected males. Annett (1999a) found a greater number of left-handed children in R × L families (than predicted by the Carter effect and the RS theory) only when parental incidences were low. It was not present in combined data when parental incidences were greater than 7%, where there was rather a shortfall of left-handers in L × R families. The apparent excess of left-handers in R × L families in combined data over all studies could be corrected by moving right-handed children from R × R to R × L families (on the assumption than right-handed children had under-reported left-handedness in mothers) such as to increase the maternal incidence by 1%. The proportion of left-handed children in R × L families was then not greater than predicted (Annett, 1999a).

These analyses suggest there is no need to look for X-linked inheritance for asymmetry. The difference between the sexes and between the families of left-handed mothers and fathers is probably due to stronger expression of the *RS+* gene in females. Stronger expression is probably a function of rates of growth and relative maturity at birth, greater in females than males, and in the singleborn than twins.

Handedness in twins

Handedness in twin pairs is often given as a reason to doubt a genetic influence (Bishop, 2001; Coren, 1992). It is clear that handedness cannot be determined directly by genes for right- and left-handedness or there would be no discordant MZ pairs, whereas about 20% are found (Collins, 1970). A similar percentage is found for DZ pairs, suggesting that similar mechanisms are at work in both types of twin. An interesting feature of the twin data is that the proportions of the three types of pairs are as expected by chance, the binomial proportions expected if right- and left-handers were represented by black and white marbles, placed in a bag, and taken out in pairs at random. This feature of the data persuaded Collins that genetic inheritance was not possible, and he suggested (Collins, 1977) that culture might explain associations between parents and children. McManus (1980) concluded that while dizygotic twin pairs were binomial, MZ twins tended to have more LL pairs and fewer RL pairs than expected.

The idea that twins are more often left-handed than singletons has been controversial (Coren, 1992; McManus, 1980; Zazzo, 1960). However, when Annett (1978) discovered that a single gene could predict handedness in families, the same model could account for handedness in twin pairs, if the extent of shift were reduced in twins compared with the singleborn. The same reduction of shift was required for MZ and DZ pairs, showing that the effect was not genetic but a function of twinning. The reduced shift implied that twins should be more often left-handed than the singleborn by about 3% to 4%. Rife (1940, 1950) found 12.4% of twins left-handed compared with 8.8% of students, on the same questionnaire. Davis and Annett (1994) examined the responses of some 30 000 people to a questionnaire on hearing disabilities, which included questions on handedness and twinning. There were more left-handers among twins in all age groups and overall there were 7.1% singleton and 11.7% twin left-handers. Sicotte *et al.* (1999) found by meta-analysis a higher incidence of left-handedness in twins than the singleborn.

The key argument, for most skeptics of genetic influence on handedness, is the discordance of MZ pairs. However, discordance is expected if the primary cause of handedness is accidental asymmetries of growth. If asymmetries arise between the two sides of the body in every individual, twin and singleton, a binomial distribution is expected in pairs of twins, or siblings. Does this mean there is no genetic influence? No, because the majority of twins are biased to the right, like the majority of singletons. The *RS+* gene influences the growth of both twins, but at most thresholds of left-handedness, twins of the same genotype may be on different sides of the threshold. The similarity of

MZ and DZ pairs is due to the fact that some 81.5% of twins of both zygosities are gene-carriers. An exaggerated analogy may help to make the point. It is not concluded that there are no genes for upright walking because MZ and DZ twins all walk upright. Similarly, most twins are influenced by the *RS+* allele.

Inheritance of brain asymmetries

An early attempt to study the inheritance of brain asymmetries used a dichotic listening test in 49 families (Bryden, 1975). Correlations were small between parents and children, and absent between siblings. Studies of cerebral asymmetries in the healthy population require reliable and non-invasive methods. Functional magnetic resonance imaging (fMRI) offered a relatively non-invasive approach (Pujol *et al.*, 1999: Szaflarski *et al.*, 2002). The assessment of language lateralization by functional transcranial Doppler ultrasonography (fTCD) allowed large numbers of healthy volunteers to be tested (Knecht *et al.*, 2000b). Right-hemisphere language dominance was found in 7.5% of healthy right-handers. Knecht *et al.* (2000a) examined atypical right hemisphere speech in relation to personal and family handedness. Incidences ranged from 4% for strong right-handers to 27% for strong left-handers. Within types of right- and left-handers there tended to be more right-hemisphere speakers if there was a left-handed parent.

Are these findings consistent with expectations for *RS--* genotypes? The numbers of left- and right-handers expected for each of the three genotypes of the RS locus, at different levels of incidence, were tabulated in terms of *N*s per 1000 (Annett, 2002, Appendix III). When 10% (100) of the population is classified as left-handed some 65/185 *RS--* genotypes are left-handed and the remaining 120 right-handed. By chance, half of *RS--* are expected to develop right-hemisphere speech, so that 32.5/100 (32.5%) of left-handers and 60/900 (6.7%) of right-handers should have right-hemisphere speech. When 20% of the population is left-handed the expected incidences of right-hemisphere speech are 26.5% in left-handers and 4.9% in right-handers. These values approximate those found by Knecht *et al.*

An association for strength of language lateralization between relatives was sought by fTCD in ten families (Anneken *et al.*, 2004). In two families where both parents were strongly lateralized three children were also strongly lateralized. By contrast in two families where neither parent was strongly lateralized none of the three children were strongly lateralized. In six families where parents differed, eight of fourteen children were strongly lateralized. Numbers were small, but this represents a first attempt to show familial segregation for strength of functional cerebral lateralization.

With regard to anatomical asymmetries Steinmetz *et al.* (1991) described the planum temporale (PT) in right- and left-handers with and without family sinistrality. The trends were as expected if presence of left-handed relatives was associated with reduced asymmetry. In left-handers with left-handed relatives overall asymmetry was absent, consistent with the hypothesized *RS--* genotype.

Is it likely that models developed for handedness are applicable to cerebral dominance? An important question is the nature of the underlying distributions, continuous or discrete? When describing relations between speech laterality and handedness it is often necessary to classify cases in discrete categories such as the presence or absence of aphasia, or handedness left or right. However, the underlying distributions of asymmetry for hand and brain are probably continuous. For over 300 cases described by Knecht *et al.* (2001) the distribution of fTCD asymmetry was continuous and approximately normal with negative skew. There was a small mode to the left of L = R but this is expected as Knecht *et al.* recruited extra left-handers. The distribution resembles that for differences in the internal lengths of the left and right halves of the cranium (Hoadley & Pearson, 1929) and asymmetry for peg moving (Annett, 1992). Other measures of hand skill for which participants use a pen or pencil give a bimodal distribution, but this is not surprising following practice in writing. The overall conclusion is that functional cerebral asymmetry resembles other asymmetry distributions in being continuous, the mean displaced in a typical direction from R = L.

What of the hypothesis that in the absence of directional shift cerebral functions assort at random? Flöel *et al.* (2001) looked for associations between language and spatial abilities, which typically lateralize to different hemispheres. In ten cases of atypical right language laterality, spatial functions were localized to the left in six and to the right in four cases. Flöel et al. (2005) examined a further sample of left- and right-handers for language and spatial laterality. They found both functions lateralized to the left in seven subjects and both to the right in eight subjects. That is, all combinations of lateralization occur, about as expected for random assortment in atypical cases.

Cerebral lateralization in twins

When large samples of twins are reliably assessed for cerebral dominance, what proportions are expected? Annett (2003) described several predictions. Normally developing MZ twins of RS++ and RS+– genotype are expected to be concordant for left cerebral speech (81.5% of pairs). Chance assortment for cerebral dominance occurs in RS–– pairs (18.5%). Pairs of MZ twins are predicted, therefore, to assort for typical (T) and atypical (A) cerebral dominance as TT, TA, and AA in the proportions 86.1%, 9.3%, and 4.6% respectively. The corresponding predictions for DZ pairs are 83.8%, 13.8%, and 2.4%.

What of the predictions for cerebral lateralization if handedness is known? If both twins are right-handed (RR pairs) or one or both twins non-right-handed (non-RR pairs) Annett (2003) estimated that in MZ twins about 92% of RR pairs and 68% of non-RR pairs would be concordant for typical cerebral asymmetry. In DZ twins there should be about 89% of RR pairs and 69% of non-RR pairs concordant.

Geschwind et al. (2002) measured the volumes of left and right cerebral cortex in 72 pairs of MZ twins and 67 pairs of DZ twins, all male veterans of World War II. Cerebral volumes were found highly heritable. In MZ twins, within pair correlations for total cerebral volumes, and also for left and right hemispheres, were significantly higher in RR than non-RR pairs. Dizygotic twins did not show this difference but the number of non-RR DZ pairs was small. The important outcome was support for the thesis that there is a genetic influence on cerebral asymmetry in right-handed twin pairs that is diminished when one of the twins is left-handed.

Sommer et al. (2002) made a similar comparison between RR and non-RR pairs of MZ twins performing language tasks while undergoing fMRI. The lateralization index of the RR pairs was significantly larger than for the non-RR pairs. The within pair correlation of RR pairs for the lateralization index was significant but not for non-RR pairs. This pattern of findings resembles that of Geschwind et al., a strong bias to typical asymmetry in RR pairs and a marked reduction in typical bias in non-RR pairs.

Steinmetz et al. (1995) measured PT asymmetries in ten RR and ten non-RR pairs of MZ twins. Within-pair correlations were low for both sets of twins but right-handers tended to show the expected leftward asymmetry while left-handers had reduced asymmetry. Annett (2003) estimated that 9/10 RR pairs and 6/10 non-RR pairs, in this study, were concordant for typical asymmetry, consistent with predictions above.

Non-genetic influences on human lateralization

It is often pointed out that growth depends on a combination of genetic and environmental influences, but arguments about human handedness have tended to emphasize one to the exclusion of the other. Evidence for environmental influences on handedness (Orlebeke et al., 1996; Tambs et al., 1987) is often interpreted as implying no genetic influence. However, the RS theory assumes accidental environmental influences for everyone, but also a genetic influence in most people.

What non-genetic theories have been offered? The main suggestions include pathology (Coren, 1992), learning (Provins, 1997) culture (Collins, 1977), or a combination of variables (Perelle & Ehrman, 2005). With regard to pathology, it is obvious that serious disorders of growth may distort the processes of lateralization, as in cerebral palsies. No clear line can be drawn between normal and pathological accidents of development. It is not justified, however, to conclude that *all* left-handedness is pathological because *some* is pathological. In studies of family handedness, the influence of pathology was likely to be negligible. Right cerebral dominance, by fTCD, was associated with no evidence of pathology (Knecht et al., 2003).

Learning and culture influence the expression of handedness for actions such as eating and writing, but do not necessarily affect other behavior. In personal testing of older people who had been forced to use the right hand for writing from childhood, relative hand skill and preference for actions other than writing remained strongly sinistral. That is, forced learning, cultural pressure, and a lifetime of practice had no discernable effect on preference and skill for the left hand. Functional neuroanatomy for writing was studied by positron emission tomography in adults who had been forced to convert to right-handed writing and had used that hand exclusively since childhood (Siebner *et al.*, 2002). There were persisting differences from natural right-handers, even after decades of using the right hand. Pressures against the use of the left hand remain strong in many cultures and probably persist to some degree in Western societies. For a typical threshold for left-handed writing (about 10% of the population) some 35% of *RS−−* genotypes are expected to be left writers, as explained above.

Yeo and Gangestad (1993) suggested that humans are designed to be moderate right-handers and that left-handedness and strong right-handedness are caused by developmental instability. They suggested that a tendency to developmental instability may be inherited. The prediction that strong right-handers have more left-handed parents than moderate right-handers (Gangestad & Yeo, 1994) was not supported in two samples of students (Annett, 1996).

A "gene-culture" theory (Laland *et al.*, 1995) has three key elements, chance asymmetries that influence everyone, an inherited bias toward right-handedness that also influences everyone but is not strong enough to induce right-handedness in all, and a cultural bias associated with the handedness of parents. The key point is that everyone has the same genotype. The gene–culture model raises the stakes for explanations of lateralization because it is necessary to look for genetic variability for traits not likely to be influenced by culture. It is not enough to cite associations between typical asymmetries and right-handedness because both might have been caused by a common directional bias.

A specific prediction of the gene–culture model is that there is no difference in concordance for handedness between MZ and DZ twins. A small but statistically significant difference was found by meta-analysis (Sicotte *et al.*, 1999). An asymmetry unlikely to be influenced by culture is eye preference. Eye preference in children varies with eye preference in parents (Brackenridge, 1982). Segregation in families follows the same rules as for handedness, on the RS model (Annett, 1999b).

The effect of parental handedness was examined by Carter-Saltzman (1980) for the biological and adoptive children of left-handed parents. There was no raised incidence of left-handedness in the adoptive children although there was for the biological children. Annett (1974, 1983) measured hand preference and hand skill in the children of L × L parents and found the expected reduction of bias to right-handedness. In the families of parents with early history of trauma that might have led to pathological left-handedness, the children were as biased to dextrality as controls. That is, the experience of being raised by two left-handed parents did not counter the effect of the *RS+* gene.

Genome-wide searches for loci associated with relative hand skill on the Annett peg-moving task found evidence for a quantitative trait locus (QTL) on chromosome 2p12-11 (Francks *et al.*, 2002; Francks *et al.*, 2003). Francks *et al.* (2007) narrowed the locus further by describing an association between hand skill in siblings and a haplotype upstream of gene *LRRTM1* (leucine-rich repeat transmembrane neuronal 1) on chromosome 2p12, which is inherited paternally.

Search for a locus for hand preference found possible linkage to markers on chromosome 12q21-23 (Warren *et al.*, 2006). Van Agtmael *et al.* (2001) found no evidence for linkage to chromosome 7 but possible linkage to chromosome 10 (Van Agtmael *et al.*, 2002; Van Agtmael *et al.*, 2003). Medland *et al.* (2006) found a genetic influence on handedness in twins along with considerable individual variability.

The conclusion from these several lines of research must be that there are genetic influences on human lateralization, against a background of accidental asymmetries. The latter mainly give variation in the normal range, but developmental accidents may in some cases be severe enough to be called pathological. Culture moderates the expression of left- and right-handedness, but this is added to genetic and epigenetic influences.

The theory of an agnosic RS+ gene in schizophrenia and autism

Crow (1997) argued that schizophrenia, and perhaps other psychoses, arise from a disorder of the mechanisms of cerebral dominance. If the RS theory is correct in suggesting that there is only one systematic influence on cerebral dominance, then psychosis might depend on disorders of the *RS+* gene. The gene is likely to be of recent origin in human evolution and might therefore be unstable and liable to mutation. Annett (1997) suggested that there could be a mutant in which directional coding is lost. Whereas the normal form of the *RS+* gene might give an instruction, "Impair the speech cortex of one cerebral hemisphere, the right", the mutant form might lose the last element and impair either hemisphere at random. When paired with a normal *RS+* allele, which impairs the right hemisphere, both hemispheres would be impaired in 50% of cases, while in 50% there would be double impairment of the right hemisphere (as in normal *RS++* genotypes).

If schizophrenia is associated with a single dose of impairment of speech cortex in both hemispheres there would be a problem with language, and also a loss of typical asymmetry. The chance rule shows how MZ twins could be concordant for schizophrenia in 50% of pairs, while the non-schizophrenic twin in discordant pairs could be normal. Working through the probabilities, using the parameters of the RS model as already developed but with the addition of an agnosic allele (frequency 0.02), it was discovered that risks to relatives approximated those estimated by Gottesman (1991).

From the frequencies deduced above, it would follow that homozygotes for the agnosic gene would be about 4 per 10 000, about the rate estimated for autistics diagnosed by strict criteria (Rutter, 1991). Random assortment of cerebral functions would allow for many patterns of strengths and weaknesses in autistics, as well as a variety of patterns of symptoms in schizophrenia, but all associated with impairments of language functions. The implications of these ideas were reviewed, along with discussion of critical commentaries (Annett, 2002, ch.14).

If there is instability of the *RS+* gene, making it liable to mutation associated with psychosis, this would be a powerful reason for limiting the spread of the gene in the population, as suggested by the balanced polymorphism hypothesis mentioned above. The idea of an agnosic *RS+* gene remains speculative but deserves further scrutiny as new evidence becomes available.

Appendix I

Predicted percentages of left-handed sons and daughters in four types of parental mating, for different levels of incidence of left-handedness in children and at two levels of incidence in parents (from Annett, 2008).

Appendix Ia. Parental incidence 10% (fathers 10.6%, mothers 9.4%)

Filial incidence		Sons				Daughters			
%	male/female	R × R	R × L	L × R	L × L	R × R	R × L	L × R	L × L
5	5.3/4.7	4.6	8.3	7.9	14.1	4.0	7.7	7.2	13.8
10	10.6/9.4	9.3	16.0	15.2	25.3	8.1	14.8	14.0	25.1
15	16.0/14.0	14.3	23.4	22.3	35.1	12.2	21.4	20.3	34.5
20	21.5/18.5	19.4	30.5	29.2	43.8	16.3	27.6	26.3	42.5
25	27.0/23.0	24.6	37.3	35.8	51.5	20.5	33.5	32.0	49.6
30	32.5/27.5	29.9	43.8	42.2	58.3	24.8	39.2	37.5	55.9
35	38.0/32.0	35.2	50.1	48.3	64.4	29.0	44.6	42.8	61.5
40	43.5/36.5	40.6	56.0	54.2	69.9	33.4	49.9	47.9	66.5

Appendix Ib. Parental incidence 20% (fathers 21.5%, mothers 18.5%)

Filial incidence		Sons				Daughters			
%	male/female	R × R	R × L	L × R	L × L	R × R	R × L	L × R	L × L
5	5.3/4.7	4.0	7.3	6.8	12.2	3.4	6.6	6.2	11.8
10	10.6/9.4	8.3	14.2	13.4	22.3	7.1	12.9	12.2	21.8
15	16.0/14.0	12.8	21.0	19.9	31.3	10.8	18.9	17.9	30.2
20	21.5/18.5	17.6	27.7	26.4	39.4	14.6	24.6	23.3	37.6
25	27.0/23.0	22.6	34.1	32.7	46.8	18.5	30.2	28.7	44.3
30	32.5/27.5	27.7	40.4	38.8	53.5	22.5	35.6	33.9	50.3
35	38.0/32.0	32.9	46.5	44.8	59.6	26.6	40.8	39.0	55.8
40	43.5/36.5	38.2	52.4	50.6	65.1	30.8	45.9	44.0	60.9

REFERENCES

Alexander, M. P. & Annett, M. (1996). Crossed aphasia and related anomalies of cerebral organization: case reports and a genetic hypothesis. *Brain and Language*, **55**, 213–39.

Anneken, K., Konrad, C., Dräger, B. *et al.* (2004). Familial aggregation of strong hemispheric language lateralization. *Neurology*, **63**, 2433–5.

Annett, M. (1972). The distribution of manual asymmetry. *British Journal of Psychology*, **63**, 343–58.

Annett, M. (1974). Handedness in the children of two left-handed parents. *British Journal of Psychology*, **65**, 129–31.

Annett, M. (1975). Hand preference and the laterality of cerebral speech. *Cortex*, **11**, 305–28.

Annett, M. (1978). *A Single Gene Explanation of Right and Left Handedness and Brainedness*. Coventry, UK: Lanchester Polytechnic.

Annett, M. (1983). Hand preference and skill in 115 children of two left-handed parents. *British Journal of Psychology*, **74**, 17–32.

Annett, M. (1992). Five tests of hand skill. *Cortex*, **28**, 583–600.

Annett, M. (1996). In defence of the right shift theory. *Perceptual and Motor Skills*, **82**, 115–37.

Annett, M. (1997). Schizophrenia and autism considered as the products of an agnosic right shift gene. *Cognitive Neuropsychiatry*, **2**, 195–240.

Annett, M. (1999a). Left-handedness as a function of sex, maternal versus paternal inheritance and report bias. *Behavior Genetics*, **29**, 103–14.

Annett, M. (1999b). Eye dominance in families predicted by the right shift theory. *Laterality*, **4**, 167–72.

Annett, M. (2002). *Handedness and Brain Asymmetry: The Right Shift Theory*. Hove, UK: Psychology Press.

Annett, M. (2003). Cerebral asymmetry in twins: predictions of the right shift theory. *Neuropsychologia*, **41**, 469–79.

Annett, M. (2004). Perceptions of the right shift theory. *Cortex*, **40**, 143–50.

Annett, M. (2008). Tests of the right shift genetic model for two new samples of family handedness and for the data of McKeever 2000. *Laterality*, **13**, 105–23.

Annett, M. & Alexander, M. P. (1996). Atypical cerebral dominance: predictions and tests of the right shift theory. *Neuropsychologia*, **34**, 1215–27.

Ashton, G. C. (1982). Handedness: an alternative hypothesis. *Behavior Genetics*, **12**, 125–47.

Bishop, D. V. M. (2001). Individual differences in handedness and specific language impairment: evidence against a genetic link. *Behavior Genetics*, **31**, 339–51.

Brackenridge, C. J. (1982). The contribution of genetic factors to ocular dominance. *Behavior Genetics*, **12**, 319–25.

Bryden, M. P. (1975). Speech lateralization in families: a preliminary study using dichotic listening. *Brain and Language*, **2**, 210–11.

Carter, C. O. (1961). Inheritance of congenital pyloric stenosis. *British Medical Bulletin*, **17**, 251–3.

Carter-Saltzman, L. (1980). Biological and sociocultural effects on handedness: comparison between biological and adoptive families. *Science*, **209**, 1263–5.

Chamberlain, H. D. (1928). The inheritance of left handedness. *Journal of Heredity*, **19**, 557–9.

Collins, R. L. (1970). The sound of one paw clapping: an inquiry into the origin of left handedness. In G. Lindzey & D. D. Thiessen (eds.) *Contribution to Behavior-Genetic Analysis – The Mouse as a Prototype*. New York: Appleton, pp. 115–36.

Collins, R. L. (1977). Origins of the sense of asymmetry: Mendelian and non-Mendelian models of inheritance. *Annals of the New York Academy of Sciences*, **299**, 283–305.

Corballis, M. C. (1997). The genetics and evolution of handedness. *Psychological Review*, **104**, 714–27.

Corballis, M. C. (2001). Is the handedness gene on the X chromosome: comment on Jones and Martin (2000). *Psychological Review*, **108**, 805–10.

Corballis, M. C. (2004). Taking your chances. *Cortex*, **40**, 115–17.

Coren, S. (1992). *The Left-Hander Syndrome: The Causes and Consequences of Left-Handedness*. London: John Murray.

Crow, T. J. (1997). Schizophrenia as a failure of hemispheric dominance for language. *Trends in the Neurosciences*. **20**, 339–43.

Crow, T. J. (2004). What Marian Annett can teach Noam Chomsky and could have taught Stephen Jay Gould if he'd had time to listen. *Cortex*, **40**, 118–32.

Davis, A. & Annett, M. (1994). Handedness as a function of twinning, age and sex. *Cortex*, **30**, 105–11.

Elias, L. (2004). Acknowledge the ambition, but look elsewhere for the alternatives. *Cortex*, **40**, 133–5.

Flöel, A., Buyx, A., Breitenstein, C., Lohman, H. & Knecht, S. (2005). Hemispheric lateralization of spatial attention in right- and left-hemispheric language dominance. *Behavioral Brain Research*, **158**, 269–75.

Flöel, A., Knecht, S., Lohman, H. *et al.* (2001). Language and spatial attention can lateralize to the same hemisphere in healthy humans. *Neurology*, **57**, 1018–24.

Francks, C., DeLisi, L. E., Fisher, S. E. *et al.* (2003). Confirmatory evidence for linkage of relative hand skill to 2p12-q11. *American Journal of Human Genetics*, **72**, 499–502.

Francks, C., Fisher, S. E., MacPhie, I. L. *et al.* (2002). A genome wide linkage screen for relative hand skill in sibling pairs. *American Journal of Human Genetics*, **70**, 800–5.

Francks, C., Maegawa, S., Laurén, J. *et al.* (2007). LRRTM1 on chromosome 2p12 is a maternally suppressed gene that is associated paternally with handedness and schizophrenia. *Molecular Psychiatry*, **12**(12), 1129–39.

Gangestad, S. W. & Yeo, R. A. (1994). Parental handedness and relative hand skill: a test of the developmental instability hypothesis. *Neuropsychology*, **8**, 572–8.

Geschwind, D. H., Miller, B. L., DeCarli, C. & Carmelli, D. (2002). Heritability of lobar brain volumes in twins supports genetic models of cerebral laterality and handedness. *Proceedings of the National Academy of Sciences*, **99**, 3176–81.

Gottesman, I. I. (1991). *Schizophrenia Genesis: The Origins of Madness*. New York: W. H. Freeman.

Hoadley, M. F. & Pearson, K. (1929). On measurement of the internal diameter of the skull in relation: I. To the prediction of its capacity, II. To the "pre-eminence" of the left hemisphere. *Biometrika*, **21**, 85–123.

Jones, G. V. & Martin, M. (2000). A note on Corballis (1997) and the genetics and evolution of handedness: developing a unified distributional model from the sex-chromosome gene hypothesis. *Psychological Review*, **107**, 213–18.

Jones, G. V. & Martin, M. (2001). Confirming the X-linked handedness gene as recessive, not additive: reply to Corballis (2001). *Psychological Review*, **108**, 811–13.

Jordan, H. E. (1911). The inheritance of left-handedness. *American Breeders Magazine*, **2**, 19–29, 113–24.

Kang, Y. & Harris, L. J. (1996). Accuracy of college students' reports of parental handedness. *Laterality*, **1**, 269–79.

Kennedy, D. N., Ocraven, K. M., Ticho, B. S. *et al.* (1999). Structural and functional brain asymmetries in human situs inversus totalis. *Neurology*, **53**, 1260–5.

Kilshaw, D. & Annett, M. (1983). Right and left-hand skill I: effects of age, sex and hand preference showing superior skill in left-handers. *British Journal of Psychology*, **74**, 253–68.

Klar, A. J. S. (1996). A single locus, RGHT, specifies preference for hand utilization in humans. *Cold Spring Harbor Symposia on Quantitative Biology*, **61**, 59–65.

Knecht, S., Dräger, B., Deppe, M. *et al.* (2000a). Handedness and hemispheric language dominance in healthy humans. *Brain*, **123**, 2512–2518.

Knecht, S., Dräger, B., Deppe, M. *et al.* (2000b). Variability of the side and extent of language lateralization in the healthy population. *Journal of Neurolinguistics*, **13**, 297–300.

Knecht, S., Dräger, B., Flöel, A. *et al.* (2001). Behavioural relevance of atypical language lateralization in healthy subjects. *Brain*, **124**, 1657–65.

Knecht, S., Jansen, A., Frank, A. *et al.* (2003). How atypical is atypical language dominance? *Neuroimage*, **18**, 917–27.

Laland, K. N., Kumm, J., Van Horn, J. D. & Feldman, M. W. (1995). A gene-culture model of human handedness. *Behavior Genetics*, **25**, 433–45.

Layton, W. M. Jr. (1976). Random determination of a developmental process. *Journal of Heredity*, **67**, 336–8.

McGee, M. G. & Cozad, T. (1980). Population genetic analysis of human hand preference: evidence for generation difference, familial resemblance and maternal effects. *Behavior Genetics*, **10**, 263–75.

McGuire, W. J. & MGuire, C. V. (1980). Salience of handedness in the spontaneous self-concept. *Perceptual and Motor Skills*, **50**, 3–7.

McKeever, W. F. (2000). A new family handedness sample with findings consistent with X-linked transmission. *British Journal of Psychology*, **91**, 21–39.

McKeever, W. F. (2004). An X-linked three allele model of hand preference and hand posture for writing. *Laterality*, **9**, 149–73.

McManus, I. C. (1980). Handedness in twins: a critical review. *Neuropsychologia*, **18**, 347–55.

McManus, I. C. (1985). Handedness, language dominance and aphasia: a genetic model. *Psychological Medicine*, Supplement 8.

McManus, I. C. (2004). Grappling with the hydra. *Cortex*, **40**, 137–9.

McManus, I. C. & Bryden, M. P. (1992). The genetics of handedness, cerebral dominance and lateralization. In I. Rapin & S. J. Segalowitz (eds.) *Handbook of Neuropsychology, vol. 6: Child Neuropsychology*. Amsterdam: Elsevier, pp. 115–44.

McManus, I. C., Martin, N., Stubbings, G. F., Chung, E. M. K. & Mitchison, H. M. (2004). Handedness and situs inversus in primary ciliary dyskinesia. *Proceedings of the Royal Society of London, Series B – Biological Sciences*, **271** (1557), 2579–82.

Medland, S. E., Duffy, D. L., Wright, M. J., Geffen, G. M. & Martin, N. G. (2006). Handedness in twins: joint analysis of data from 35 samples. *Twin Research and Human Genetics*, **9**, 46–53.

Nonaka, S., Tanaka, Y., Okada, Y. *et al.* (1998). Randomization of left-right asymmetry due to loss of nodal cilia generating leftward flow of extraembryonic fluid in mice lacking KIF3B motor protein. *Cell*, **95**, 829–37.

Okada, Y., Nonaka, S., Tanaka, Y. *et al.* (1999). Abnormal nodal flow precedes situs inversus in iv and inv mice. *Molecular Cell*, **4**, 459–68.

Orlebeke, J. F., Knol, D. L., Koopmans, J. R., Boomsma, D. I. & Bleker, O. P. (1996). Left-handedness in twins – genes or environment. *Cortex*, **32**, 479–90.

Pedersen, P. M., Jorgensen, H. S., Nakayama, H., Raaschou, H. O. & Olsen, T. S. (1995). Aphasia in acute stroke: incidence, determinants and recovery. *Annals of Neurology*, **38**, 659–66.

Perelle, I. B. & Erhman, L. (2005). On the other hand. *Behavior Genetics*, **35**, 343–50.

Porac, C. & Coren, S. (1979). A test of the validity of offsprings' report of parental handedness. *Perceptual and Motor Skills*, **49**, 227–31.

Provins, K. A. (1997). Handedness and speech: a critical reappraisal of the role of genetic and environmental factors in the cerebral lateralization of function. *Psychological Review*, **104**, 554–71.

Pujol, J., Deus, J., Losilla, J. M. & Capdevila, A. (1999). Cerebral lateralization of language in normal left-handed people studied by functional MRI. *Neurology*, **52**, 1038–43.

Ramaley, F. (1913). Inheritance of left-handedness. *The American Naturalist*, **47**, 730–8.

Rife, D. C. (1940). Handedness with special reference to twins. *Genetics*, **25**, 178–86.

Rife, D. C. (1950). An application of gene frequency analysis to the interpretation of data from twins. *Human Biology*, **22**, 136–45.

Rutter, M. (1991). Autism as a genetic disorder. In P. McGuffin & R. Murray (eds.) *The New Genetics of Mental Illness*. London: Butterworth-Heineman, pp. 223–44.

Rutter, M., Moffitt, T. E. & Caspi, A. (2006). Gene – environment interplay and psychopathology: multiple varieties but real effects. *Journal of Child Psychology and Psychiatry*, **47**, 226–61.

Sicotte, N. L., Woods, R. P. & Mazziotta, J. C. (1999). Handedness in twins: a meta-analysis. *Laterality*, **4**, 265–86.

Siebner, H. R., Limmer, C., Peinemann, A. *et al.* (2002). Long-term consequences of switching handedness: a positron emission tomography study on handwriting in "converted" left-handers. *Journal of Neuroscience*, **22**, 2816–25.

Smythe, P. & Annett, M. (2006). Phonology and handedness in primary school: predictions of the right shift theory. *Journal of Child Psychology and Psychiatry*, **47**, 205–12.

Sommer, I. E. C., Ramsey, N. F., Mandl, R. C. W. & Kahn, R. S. (2002). Language lateralization in monozygotic twin pairs concordant and discordant for handedness. *Brain*, **125**, 2710–18.

Steinmetz, H., Herzog, A., Schlaug. G., Huang, Y. & Jäncke, L. (1995). Brain (a)symmetry in monozygotic twins. *Cerebral Cortex*, **5**, 296–300.

Steinmetz, H., Volkman, J., Jäncke, L. & Freund, H-J. (1991). Anatomical left-right asymmetry of language-related temporal cortex is different in left- and right-handers. *Annals of Neurology*, **29**, 315–19.

Szaflarski, J. P., Binder, J. R., Possing, E. T. *et al.* (2002). Language lateralization in left-handed and ambidextrous people: fMRI data. *Neurology*, **59**, 238–44.

Tambs, K., Magnus, P. & Berg, K. (1987). Left-handedness in twin families: support of an environmental hypothesis. *Perceptual and Motor Skills*, **64**, 155–70.

Tanaka, S., Kanzaki, R., Yoshibayashi, M., Kamiya, T. & Sugishita, M. (1999). Dichotic listening in patients with situs inversus: brain asymmetry and situs asymmetry. *Neuropsychologia*, **37**, 869–74.

Trankell, A. (1955). Aspects of genetics in psychology. *American Journal of Human Genetics*, **7**, 264–76.

Van Agtmael, T., Forrest, S. M., Del-Favero, J., Van Broeckhoven, C. & Wlilliamson, R. (2003). Parametric and non-parametric genome scan analyses for human handedness. *European Journal of Human Genetics*, **11**, 779–83.

Van Agtmael, T., Forrest, S. M. & Williamson, R. (2001). Genes for left-handedness: how to search for the needle in the haystack? *Laterality*, **6**, 149–64.

Van Agtmael, T., Forrest, S. M. & Williamson, R. (2002). Parametric and non-parametric linkage analysis of several candidate regions for genes for human handedness. *European Journal of Human Genetics*, **10**, 623–30.

Warren, D. M., Stern, M., Ravindranath, D., Dyer, T. D. & Almasy, L. (2006). Heritability and linkage analysis of hand, foot and eye preference in Mexican Americans. *Laterality*, **11**, 508–24.

Yeo, R. A. & Gangestad, S. W. (1993). Developmental origins of variations in human hand preference. *Genetics*, **89**, 281–96.

Zazzo, R. (1960). *Les Jumeaux: Le Couple et la Personne*. Paris: Presses Universitaire de France.

6

Language lateralization and handedness in twins; an argument against a genetic basis?

Iris E. C. Sommer and René S. Kahn

Summary

There is ample evidence that both handedness and language lateralization have a genetic basis. A first argument is that left-handedness tends to run in families. A second piece of evidence is derived from adoption studies. Handedness of a child is strongly related to handedness of the biological parents, while handedness of the adoption parents is not correlated to the child's handedness. Twin studies, however, appear to provide evidence against a genetic basis for handedness. Concordance rates for handedness in monozygotic (identical) twins are low and hardly exceed those in dizygotic (fraternal) twins. Similar concordance rates in monozygotic and dizygotic twins would suggest that handedness is almost completely determined by environmental factors. However, this conclusion is not in line with family and adoption studies. This chapter discusses several twin-specific factors that could affect handedness in twins and thereby decrease concordance rates in twins.

Handedness and language lateralization in twins appear to be different from those in singletons. Both monozygotic and dizygotic twins have a higher prevalence of left-handedness than singletons. First-degree relatives of twins are also more frequently left-handed than subjects without twin relatives, which suggests a genetic predisposition for left-handedness in twins.

The mode of inheritance for handedness probably includes a random factor. In the absence of a dominant allele, hand preference and cerebral lateralization probably results from enlargement of stochastic variance. Concordance for left-handedness will therefore never be higher than 50% in monozygotic twins, even when the phenotype would completely be defined by the genotype. This could explain the relatively low concordance rate for handedness in twins. However, this genetic model would still predict higher concordance for handedness in monozygotic than in dizygotic twins. A possible explanation for the low concordance in monozygotic twins, which hardly exceeds that of dizygotic twins, is the monozygotic twinning process itself, which may also affect the phenotype. Early embryonic division to form twins may disrupt the developmental pathways that normally induce lateralization. This phenomenon is called "mirror-imaging", and may produce twin pairs with opposite handedness and lateralization.

In addition, twin birth carries an increased risk for perinatal brain damage as compared to singleton birth. Twins with perinatal damage to the left hemisphere may develop right cerebral dominance for language and left-handedness, while their unaffected co-twins develop the genetically predisposed right-handedness. This mechanism may act to increase the prevalence of left-handedness in dizygotic and monozygotic twins and decrease concordance for handedness in both types of twins.

The exact contribution of mirror-imaging and perinatal brain damage to the distribution of handedness in twins is yet to be determined. It is therefore premature to conclude that handedness and lateralization are not genetically determined on the basis of concordance rates in twin studies.

Introduction

Like most other physical and cerebral human traits, hand preference and cerebral lateralization are expected to be, at least in part, determined by genetic information. Indeed, there is ample evidence that both handedness and language lateralization have a genetic basis. A first argument is that left-handedness tends to run in families (Annett, 1970; 2004). Children from two left-handed parents have a 50% chance of becoming left-handed (Annett, 1979; Annett, 2003; McManus, 1985), while the chance to become left-handed for children of right-handed parents is less than 10%. In parallel, language lateralization is also determined to a large extent by the lateralization pattern of the parents (Bryden, 1976; Anneken *et al.*, 2004). A second piece of evidence is derived from adoption studies. Handedness of a child is strongly related to handedness of the biological parents, while handedness of the adoption parents is not correlated to the child's handedness (Hicks & Kinsbourne, 1976).

The classical method to determine the genetic contribution to a trait is to compare concordance for that trait between monozygotic (identical) and dizygotic (fraternal) twins. "Concordance" implies that both twins of a pair have the same trait. The basic assumption of the twin method is that both types of twins share several environmental influences (both prenatal and postnatal), while the genotype is 100% shared in monozygotic, but only 50% in dizygotic twins. Remarkably, most twin studies on handedness found no difference in concordance between monozygotic and dizygotic twins (reviewed by Coren & Halpern, 1991). If similar concordance rates are found in monozygotic and dizygotic twins, this generally implies that the contribution of genes to that trait is minimal. This conclusion would be in sharp contrast to the above-mentioned findings of family and adoption studies.

An alternative explanation for the results of the twin studies is that certain factors, that are present in twins but not in singletons, may affect their handedness and lateralization. These factors may affect only one twin of a pair, thereby decreasing concordance for handedness and lateralization in twins. When such a factor affects monozygotic, but not dizygotic, twins it may decrease concordance for handedness only in monozygotic pairs. This would give the impression that monozygotic twins are no more similar for that trait than dizygotic twins. An example of such a factor is the monozygotic twinning process itself, which may alter the genetically pre-programmed pattern of lateralization.

In this chapter we will discuss which implications the model of inheritance for handedness has on concordance rates in twins. The effect of special twin factors, such as perinatal trauma and mirror-imaging on concordance rates in twins is investigated. Understanding the role of these factors in twins will help to interpret the results of twins studies and may resolve part of the controversy about genetic aspects of handedness and lateralization.

Handedness and lateralization in twins

The distribution of handedness in twins, irrespective of zygosity, appears to be different from that in singletons. Davis and Annett (1994) reported 12% left-handedness in a sample of twins, against 7% left-handedness in the singleton population. A later meta-analysis on 12 studies that assessed handedness in twins and singletons (Sicotte *et al.*, 1999), found that twins are indeed more frequently left-handed than singletons, the mean odds ratio being 1.73. This study also investigated the prevalence of left-handedness in monozygotic and dizygotic twins and found no difference between the two twin types. The increased left-handedness in both types of twins may partly be caused by environmental factors, such as increased rates of birth trauma in twins, but there is also some evidence suggesting a genetic cause. Tambs *et al.* (1987) noted that the increased rate of left-handedness was not only present in twins, but also in single born subjects with twin siblings. Medland *et al.* (2006) merged data from four twin studies and replicated this finding in a large sample. They reported increased left-handedness as compared to singletons both in twins (14.0%) and in their single-born siblings (13.5%). In parallel, parents of twins were more often left-handed than parents without twin children (Boklage, 1981). Though environmental factors may be an obvious explanation for the increased left-handedness in twins, genetic factors appear to play an even more important role in increasing left-handedness in twins. The presence of increased left-handedness in first-degree relatives of twins suggests a common genetic factor that may predispose for both twinning and left-handedness. This suggestion may sound curious, but both the development of left-handedness (or cerebral dominance) and twinning can be considered as deviations from the normal development of embryonic chirality. It can be hypothesized that alterations in molecular mechanisms that pattern the embryonic development of left–right asymmetry along the head–tail axis may induce both twinning and abnormal asymmetry. In fact, the monozygotic twinning process involves a duplication of structures along this head–tail axis (Steinman, 2001), which can be viewed as a major deviation from normal development of bilateral asymmetry. Other findings appear to support this hypothesis, as there is an association between twinning, left-handedness, and midline fusion malformations, such as cleft-palate and neural tube defects (Boklage, 1987; Luke & Keith, 1990). As is the case for left-handedness, midline fusion malformations are also more prevalent in twins *and* in their siblings in comparison to singletons without twin siblings.

In sum, twins are more frequently left-handed than singletons, which may in part result from a genetic predisposition. Therefore, findings on handedness in twins should not be extrapolated to singletons without caution.

There is much less information on language lateralization in twins and their relatives than there is on handedness in these groups. Springer and Searleman (1978) measured language lateralization in twins and unrelated singletons by applying a verbal dichotic listening test. This test elicits a right-ear advantage in most right-handed subjects, reflecting left cerebral dominance for language. Springer and Searleman found similar language lateralization in right-handed twin pairs as compared to right-handed singletons. Twin pairs with discordant (unequal) handedness showed decreased language lateralization in both the right-handed and the left-handed twins. Jäncke and Steinmetz (1994) also applied verbal dichotic listening to 20 monozygotic twin pairs and their singleton siblings. They found lower language lateralization in the twins, even in the concordant right-handed pairs than in their singleton siblings. Though suggestive, sample sizes of these two studies are too small to draw any general conclusions on a possible difference in language lateralization between twins, singletons, and singletons with twin siblings.

Concordance for handedness and language lateralization in monozygotic and dizygotic twins

As mentioned in the introduction, many large studies on handedness found similar concordance for handedness in monozygotic twin pairs in comparison with dizygotic pairs (McManus, 1980; Coren & Halpern, 1991; Orlebeke *et al.*, 1996; Reiss *et al.*, 1999; Ross, 1999). The only study that found significantly higher concordance for handedness in monozygotic twins is a meta-analysis that pooled handedness data of 9969 twin pairs from 28 studies (Sicotte *et al.*, 1999). Thus, concordance for handedness in monozygotic twins may be higher than in dizygotic twins, but samples of 10 000 twin pairs are needed to reach statistical significance. This may yield the impression that there is some genetic influence on handedness, but of negligible size.

Several studies assessed language lateralization in twin pairs, but all used much smaller samples than the studies on handedness (Springer & Searleman, 1978; Jäncke & Steinmetz, 1994; Steinmetz *et al.*, 1995; Geschwind *et al.*, 2002; Sommer *et al.*, 2004). Springer and Searleman assessed 88 twin pairs and found that intra-pair correlations were significant in right-handed twin pairs, but insignificant in twin pairs with one left-hander. They also found that the intra-pair difference in language lateralization was much larger in monozygotic pairs with one left-hander than in dizygotic pairs of unequal handedness. Jäncke and Steinmetz (1994) assessed lateralization in 20 monozygotic twin pairs, of whom 10 pairs differed for handedness. The intra-pair correlation for lateralization of all 20 pairs was not significant, indicating that concordance for language lateralization was low.

The findings of these two dichotic listening studies are in line with studies on handedness; monozygotic twin pairs do not resemble each other very much for both traits.

Another way to study language lateralization is to measure asymmetry of the temporal planes using magnetic resonance imaging (MRI). The temporal plane is the upper surface of the posterior temporal lobe, which overlaps with Wernicke's area. Asymmetry of this plane provides a reflection of cerebral dominance for language (Shapleske *et al.*, 1999). Following this method, Steinmetz *et al.*, (1995) measured asymmetry in 20 monozygotic twin pairs, 10 of which were discordant for handedness. As in the dichotic listening study by Jäncke and Steinmetz (1994), which included the same participants, a low within-pair correlation for temporal plane asymmetry was observed for the whole sample. Interestingly, however, seven pairs had almost identical asymmetry, while five pairs showed completely opposite cerebral asymmetry.

In a similar manner, Geschwind *et al.* (2002) assessed anatomical asymmetry of the frontal and temporal lobes in 72 monozygotic and 67 dizygotic twin pairs. They found significant intra-pair correlations in monozygotic twins who were both right-handed, but monozygotic twin pairs with one left-hander showed large intra-pair differences in asymmetry. In contrast, dizygotic twin pairs with one left-hander showed similar intra-pair correlations to dizygotic pairs who were both right-handed. A similar pattern was demonstrated in the dichotic listening study by Springer and Searleman (1978) who also found large intra-pair differences in *monozygotic* twins of unequal handedness and much smaller intra-pair differences in *dizygotic* twins of unequal handedness. It appears that discordant handedness in monozygotic twins is associated with large intra-pair differences in lateralization, while discordant handedness in dizygotic twins is not.

In a study by our group (Sommer *et al.*, 2002), language lateralization was measured with functional MRI in 25 monozygotic twin pairs, from which 13 pairs included one left-hander. The intra-pair correlation for language lateralization was significant (rho = 0.74, $p < 0.01$) in pairs who were both right-handed. This correlation is only slightly lower than the correlation of 0.79, which we found when the same 12 subjects were measured twice to test the reproducibility of our fMRI paradigm (Rutten *et al.*, 2002). This clearly suggests that monozygotic twins do resemble each other for language lateralization, at least when both twins are right-handed. Pairs with one left-hander, however, showed no intra-pair correlation for language lateralization (rho = 0.18, not significant). Among the 13 pairs with unequal handedness, six pairs had almost identical lateralization, while the other five pairs had opposite cerebral

dominance; left cerebral dominance in the right-handed twin and right cerebral dominance in the left-hander. Examples of language activation patterns of a monozygotic pair consisting of a left-hander and a right-hander with opposite language lateralization are shown in Figs. 6.1a and b. Another monozygotic twin pair of unequal handedness, but with almost identical language lateralization is shown in Figs. 6.2a and b.

Among the twin pairs of unequal handedness, pairs with familial left-handedness had lower intra-pair differences in lateralization than pairs without familial left-handedness. This may suggest that two different causes can induce discordance for handedness in monozygotic twins. First, both twins may be homozygote recessive for right-handedness, and thus have the genetic predisposition for left-handedness. By chance (50%), one twin became left-handed and the other right-handed. These twins are likely to have left-handed family. Since they are both genetically predisposed for low degrees of language lateralization, lateralization may be reduced in both twins. Alternatively, handedness discordance may arise from non-genetic factors, for example from the monozygotic twinning process itself, as will be explained later in this chapter. These twins may have been genetically predisposed to be right-handed and to have strong left-cerebral dominance, but the twinning process disrupted cerebral lateralization in one twin of the pair. These twins are less likely to have left-handed family and may display a large difference in lateralization. The first type of discordant handedness is also observed in dizygotic twins, but the latter type may be specific for monozygotic twins. The existence of this subgroup of monozygotic twins with high intra-pair differences in lateralization may decrease the concordance rates for handedness and lateralization in monozygotic twins.

In sum, concordance for handedness in monozygotic twin pairs is only slightly higher than concordance in dizygotic twin pairs. The intra-pair correlations for language lateralization in monozygotic twin pairs are low. Monozygotic pairs of unequal handedness have larger differences in lateralization than dizygotic twin pairs of unequal handedness. This may be caused by a subgroup of monozygotic twins with extremely discordant language lateralization, perhaps resulting from the twinning process itself.

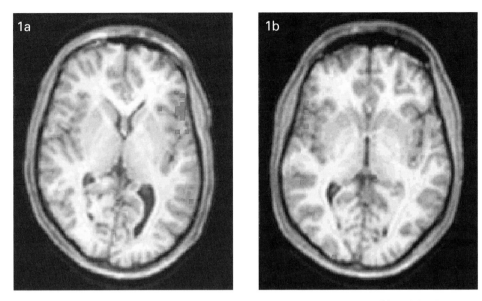

Figure 6.1 Examples of language activation patterns of a monozygotic pair consisting of (a) a left-hander and (b) a right-hander with opposite language lateralization. (See color plate section.)

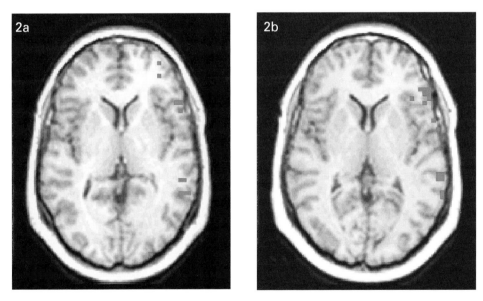

Figure 6.2 Another monozygotic twin pair of unequal handedness, but with almost identical language lateralization to those shown in Fig. 6.1. (See color plate section.)

Predictions from genetic models on handedness

In most models of inheritance (Annett, 1964; McManus, 1985), handedness is defined by a genetic predisposition, *plus* the influence of a stochastic variable. Thus, when two subjects are genetically identical (as in monozygotic twins) the random variable (or "chance") defines whether they will develop similar or different handedness.

The models by Annett (1964) and by McManus (1985) propose that a dominant allele with partial penetration increases the chance of developing right-handedness. In the absence of this allele, as in the homozygote recessive genotype, handedness is determined by chance alone, resulting in a 50% chance of either left- or right-handedness. These models are in line with data on handedness in children of two left-handed parents; only 50% of these children are left-handed themselves (Annett, 1974). According to these models, language lateralization is influenced by the same gene, inducing left-cerebral dominance for language and motor control. This dominant allele hypothesized to induce right-handedness and left-cerebral dominance has not yet been identified in linkage studies (Geschwind & Miller, 2001; Francks *et al.*, 2002; Van Aegtmaal *et al.*, 2003; Warren *et al.*, 2006). This may suggest that handedness and cerebral lateralization are polygenic rather than monogenic traits (Francks *et al.*, 2002; Van Aegtmaal *et al.*, 2003; Sun *et al.*, 2005). While the gene(s) for handedness and cerebral lateralization remain elusive, several genes have been discovered that play a pivotal role in the development of bodily left–right asymmetry (Levin & Mercola, 1998; Schneider & Brueckner, 2000). When asymmetrical expression of these patterning genes is blocked, for example in knock out mouse models, bodily asymmetry of the embryo develops in a random fashion, with 50% of embryos developing situs solitus (normal asymmetry of the internal organs) and 50% developing situs inversus (complete reversion of visceral asymmetry). In the absence of asymmetric gene expression, left–right asymmetry is obviously derived from a feed-forward mechanism that enlarges stochastic differences between the two sides. Possibly, randomness is the underlying substrate of all lateral asymmetries (Davis & Annett, 1994).

It is presently assumed that discrete mechanisms regulate visceral and cerebral asymmetry and that the gene(s) for cerebral lateralization are probably different from the genes that regulate bodily asymmetry. Evidence for this assumption is derived from studies in humans with situs inversus, who showed no reversal of structural (Kennedy *et al.*, 1999) or functional (Tanaka *et al.*, 1999; Kennedy *et al.*, 1999) brain asymmetry, nor were they more likely to be left-handed (McManus *et al.*, 2004). Though cerebral lateralization in humans may be independent of visceral asymmetry, the mechanism of asymmetric gene expression overruling a basic system of random asymmetry is probably the same in the brain.

The genetic models for handedness predict that twice as many subjects in a population will have the genetic predisposition for left-handedness (the homozygote recessives for the allele that determines right-handedness), than the actual prevalence of left-handed subjects. In a population with 10% left-handedness, approximately 20% will be homozygote recessive for the right-handedness gene and thus genetically predisposed for left-handedness. In subjects with this genotype, hand preference will develop at random, with a 50% chance for left-handedness. In monozygotic twins, the prevalence of the homozygote recessive genotype is probably higher, since twins and their siblings have a higher prevalence of left-handedness. In twins of this genotype, concordance for handedness is expected in only 50% of pairs, despite the fact that they share exactly the same genetic information and without taking non-genetic factors into account. This may explain why concordance for handedness is relatively low, even in monozygotic twins.

Studies on language lateralization in twins have generally included small samples. All studies have therefore enriched their samples by including an over-representation of left-handed twins (Springer & Searleman, 1978; Jäncke & Steinmetz, 1994; Steinmetz *et al.*, 1995; Geschwind *et al.*, 2002; Sommer *et al.*, 2004). These selected samples have a prevalence of left-handedness of approximately 25% (Jäncke & Steinmetz, 1994; Steinmetz *et al.*, 1995; Geschwind *et al.*, 2002; Sommer *et al.*, 2004), and therefore a large part of their sample will have the homozygote recessive genotype. In this genotype, chance determines both handedness and language lateralization. It can therefore be expected that concordance for language lateralization is low in samples of monozygotic twins that include many pairs of the homozygote recessive genotype. Thus, even when handedness and lateralization would be completely genetically determined, concordance for *left*-handedness in monozygotic twins will never exceed 50% and samples with many left-handers will never reach high concordance rates for language lateralization.

On the other hand, in a sample with few left-handed twins, concordance for *right*-handedness may be rather high, since the random factor is overruled by a dominant allele that induces right-handedness and left cerebral dominance. Indeed, when analysis is restricted to right-handed monozygotic twin pairs, all studies observed high concordance for language lateralization.

In sum, the proposed models of inheritance can explain both the relatively low concordance for handedness in monozygotic twins and the low concordance for lateralization in samples with many left-handers. However, the models still predict higher concordance for both traits in monozygotic than in dizygotic twins, which does not fit the data. An explanation for the similar concordance in monozygotic and dizygotic twins may be found in non-genetic factors, such as the monozygotic twinning process itself.

Non-genetic factors affecting handedness and language lateralization in twins

An explanation for the low concordance for handedness and lateralization in twin pairs could be the presence of a non-genetic factor that affects twins more than singletons (Derom *et al.*, 1996; Sicotte *et al.*, 1999). An obvious difference in environmental influences is that twin birth is more difficult than singleton

birth. Birth complications may cause trauma to the developing brain, which may lead to "pathologic left-handedness", i.e. left-handedness as a result of a shift to right-cerebral dominance after injury of the left hemisphere (Annett, 1974; Annett & Ockwell, 1980). Twins are at increased risk for low birth weight, preterm birth, prolonged labor, aberrant fetal position at birth, bleeding complications, and asphyxia (Norwitz *et al.*, 2005). Left-handedness in twins could thus be viewed as a "soft-sign" of clinical or sub-clinical neuropathology resulting from birth stress. Indeed, subjects who have suffered traumatic brain insults early in life have a higher prevalence of left-handedness than subjects without such a history (Satz *et al.*, 1985). Several functional imaging studies reported reorganization of motor dominance following perinatal brain lesion of the left hemisphere, with activation of the motor cortex in the right hemisphere for tasks with the right hand (Müller *et al.*, 1997; Müller *et al.*, 1998; Cao *et al.*, 1998; Chu *et al.*, 2000). Cioni *et al.* (2001) assessed cortical reorganization with fMRI in two monozygotic twin pairs, from which one twin of each pair had suffered early injury of the left hemisphere. The twins with lesioned left hemispheres showed significant activation of the right motor cortex during tasks with the right hand, in contrast to their unaffected co-twins who only showed activation in the left motor cortex. These studies demonstrate that left hemisphere lesions after perinatal complications can affect cerebral lateralization of motor functions and lead to discordance for handedness and lateralization in twins. However, the switching of motor dominance to the right hemisphere is demonstrated only in subjects with a clinical picture of hemiplegia or hemiparesis. It is unknown whether these findings can be extrapolated to sub-clinical cases, without overt neurological impairments, who have suffered milder perinatal complications.

A large-scale study in singletons tested the association between handedness of a child and the mother's report regarding the presence or absence of 25 possible pregnancy and birth complications (Bailey & McKeever, 2004). Of these 25 complications, only "maternal age" was associated with left-handedness of the child. This association accounted for no more than

1% of the prevalence of left-handedness. Thus, at least in singletons, birth complication is not an important determinant of handedness. However, twins have a higher rate of severe birth complications, and may therefore have a higher incidence of pathologic left-handedness than singletons.

The association between birth complications and left-handedness in twins can be assessed by studying the influence of birth order on handedness. Second-born twins have a much higher risk for birth complications than first-born twins (Sheay *et al.*, 2004; Kor-anantakul *et al.*, 2007; Edris *et al.*, 2006). The second-born twin is thus expected to be more frequently left-handed than his first-born co-twin. Six studies assessed the association between birth order and handedness in twins, but none of them found that left-handedness is more frequent in second-born than in first-born twins (Nachshon & Denno, 1986; Nachshon & Denno, 1987; Orlebeke *et al.*, 1996; Christian *et al.*, 1979; Segal, 1989; Medland *et al.*, 2006). This quite consistent finding indicates that birth complications have probably no major effect on handedness in twins.

There is yet another way to assess the association between handedness and birth trauma in twins. Twins with brain lesions severe enough to cause a shift in cerebral dominance are also expected to be hampered by other cerebral impairment. When left-handedness is caused by birth trauma, the left-handed twins will be expected to have some shortcomings in cognitive and manual performance in comparison to their right-handed twins. Gurd *et al.* (2006) assessed performance on three manual tasks (dot filling, finger tapping, and peg moving) in 20 monozygotic twin pairs of discordant handedness. They found no evidence of impaired performance on any of the three manual tasks in the left-handed twins as compared to their right-handed co-twins. Kee *et al.* (1998) tested 13 monozygotic twin pairs of discordant handedness on verbal, spatial, and motor tasks. In line with the findings of Gurd *et al.* (2006), left-handed twins did not have lower performance than their right-handed co-twins on any of these tasks. Only one study assessed cognitive functions and handedness in both monozygotic and dizygotic twins. This study applied several cognitive

tasks to test 46 handedness discordant monozygotic and 54 handedness discordant dizygotic twin pairs. They found that the *monozygotic* left-handed twins outperformed their right-handed co-twins on all tests, while the left-handed *dizygotic* twins performed worse than their right-handed co-twins. This last study suggests that pathologic left-handedness may explain part of the left-handedness in dizygotic discordant twin pairs, but not in the monozygotic twin pairs, though replication of this finding is needed.

In sum, pathologic left-handedness is indeed observed in subjects with brain injury after severe birth complications, but it is uncertain if it also occurs in milder cases of birth trauma. Birth complications probably do not have much influence on the prevalence of left-handedness in twins nor on the concordance rate for handedness and lateralization.

The influence of the monozygotic twinning process itself

A possible explanation for the low concordance for handedness and language lateralization in monozygotic twin pairs is a phenomenon called "mirror-imaging" (Newman, 1937; Keeler, 1929). The existence of this phenomenon is much disputed and controversy still remains. In the first half of the twentieth century, the idea of mirror-imaging in monozygotic twins was so influential that monozygosity of a twin pair was frequently diagnosed on the basis of discordant handedness (McManus, 1980). In the second half of that century, most scientists were rather skeptic about the existence of mirror-imaging in twins (James, 1983). However, discoveries on bodily left–right asymmetry in animal embryos have revived the old idea (Boklage, 1987; Levin, 1999).

Mirror-imaging is thought to arise when the split of one original embryo to form two monozygotic twins disrupts early development of left–right asymmetry. The resulting twin pair will be discordant for several asymmetric traits and may thus be mirror-images of each other. It can be assumed that monozygotic twinning occurs after the first establishments of bilateral asymmetry. Several asymmetrical phenomena, such as asymmetric ion fluxes and asymmetric distribution of mRNA for ion exchangers, are already observed during the first few cell divisions (Levin, 2004). Interruption of these early asymmetric developments may lead to unequal division of left–right signaling pathways over the two developing twin embryos (Flannery, 1987). After the twinning process, left–right asymmetry may become deviant in the embryo that develops from the side that lacks important signaling molecules. Deviant asymmetry in only one of the pair will increase discordance for asymmetrical traits, such as visceral asymmetry, handedness, and cerebral dominance in monozygotic twin pairs.

Several congenital heart malformations such as tetralogy of Fallot, hypoplastic left heart, and abnormal great vessel implantation can be viewed as incomplete reversions of visceral laterality (Burn & Corney, 1984). These malformations significantly more frequently affect monozygotic twins than singletons, typically affecting only one of the pair (Burn, 1991). Other congenital malformations that stem from disturbances in visceral left–right asymmetry, such as asplenia (absent spleen, as if two right halves have fused), polysplenia (two or more spleens, as if two left halves have fused) and malrotation of the alimentary tract are also more frequent in monozygotic twins than in dizygotic twins or in singletons, again affecting only one twin of a pair (reviewed by Luke & Keith, 1990).

Mirror-imaging in monozygotic twins is frequently described for hair whorls, eyes, eye nerves, and teeth (Golbin et al., 1993; Brown, 1995; Townsend et al., 1985; Townsend & Richards, 1990; Cidis et al., 1997). Results from studies on language lateralization suggest that mirror-imaging of the cerebral hemispheres may also be rather common (Steinmetz et al., 1995; Sommer et al., 2004).

It is difficult to test whether mirror-imaging in monozygotic twins is indeed a reason for the low concordance for language lateralization and handedness in monozygotic twins. In support of this hypothesis, studies that assessed language lateralization in monozygotic and dizygotic twins found that monozygotic twin pairs with one left-hander show a much larger intra-pair difference than dizygotic pairs with one left-hander (Springer & Searleman, 1978; Geschwind

et al., 2002). This could indicate that monozygotic twins of discordant handedness include several cases of mirror-imaged twin pairs, who show opposite patterns of language lateralization. Steinmetz et al. (1995) included ten handedness discordant monozygotic twins and found three pairs with opposite cerebral asymmetry, possibly resulting from mirror-imaging, and seven pairs with small intra-pair differences, possibly resulting from a homozygote recessive genotype. In parallel, from thirteen handedness discordant monozygotic twins in our study, five pairs showed opposite patterns of language lateralization, while the other eight pairs of discordant handedness had quite similar degrees of language lateralization (Sommer et al., 2004). These studies suggest that opposite patterns of lateralization, possibly resulting from mirror-imaging, may be present in 30% to 40% of monozygotic twin pairs with one left-hander.

It could be hypothesized that twins resulting from a relatively late monozygotic twinning process (occurring four or more days after fertilization) may be most liable to the influence of mirror-imaging than twins who have split early, since the original embryo may have developed a higher degree of left–right asymmetry at a later time of splitting. If this hypothesis is true, concordance for handedness and lateralization is expected to be lower in twins who separated late than in twins with earlier separation. The time of splitting of a human embryo into monozygotic twins can be deduced from the anatomy of the placenta. Approximately one-third of monozygotic twins are dichorionic, which means that they have separate birth fleeces and placentas. The twinning process of these dichorionic twins probably occurs before blastocyst formation, when the embryo is still massive and homogeneous. Two-thirds of monozygotic twins are monochorionic, which means that they share the placenta and the outer fleece (Bryan, 1992). Monochorionic twin pairs split after formation of the chorion at least four days after fertilization (Bulmer, 1970). The assumption that twins with a late split are more likely to be discordant for handedness can thus be tested by comparing monochorionic twin pairs to dichorionic twin pairs. Medland et al. (2006) merged data from four twin studies and found no difference between mono- and dichorionic twin pairs on the prevalence of left-handedness in 3657 monozygotic pairs. Thus, the hypothesis that mirror-imaging has more impact when the twins separate later in embryogenesis is not supported. This may imply that mirror-imaging is not an important determinant of handedness in monozygotic twins, or it may suggest that both monochorionic and dichorionic twins are liable to mirror-imaging to a similar degree. At this point, there are no studies to distinguish between these two possibilities.

In sum, the monozygotic twinning process itself may affect handedness and lateralization of the resulting twins. This could decrease concordance for both traits in monozygotic twin pairs only. It can as yet not be concluded whether the hypothesized process of mirror-imaging has indeed an important impact on lateralization and handedness in monozygotic twins.

Conclusion

Both monozygotic and dizygotic twins have a higher prevalence of left-handedness than single-born subjects. First-degree relatives of twins also have a higher prevalence of left-handedness, which suggests a common genetic predisposition for both twinning and deviant lateralization. Furthermore, the concordance rate for handedness and language lateralization in monozygotic twins is rather low, hardly exceeding that of dizygotic twins. This finding has led to the conclusion that handedness and lateralization are exclusively defined by environmental factors. However, this conclusion may be precarious since several other factors may affect handedness and lateralization in twins. For example, the genetic models for handedness and lateralization involve a random factor, which produces low concordance for handedness and cerebral lateralization even in monozygotic twin pairs. This effect specifically reduces concordance for language lateralization in "enriched" samples with many left-handers.

Twins have more perinatal complications than singletons, which may produce more cases of "pathologic left-handedness", thereby increasing the prevalence of left-handedness and reducing concordance rates in both types of twins. Severe birth complications

can indeed affect cerebral motor dominance. Nevertheless, the influence of "pathologic left-handedness" on the handedness distribution in twins is probably not high, since left-handed twins do not have lower scores on manual ability and IQ tests than their right-handed co-twins.

Discordance for handedness and language lateralization in some monozygotic twin pairs may result from disruption of embryonic asymmetry development by the twinning process itself, a phenomenon called "mirror-imaging". Though the concept of mirror-imaging in monozygotic twins is difficult to investigate, it is obvious that monozygotic twinning is a very different process than dizygotic twinning, and much more susceptible to developmental deviations. Possibly, some 30% to 40% of discordant handedness in monozygotic twins results from mirror-imaging. Though twins who have separated late, e.g., monochorionic twins, may be expected to be more liable to mirror-imaging, there was no difference in concordance rates for handedness between monochorionic and dichorionic twins. Mirror-imaging may affect handedness and laterality in twins, but the extent of its influence has yet to be defined.

We can conclude that handedness and lateralization in twins are affected by factors that are either absent (mirror-imaging) or less frequent (birth trauma) in singletons. Findings on heredity of these traits in twins can therefore not be extrapolated to predict heredity in singletons. The classic twin study design may therefore not be the ideal method to test heredity of handedness and language lateralization. Since cerebral lateralization is related to several cognitive and psychiatric traits, twin studies on these traits may also be influenced by the special aspects of lateralization in twins.

REFERENCES

Anneken, K., Konrad, C., Dräger, B. *et al.* (2004). Familial aggregation of strong hemispheric language lateralization. *Neurology*, **63**(12), 2433–5.

Annett, M. (1964). A model of the inheritance of handedness and cerebral dominance. *Nature*, **3**(204), 59–60.

Annett, M. (1974). Handedness in the children of two left-handed parents. *Br J Psychol*, **65**(1), 129–31.

Annett, M. (1979). Family handedness in three generations predicted by the right shift theory. *Ann Hum Genet*, **42**(4), 479–91.

Annett, M. (2003). Cerebral asymmetry in twins: predictions of the right shift theory. *Neuropsychologia*, **41**(4), 469–79.

Annett, M. (2004). Hand preference observed in large healthy samples: classification, norms and interpretations of increased non-right-handedness by the right shift theory. *British Journal of Psychology*, **95**(3), 339–53.

Annett, M. & Ockwell, A. (1980). Birth order, birth stress and handedness. *Cortex*, **16**(1), 181–7.

Bailey, L. M. & McKeever, W. F. (2004). A large-scale study of handedness and pregnancy/birth risk events: implications for genetic theories of handedness. *Laterality*, **9**(2), 175–88.

Boklage, C. E. (1981). On the distribution of nonrighthandedness among twins and their families. *Acta Genet Med Gemellol*, **30**(3), 167–87.

Boklage, C. E. (1987). Twinning, nonrighthandedness, and fusion malformations: evidence for heritable causal elements held in common. *Am J Med Genet*, **28**(1), 67–84.

Brown, D. C. (1995). Twin-to-twin atopy. *Lancet*, **345**(8956), 1053.

Bryan, E. M. (1992). The role of twins in epidemiological studies. *Paediatr Perinat Epidemiol*, **6**(4), 460–4.

Bryden, M. P. (1976). Speech lateralization in families: a preliminary study using dichotic listening. *Brain Lang*, **2**(2), 201–11.

Bulmer, M. G. (1970). *The Biology of Twinning in Man*. Oxford: Clarendon Press.

Burn, J. (1991). Disturbance of morphological laterality in humans. *Ciba Found Symp*, **162**, 282–96; discussion 296–9.

Burn, J. & Corney, G. (1984). Congenital heart defects and twinning. *Acta Genet Med Gemellol*, **33**(1), 61–9.

Cao, Y., D'Olhaberriague, L., Vikingstad, E. M., Levine, S. R. & Welch, K. M. (1998). Pilot study of functional MRI to assess cerebral activation of motor function after poststroke hemiparesis. *Stroke*, **29**(1), 112–22.

Carton, A. & Rees, R. T. (1987). Mirror image dental anomalies in identical twins. *Br Dent J*, **162**(5), 193–4.

Christian, J. C., Hunter, D. S., Evans, M. M. & Standeford, F. M. (1979). Association of handedness and birth order in monozygotic twins. *Acta Genet Med Gemellol*, **28**(1), 67–8.

Chu, D., Huttenlocher, P. R., Levin, D. N. & Towle, V. L. (2000). Reorganization of the hand somatosensory cortex following perinatal unilateral brain injury. *Neuropediatrics*, **31**(2), 63–9.

Cidis, M. B., Warshowsky, J. H., Goldrich, S. G. & Meltzer, C. C. (1997). Mirror-image optic nerve dysplasia with associated anisometropia in identical twins. *J Am Optom Assoc*, **68**(5), 325–9.

Cioni, G., Montanaro, D., Tosetti, M., Canapicchi, R. & Ghelarducci, B. (2001). Reorganisation of the sensorimotor cortex after early focal brain lesion: a functional MRI study in monozygotic twins. *NeuroReport*, **12**(7), 1335–40.

Coren, S. & Halpern, D. F. (1991). Left-handedness: a marker of decreased survival fitness. *Psychol Bull*, **109**, 90–106.

Davis, A. & Annett, M. (1994). Handedness as a function of twinning, age and sex. *Cortex*, **30**(1), 105–11.

Derom, C., Thiery, E., Vlietinck, R., Loos, R. & Derom, R. (1996). Handedness in twins according to zygosity and chorion type: a preliminary report. *Behav Genet*, **26**(4), 407–8.

Edris, F., Oppenheimer, L., Yang, Q. *et al.* (2006). Relationship between intertwin delivery interval and metabolic acidosis in the second twin. *Am J Perinatol*, **23**(8), 481–5.

Flannery, D. B. (1987). The possible role of homeotic genes in the causation of malformations in monozygotic twins. *Acta Genet Med Gemellol*, **36**(3), 433–6.

Francks, C., Fisher, S. E., MacPhie, I. L. *et al.* (2002). A genome-wide linkage screen for relative hand skill in sibling pairs. *Am J Hum Genet*, **70**(3), 800–5. Erratum in: *Am J Hum Genet*, **70**(4), 1075.

Geschwind, D. H., Miller, B. L., DeCarli, C. & Carmelli, D. (2002). Heritability of lobar brain volumes in twins supports genetic models of cerebral laterality and handedness. *Proc Natl Acad Sci USA*, **99**(5), 3176–81

Geschwind, D. H. & Miller, B. L. (2001). Molecular approaches to cerebral laterality: development and neurodegeneration. *Am J Med Genet*, **101**(4), 370–81.

Golbin, A., Golbin, Y., Keith, L. & Keith, D. (1993). Mirror imaging in twins: biological polarization – an evolving hypothesis. *Acta Genet Med Gemellol*, **42**(3–4), 237–43.

Gurd, J. M., Schulz, J., Cherkas, L. & Ebers, G. C. (2006). Hand preference and performance in 20 pairs of monozygotic twins with discordant handedness. *Cortex*, **42**(6), 934–45.

Hicks, R. E. & Kinsbourne, M. (1976). Human handedness: a partial cross-fostering study. Interpretations of increased non-right-handedness by the right shift theory. *Science*, **192**(4242), 908–10.

Jäncke, L. & Steinmetz, H. (1994). Auditory lateralization in monozygotic twins. *Int J Neurosci*, **75**(1–2), 57–64.

James, W. H. (1983). Twinning handedness and embryology. *Percept Mot Skills*, **56**(3), 721–2.

Keeler, C. E. (1929). On the amount of external mirror imagery in double monsters and identical twins. *Proc Natl Acad Sci USA*, **15**(11), 839–42.

Kee, D. W., Cherry, B. J., Neale, P. L., McBride, D. M. & Segal, N. L. (1998). Multitask analysis of cerebral hemisphere specialization in monozygotic twins discordant for handedness. Monozygotic twin pairs. *Neuropsychology*, **12**(3), 468–78.

Kennedy, D. N., O'Craven, K. M., Ticho, B. S. *et al.* (1999). Structural and functional brain asymmetries in human situs inversus totalis. *Neurology*, **53**(6), 1260–5.

Kor-anantakul, O., Suwanrath, C., Suntharasaj, T., Getpook, C. & Leetanaporn, R. (2007). Outcomes of multifetal pregnancies. *J Obstet Gynaecol Res*, **33**(1), 49–55.

Levin, M. (1999). Twinning and embryonic left-right asymmetry. *Laterality*, **4**(3), 197–208.

Levin, M. (2004). The embryonic origins of left-right asymmetry. *Crit Rev Oral Biol Med*, **15**(4), 197–206.

Levin, M. & Mercola, M. (1998). The compulsion of chirality: toward an understanding of left-right asymmetry. *Genes Dev*, **12**(6), 763–9.

Luke, B. & Keith, L. G. (1990). Monozygotic twinning as a congenital defect and congenital defects in monozygotic twins. *Fetal Diagn Ther*, **5**(2), 61–9.

McManus, I. C. (1980). Handedness in twins: a critical review. *Neuropsychologia*, **18**(3), 347–55.

McManus, I. C. (1985). Handedness, language dominance and aphasia: a genetic model. *Psychol Med Monogr Suppl*, **8**, 1–40.

McManus, I. C., Martin, N., Stubbings, G. F., Chung, E. M. & Mitchison, H. M. (2004). Handedness and situs inversus in primary ciliary dyskinesia. *Proc Biol Sci*, **271**(1557), 2579–82.

Medland, S. E., Duffy, D. L., Wright, M. J., Geffen, G. M. & Martin, N. G. (2006). Handedness in twins: joint analysis of data from 35 samples. *Twin Res Hum Genet*, **9**(1), 46–53.

Müller, R. A., Rothermel, R. D., Behen, M. E. *et al.* (1997). Plasticity of motor organization in children and adults. *NeuroReport*, **8**(14), 3103–8.

Müller, R. A., Rothermel, R. D., Behen, M. E. *et al.* (1998). Differential patterns of language and motor reorganization following early left hemisphere lesion: a PET study. *Arch Neurol*, **55**(8), 1113–19.

Nachshon, I. & Denno, D. (1986). Birth order and lateral preferences. *Cortex*, **22**(4), 567–78.

Nachshon, I. & Denno, D. (1987). Birth stress and lateral preferences. *Cortex*, **23**(1), 45–58.

Newman, H. H. *et al.* (1937). *Twins: A Study of Heredity and Environment*, 1st edn. Chicago: University of Chicago Press.

Norwitz, E. R., Edusa, V. & Park, J. S. (2005). Maternal physiology and complications of multiple pregnancy. *Semin Perinatol*, **29**(5), 338–48.

Orlebeke, J. F., Knol, D. L., Koopmans, J. R., Boomsma, D. I. & Bleker, O. P. (1996). Left-handedness in twins: genes or environment? *Cortex*, **32**(3), 479–90.

Reiss, M., Tymnik, G., Kögler, P., Kögler, W. & Reiss, G. (1999). Laterality of hand, foot, eye, and ear in twins. *Laterality*, **4**(3), 287–97.

Ross, C. N. (1999). Twins and the fetal origins hypothesis. Fetal insult may cause vascular changes and growth retardation. *B M J*, **319**(7208), 517–8.

Rutten, G. J., Ramsey, N. F., van Rijen, P. C. & van Veelen, C. W. (2002). Reproducibility of fMRI-determined language lateralization in individual subjects. *Brain Lang*, **80**(3), 421–37.

Satz, P., Orsini, D. L., Saslow, E. & Henry, R. (1985). The pathological left-handedness syndrome. *Brain Cogn*, **4**(1), 27–46.

Schneider, H. & Brueckner, M. (2000). Of mice and men: dissecting the genetic pathway that controls left–right asymmetry in mice and humans. *Am J Med Genet*, **97**(4), 258–70.

Segal, N. L. (1989). Origins and implications of handedness and relative birth weight for IQ in monozygotic twin pairs. *Neuropsychologia*, **27**(4), 549–61.

Shapleske, J., Rossell, S. L., Woodruff, P. W. & David, A. S. (1999). The planum temporale: a systematic, quantitative review of its structural, functional and clinical significance. *Brain Res Brain Res Rev*, **29**(1), 26–49.

Sheay, W., Ananth, C. V. & Kinzler, W. L. (2004). Perinatal mortality in first- and second-born twins in the United States. *Obstet Gynecol*, **103**(1), 63–70.

Sicotte, N. L., Woods, R. P. & Mazziotta, J. C. (1999). Handedness in twins: a meta-analysis. *Laterality*, **4**(3), 265–86

Sommer, I. E., Ramsey, N. F., Mandl, R. C. & Kahn, R. S. (2002). Language lateralization in monozygotic twin pairs concordant and discordant for handedness. *Brain*, **125**(12), 2710–18.

Sommer, I. E., Ramsey, N. F., Mandl, R. C., van Oel, C. J. & Kahn, R. S. (2004). Language activation in monozygotic twins discordant for schizophrenia. *Br J Psychiatry*, **184**, 128–35.

Springer, S. P. & Searleman, A. (1978). The ontogeny of hemispheric specialization: evidence from dichotic listening in twins. *Neuropsychologia*, **16**(3), 269–81.

Steinman, G. (2001). Mechanisms of twinning. II. Laterality and intercellular bonding in monozygotic twinning. *J Reprod Med*, **46**(5), 473–9.

Steinmetz, H., Herzog, A., Schlaug, G., Huang, Y. & Jäncke, L. (1995). Brain (A) symmetry in monozygotic twins. *Cereb Cortex*, **5**(4), 296–300.

Sun, T., Patoine, C., Abu-Khalil, A. *et al.* (2005). Early asymmetry of gene transcription in embryonic human left and right cerebral cortex. *Science*, **308**(5729), 1794–8.

Tambs, K., Magnus, P. & Berg, K. (1987). Left-handedness in twin families: support of an environmental hypothesis. *Percept Mot Skills*, **64**(1), 155–70.

Tanaka, S., Kanzaki, R., Yoshibayashi, M., Kamiya, T. & Sugishita, M. (1999). Dichotic listening in patients with situs inversus: brain asymmetry and situs asymmetry. *Neuropsychologia*, **37**(7), 869–74.

Townsend, G. & Richards, L. (1990). Twins and twinning, dentists and dentistry. *Aust Dent J*, **35**(4), 317–27.

Townsend, G., Rogers, J., Richards, L. & Brown, T. (1995). Agenesis of permanent maxillary lateral incisors in South Australian twins. *Aust Dent J*, **40**(3), 186–92.

Usta, I. M., Nassar, A. H., Awwad, J. T. *et al.* (2002). Comparison of the perinatal morbidity and mortality of the presenting twin and its co-twin. *J Perinatol*, **22**(5), 391–6.

Van Agtmael, T., Forrest, S. M. & Williamson, R. (2002). Parametric and non-parametric linkage analysis of several candidate regions for genes for human handedness. *Eur J Hum Genet*, **10**(10), 623–30.

Van Agtmael, T., Forrest, S. M., Del-Favero, J., Van Broeckhoven, C. & Williamson, R. (2003). Parametric and nonparametric genome scan analyses for human handedness. *Eur J Hum Genet*, **11**(10), 779–83.

Warren, D. M., Stern, M., Duggirala, R., Dyer, T. D. & Almasy, L. (2006). Heritability and linkage analysis of hand, foot, and eye preference in Mexican Americans. *Laterality*, **11**(6), 508–24.

West, V. C. (1985). Case reports. Mirror image twins. *Aust Orthod J*, **9**(2), 243.

7

Sex differences in handedness and language lateralization

Iris E. C. Sommer and René S. Kahn

Summary

This chapter provides a quantitative review of sex differences in handedness, asymmetry of the planum temporale (PT), and cerebral lateralization of language. We have reviewed two reflections of language lateralization: asymmetric performance on dichotic listening tests (right-ear advantage) and asymmetry of functional language activation as measured with functional imaging techniques.

Meta-analysis of studies that assessed handedness in males and females yielded a higher prevalence of left-handedness in males, with a mean weighted odds ratio of 1.29 ($p < 0.000$).

Studies on anatomical asymmetry and functional language lateralization were less abundant and generally assessed much smaller samples than studies on handedness. Meta-analysis of studies on PT asymmetry yielded no sex difference in asymmetry (Hedge's $g = -0.05$, $p = 0.47$). Results of the meta-analysis on dichotic listening studies were consistent with the findings for PT asymmetry; no sex difference in lateralization (Hedge's $g = 0.04$, $p = 0.33$). When the studies were subdivided according to the paradigm they applied, meta-analysis of studies that used the consonant–vowel task yielded significant sex differences favoring males. Meta-analyses of studies that applied other dichotic listening tasks yielded no sex difference. The subdivision into studies applying a certain paradigm largely overlapped with the subdivision into studies that did or did not focus on sex differences as their main topic. Analysis of an unpublished database that also used a consonant–vowel task and included three times as many subjects as our sub-analysis found no sex difference. It appears, therefore, more likely that the significant sex effect observed in a sub-analysis is caused by publication bias, than that the applied paradigm produces a sex difference in language lateralization.

Consistent with the meta-analyses on PT asymmetry and on dichotic listening studies, analysis of functional imaging studies yielded no significant sex difference (Hedge's $g = 0.01$, $p = 0.73$) in language lateralization. Sub-analyses of studies that applied word generation tasks, semantic decision tasks, or listening tasks all yielded no sex difference.

In conclusion, males are more frequently left-handed than females, but there is no significant difference in cerebral asymmetry or in language lateralization between the sexes.

Several factors may cause the increased left-handedness in males in the absence of decreased asymmetry or language lateralization. Higher antenatal testosterone levels appear to increase the chance for left-handedness. Alternatively, genetic factors could also lead to increased left-handedness in males. Left-handed mothers are more likely to have left-handed offspring than left-handed fathers. This suggests that sex-linked transmission, for example through an imprinted gene or a locus on the X-chromosome, may play a role in the genetics of handedness. Finally, sex differences in social pressure to use the right hand for writing and eating may explain the increased left-handedness in males. Females more frequently report to have switched in hand preference than males. Social factors would offer a valid explanation for the sex difference in handedness in the absence of associated sex differences in asymmetry and lateralization.

Introduction

In 1980, Harris wrote the first review on sex differences in lateralization, in which he concluded that females are less lateralized than men. Reviews conducted in the years since have generally agreed with Harris' conclusion that females have lower degrees of language lateralization than males (Bryden, 1982; McGlone, 1980). An early dissenting view was expressed by Fairweather *et al.* (1982). Boles (1984) also failed to find a sex difference in lateralization in a meta-analysis on studies that applied visual half-field paradigms. Another review by Hiscock and Mackay (1985) also failed to find a sex difference in lateralization assessed with dichotic listening. In line with these findings, a meta-analysis on functional imaging studies applying language tasks yielded no sex difference (Sommer *et al.*, 2004). Thirty years after the first review on this topic, there is still no consensus about sex differences in lateralization and it remains a much debated topic (Clements *et al.*, 2006; Plante *et al.*, 2006).

There are several reasons why this topic remains in the center of attention for so many years. First, there are considerable differences between girls and boys in the development of language abilities. When speaking first begins, girls generally articulate better than boys and produce longer sentences (Maccoby & Konrad, 1966). Perhaps as a consequence of this advantage, girls tend to have larger working vocabularies and better use of grammar than boys. Some years later, girls typically have superior reading abilities than boys. Part of this verbal advantage for females survives into adult age, especially in the domain of verbal fluency and use of grammar. Furthermore, language disabilities, both of severe and mild type, affect boys more frequently than girls, with reported sex ratios between 3:1 and 7:1 (reviewed by Liederman *et al.*, 2005). Psychiatric disorders, such as autism, attention deficit hyperactivity disorder (ADHD), and schizophrenia all have higher prevalences in males as compared to females (reviewed by Afifi, 2007). Finally, women appear to recover better from aphasia than males after left cerebral stroke (Pedersen *et al.*, 1995). If women indeed have more bilateral language lateralization than men, this could provide an explanation for all these observed sex differences. This meta-analysis aims to provide an overview of the current literature on sex differences in cerebral dominance, as reflected in handedness, asymmetry of the planum temporale, and functional language lateralization.

Methods

Handedness is associated with language lateralization, though this correlation is complex (Pujol *et al.*, 1999). Handedness therefore provides a reflection of language

lateralization. Though this reflection is not very accurate, it can be observed easily and has been assessed in large samples of males and females. We have selected three other measurement methods that correlate to language lateralization and have frequently been applied in the study of healthy males and females, these are as follows.

1. Asymmetry of the planum temporale (PT) – measured with MRI or directly in post-mortem brains
2. Right ear advantage (REA) – measured with dichotic presentation of verbal stimuli
3. Asymmetry of language activation – as assessed with functional imaging techniques (functional magnetic resonance imaging, positron emission tomography, and functional transcranial Doppler) using verbal stimuli (words, phonemes, sentences, or stories).

Search criteria

The literature on handedness and language lateralization comprises more than forty years of research and is estimated to consist of over 10 000 studies. This meta-analysis cannot, therefore, provide a complete review of all studies reporting sex differences in handedness or lateralization. Explored databases were Embase, PsychLit, PubMed, and Science Direct, using combinations of the following search terms: "handedness", "sex", "left-handed", "gender", "planum temporale", "REA", "dichotic listening", "fMRI", "language lateralization", "fTCD", and "PET". Reference lists from retrieved articles were also assessed for cross-references. Only English publications from international journals were selected. In addition, the last five volumes of three journals (*Brain and Language*, *NeuroImage* and *Human Brain Mapping*) were searched manually to check for other suitable studies.

Papers were included if they met the following criteria:

- The study used exactly the same method to assessed handedness, asymmetry of the PT, or functional language lateralization as measured either with dichotic listening or with functional imaging in males and females.
- The study included individuals who were not selected on the basis of a special condition that may be related to language lateralization (such as

dyslexia, schizophrenia, epilepsy, professional mathematicians, homosexuals, or subjects with a history of birth trauma). The unselected control groups for specific population subsets were, however, included.

- Twin studies were excluded, since there is reason to assume that handedness and lateralization in twins is different from that in singletons (see Chapter 6).
- Sufficient exact data were available in the paper to calculate effect sizes for the sex difference, or could be provided post hoc by the corresponding author.

More than 1000 studies were selected and screened for suitability. Approximately half of these articles did not assess sex differences in their sample. From the studies that did mention a sex effect, the majority reported that there were no significant sex differences. These studies could have been included by presuming that the main effect of sex would have an F-value of zero. This would have been a quite conservative approach and may have led to an underestimation of the sex effect. We therefore preferred to exclude these studies, at the disadvantage of overestimating the true sex effect. Only studies that provided percentages (for handedness) or means and standard deviations per sex (PT asymmetry, language lateralization) or exact F-, t-, or p- values for the main effect for sex were included.

Combination of measurement methods

Handedness

Studies that assessed handedness have used a variety of handedness scales. A large unpublished, but frequently cited, meta-analysis by McManus found that the incidence of left-handedness was not related to the method of measurement, or the length or number of response items included in handedness inventories. Whether handedness is assessed by a questionnaire, a performance measurement, or a simple question (such as "writing hand" or "handedness of the subject") appears not to affect the observed incidence of left-handedness. We therefore felt confident to combine percentages of right-handedness obtained with different methods. When several handedness criteria were provided, we selected data based on writing hand in order to increase uniformity among studies.

Planum temporale

Studies assessing asymmetry of the PT also applied different methods of measurement. Some studies measured the surface of the PT, while others measured PT volume. Determination of the borders of the PT also showed minor differences between studies. However, in all studies right and left PT were measured in a similar fashion. The effect size for asymmetry that was calculated from PT sizes may therefore be better comparable between studies than the absolute data of the size of right and left PT. In addition, effect sizes for asymmetry were compared between men and women from the same study before combining them with other studies to calculate a mean weighted effect size.

Dichotic listening

Studies that measured language lateralization with the dichotic listening paradigm applied several different stimuli. Studies were included that used either a Consonant–Vowel(–Consonant) (CV or CVC) task, a fused word, or a rhyme word task, or binaural presentation of different digits or words (triad task and other recall tasks), to elicit an REA. One study (Lamm & Epstein, 1997) provided data on two different paradigms. Data sets from these tasks were entered as separate studies. The type of paradigm applied to elicit an REA may affect the degree of language lateralization. It is therefore possible that the paradigm also affects the sex difference in perceptual asymmetry. In order to assess this possibility, paradigm was entered in the analysis as a potential moderator.

Functional imaging

In parallel to dichotic listening studies, studies applying functional imaging to assess language lateralization have used several different language paradigms, such as verb generation, story listening, picture naming, and semantic decision making. One study (Plante *et al.*, 2006) provided data on four different paradigms. Data sets from these paradigms were entered as separate studies. Again, the type of language paradigm was entered as a potential moderator.

Children and adults

Handedness is a rather stable individual characteristic, from about 7 years of age (Michel & Harkins, 1986). We have therefore included handedness data from both children (above age 7) and adults. Subject's age may, however, be a factor to affect language lateralization (Holland *et al.*, 2001) and possibly asymmetry of the PT. A significant interaction between age and sex has frequently been described in studies on language lateralization (Plante *et al.*, 2006; Gaillard *et al.*, 2001, 2003). We therefore marked whether data were obtained from children, from adults, or from a mixed group. An additional analysis was performed to assess possible differences in the sex difference in lateralization between children and adults.

Percentage left-handed subjects

Many studies on PT asymmetry and on language lateralization selected inclusion to right-handed subject. Selection of only right-handed subjects may affect the sex differences in PT asymmetry or in language lateralization. The percentage of left-handed subjects per study was correlated to the effect size for the sex difference to assess the potential influence of this factor.

File drawer problem

One of the main pitfalls of meta-analyses is the "file drawer problem" (Rosenthal, 1991), i.e., the possibility that published studies are a biased sample of the studies that are actually carried out, as it is presumed that only experiments with significant results are published. This problem is associated with the inclusion of only published studies in a meta-analysis. The exclusive use of published studies is likely to result in an overestimation of the effects under study. In the present meta-analysis we emphasized the inclusion of studies that did not focus on sex differences, but rather reported information on sex differences as a by product, in order to minimize the file drawer problem. For example, studies that examined the effect of age or occupation were included, as well as data from control groups of studies examining the effects of schizophrenia or epilepsy on lateralization.

It was noted whether or not sex differences were the main objective of a study and this variable was entered as a potential moderator to obtain a reflection of the influence of publication bias. Furthermore, for the meta-analysis on dichotic listening studies, we could compare the included data to the unpublished data on sex differences from the Bergen Dichotic Listening Database (courtesy of Professor K. Hugdahl). Comparing the results of our meta-analysis on published dichotic listening studies to the large database of Professor Hugdahl, provides a reflection of the impact of the file drawer problem.

Meta-analytic techniques

Handedness

From the handedness studies, odds ratios were calculated from the percentage right-handed women compared to the percentage right-handed men. Odds ratios of all studies were combined to calculate a mean weighted odds ratio and a corresponding p-value using the program Comprehensive Meta-analysis (www.meta-analysis.com/). We used random effects, since handedness assessment and study population differed between studies. In addition, a homogeneity statistic (I^2) was calculated, to assess the heterogeneity of results across studies. I^2 quantifies the effect of heterogeneity, providing a measure of the degree of inconsistency in the studies' results (Higgins *et al.*, 2003). Negative values of I^2 are put equal to zero so that I^2 lies between 0% and 100%. I^2 describes the percentage of total variation across studies that is due to heterogeneity rather than chance; a value of 0% indicates no observed heterogeneity, and larger values show increasing heterogeneity (Higgins *et al.*, 2003). Since nationality of the study sample may influence the sex difference in handedness, this factor was entered as a potential moderator.

Planum temporale

From studies on PT asymmetry, a mean weighted effect size for asymmetry was first calculated from the right and left PT size for males and females separately. In a third meta-analysis, effect sizes of females' asymmetry were compared to those of males. If means and standard deviations were not provided per sex in the study, exact F-, t-, or p- values were transformed into effect sizes using Rosenthal's (1991) formula. Effect sizes for sex differences in asymmetry of all studies were combined and weighted for sample size of the studies to obtain a mean weighted effect size "Hedge's g" (Hedges & Olkin, 1985) and p-values using the random effects module of Comprehensive Meta-analysis software. Homogeneity statistic (I^2) was calculated, to assess the heterogeneity of results across studies (Higgins *et al.*, 2003).

Dichotic listening

From each study an effect size was calculated, "Hedge's g" (Hedges & Olkin, 1985). When means and standard deviations were not available, effect sizes were computed from exact p-values, t-values, or F-values (cf. Lipsey & Wilson, 2001). After computing effect sizes for each study, the meta-analytic method was applied to obtain a combined effect size (Hedge's g), which indicated the magnitude of the association across all studies. Effect sizes were weighted for sample size, in order to correct for upwardly biased estimation of the effect in small sample sizes using the random effects module of Comprehensive Meta-analysis software. A homogeneity statistic (I^2) was calculated, to assess the heterogeneity of results across studies (Higgins *et al.*, 2003).

Functional imaging

From studies on language lateralization measured with functional imaging, the mean and standard deviation of the lateralization index was compared between the sexes. The lateralization index is defined as language activity in the left hemisphere minus language activity in the right hemisphere, divided by the total activity in both hemispheres. Language activity was measured as the number of "active" voxels in brain regions involved in language processing. If means and standard deviations of the lateralization indices were not provided per sex, exact F-, t-, or p- values for the main effect of sex on asymmetry were transformed into effect sizes using Rosenthal's (1991) formula. Effect sizes of all studies

were combined and weighted for sample size to obtain a mean weighted effect size (Hedge's g) using the random effects module of Comprehensive Meta-analysis software. A homogeneity statistic (I^2) was calculated, to assess the heterogeneity of results across studies (Higgins *et al.*, 2003).

Results

Sex differences in handedness

We included 43 studies on handedness providing information on 241 573 subjects. Figure 7.1 shows the included studies assessing handedness for males and females from several countries. The mean weighted odds ratio was 1.25 ($p < 0.0001$), indicating a 25% higher prevalence of non-right-handedness in males. The I^2-value for heterogeneity was 78%, indicating large variability among studies that cannot be explained by chance alone. Since culture or race may be involved in this sex difference in handedness, studies that assessed handedness in Western countries (European countries, Australia, Canada, and the USA) were compared to those assessing handedness in non-Western countries (Asia, Africa, Near East). The mean weighted odds ratio of 31 studies assessing Western populations was 1.19 ($p < 0.0001$), while the mean odds ratio of 12 studies assessing non-Western populations was 1.5 ($p < 0.0001$). The difference in odds ratios for sex differences between Western and non-Western countries was significant ($Q = 5.0$, $p = 0.03$).

Sex differences in asymmetry of the temporal plane

Thirteen studies could be included that provided data of right and left PT size per sex. Twelve studies applied MRI measurements and one study measured postmortem brains. All studies included only adult right-handed subjects. Meta-analyses of the PT asymmetry per sex showed that there was significant leftward asymmetry of the PT, both in males (Hedge's $g = 0.98$, $p < 0.001$) and in females (Hedge's $g = 0.98$, $p < 0.001$). The meta-analysis comparing asymmetry between

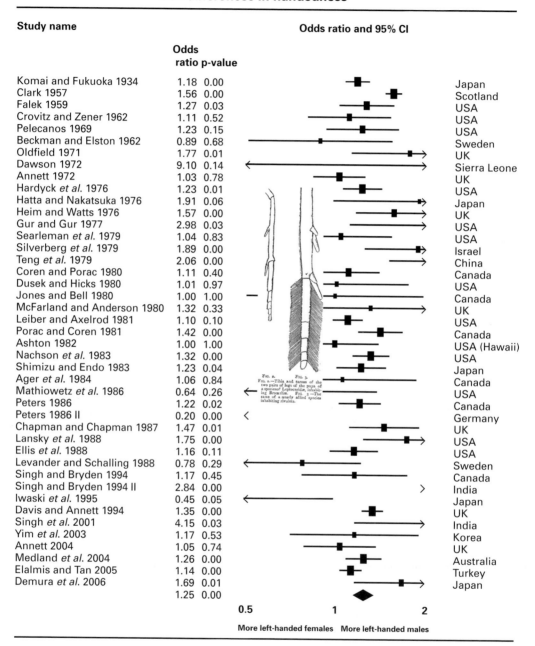

Sex differences in handedness

Study name	Odds ratio	p-value		Country
Komai and Fukuoka 1934	1.18	0.00		Japan
Clark 1957	1.56	0.00		Scotland
Falek 1959	1.27	0.03		USA
Crovitz and Zener 1962	1.11	0.52		USA
Pelecanos 1969	1.23	0.15		USA
Beckman and Elston 1962	0.89	0.68		Sweden
Oldfield 1971	1.77	0.01		UK
Dawson 1972	9.10	0.14		Sierra Leone
Annett 1972	1.03	0.78		UK
Hardyck et al. 1976	1.23	0.01		USA
Hatta and Nakatsuka 1976	1.91	0.06		Japan
Heim and Watts 1976	1.57	0.00		UK
Gur and Gur 1977	2.98	0.03		USA
Searleman et al. 1979	1.04	0.83		USA
Silverberg et al. 1979	1.89	0.00		Israel
Teng et al. 1979	2.06	0.00		China
Coren and Porac 1980	1.11	0.40		Canada
Dusek and Hicks 1980	1.01	0.97		USA
Jones and Bell 1980	1.00	1.00		Canada
McFarland and Anderson 1980	1.32	0.33		UK
Leiber and Axelrod 1981	1.10	0.10		USA
Porac and Coren 1981	1.42	0.00		Canada
Ashton 1982	1.00	1.00		USA (Hawaii)
Nachson et al. 1983	1.32	0.00		USA
Shimizu and Endo 1983	1.23	0.04		Japan
Ager et al. 1984	1.06	0.84		Canada
Mathiowetz et al. 1986	0.64	0.26		USA
Peters 1986	1.22	0.02		Canada
Peters 1986 II	0.20	0.00		Germany
Chapman and Chapman 1987	1.47	0.01		UK
Lansky et al. 1988	1.75	0.00		USA
Ellis et al. 1988	1.16	0.11		USA
Levander and Schalling 1988	0.78	0.29		Sweden
Singh and Bryden 1994	1.17	0.45		Canada
Singh and Bryden 1994 II	2.84	0.00		India
Iwaski et al. 1995	0.45	0.05		Japan
Davis and Annett 1994	1.35	0.00		UK
Singh et al. 2001	4.15	0.03		India
Yim et al. 2003	1.17	0.53		Korea
Annett 2004	1.05	0.74		UK
Medland et al. 2004	1.26	0.00		Australia
Elalmis and Tan 2005	1.14	0.00		Turkey
Demura et al. 2006	1.69	0.01		Japan
	1.25	0.00		

Odds ratio and 95% CI

0.5   1   2

More left-handed females   More left-handed males

Figure 7.1 Meta-analysis of sex differences in handedness.

Sex differences in planum temporale asymmetry

Study name	Hedges's g	p-value	Hedges's g and 95% CI
Wada et al. 1975	0.42	0.04	
DeLisi et al. 1994	−0.23	0.47	
Kulynych et al. 1994	3.13	0.00	
Preis et al. 1999	−3.04	0.00	
Watkins et al. 2001	0.56	0.00	
Foundas et al. 2002	0.19	0.44	
Knaus et al. 2004	−2.47	0.00	
Chance et al. 2006	0.89	0.07	
Eckert et al. 2006	−0.22	0.27	
Dos Santos Sequira et al. 2006	−0.48	0.02	
Takahashi et al. 2006	−0.13	0.56	
Vadlamudi et al. 2006	−0.44	0.15	
Walder et al. 2007	0.83	0.11	
	−0.11	0.68	

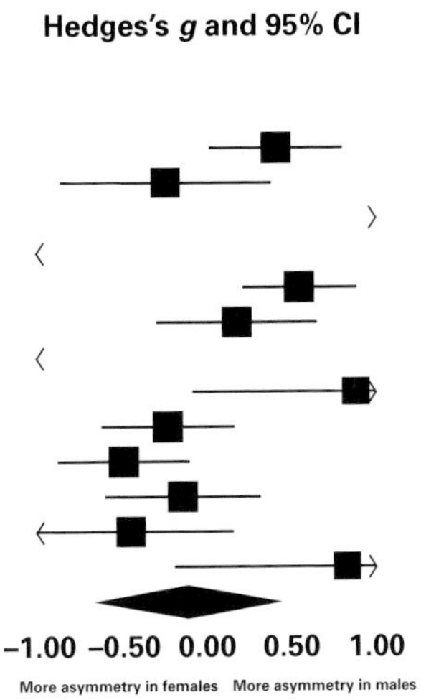

−1.00 −0.50 0.00 0.50 1.00

More asymmetry in females   More asymmetry in males

Figure 7.2 Meta-analysis of sex differences in asymmetry of the planum temporale.

males and females included 807 subjects and yielded no significant sex difference: Hedge's $g = -0.11$, $p = 0.68$. The I^2-value for heterogeneity was high: 92%. The same analysis was repeated after exclusion of the post-mortem study in an attempt to reduce heterogeneity, but the results were rather similar: Hedge's $g = -0.16$, $p = 0.6$, $I^2 = 92\%$. Separate analyses were run for studies measuring surface of the PT ($n = 5$) and those measuring volume of the PT ($n = 3$). Hedge's g for the surface measurements was -0.19, $p = 0.25$ and 0.19, $p = 0.14$ for the volume measurements. However, heterogeneity in the separate analyses remained high: 94% for the surface measurements and 81% for the volume measurements).

In order to assess the possible influence of publication bias, studies that focused on sex differences were compared to studies that reported sex differences as a by product. Five studies reported sex differences as their main topic, including a total of 184 subjects. Hedge's g of these studies was 0.35, $p = 0.64$. The I^2-value for heterogeneity increased to 93%, indicating that the studies of this sub-analysis are even more heterogeneous. Eight studies provided the sex differences in PT asymmetry

as a by product. These studies included a total of 623 subjects and Hedge's g was -0.32, $p = 0.28$. Again, studies remained highly heterogeneous ($I^2 = 91\%$). See Fig. 7.2.

Sex differences in language lateralization measured with verbal dichotic listening tests

For the meta-analysis on language lateralization measured with dichotic listening techniques, 12 studies could be included that provided mean and standard deviations of the right ear advantage (REA) for both sexes separately. All studies included adult subjects. Several studies included both right- and non-right-handed subjects. Data were available from a total of 3822 subjects. The mean weighted effect size for a sex difference in lateralization was 0.09 ($p = 0.18$), indicating no significant difference. The heterogeneity value I^2 was 35%. Several potential moderators were assessed. First, a correlation was calculated between the percentage of non-right-handed subjects per study and the effect size for sex, which was not significant (Pearson's rho $= -0.07$, $N = 12$, $p = 0.82$). This indicates that the inclusion of non-right-handed subjects

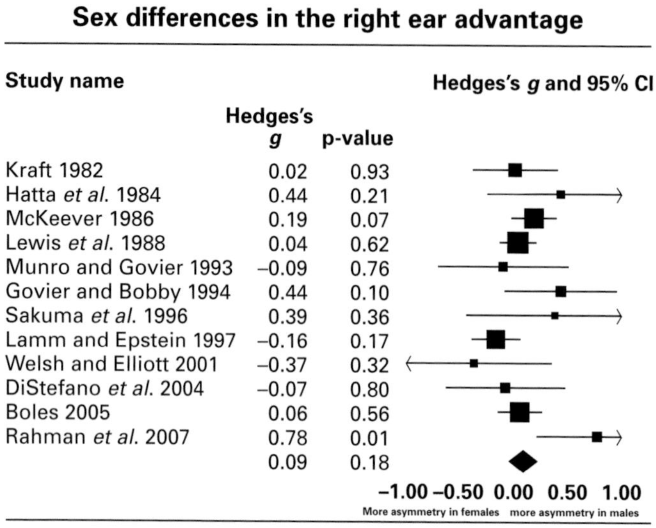

Sex differences in the right ear advantage

Study name	Hedges's g	p-value	Hedges's g and 95% CI
Kraft 1982	0.02	0.93	
Hatta *et al.* 1984	0.44	0.21	
McKeever 1986	0.19	0.07	
Lewis *et al.* 1988	0.04	0.62	
Munro and Govier 1993	−0.09	0.76	
Govier and Bobby 1994	0.44	0.10	
Sakuma *et al.* 1996	0.39	0.36	
Lamm and Epstein 1997	−0.16	0.17	
Welsh and Elliott 2001	−0.37	0.32	
DiStefano *et al.* 2004	−0.07	0.80	
Boles 2005	0.06	0.56	
Rahman *et al.* 2007	0.78	0.01	
	0.09	0.18	

−1.00 −0.50 0.00 0.50 1.00

More asymmetry in females   more asymmetry in males

Figure 7.3 Meta-analysis of sex differences in the right-ear advantage.

has no major influence on the sex difference in language lateralization measured with dichotic listening techniques. We also assessed type of paradigm as a possible moderator. Studies were divided into three categories: those using consonant–vowel(–consonant) (CV(C)) tasks, studies applying rhyme words or fused words, and studies using sets of digits or words (including triad tasks). Seven studies applied a digit or word task, including a total of 1762 subjects. The sex difference was not significant (Hedge's $g = -0.02$, $p = 0.72$) and studies were homogeneous (I^2-value = 6%). Four studies applied the CV(C) task including 506 subjects. A significant sex difference was observed favoring larger asymmetry in males (Hedge's $g = 0.30$, $p = 0.05$) but studies were more heterogeneous than in the total analysis ($I^2 = 45\%$). Only one study applied the fused word task ($n = 48$), which yielded no significant sex difference (Hedge's $g = -0.07$, $p = 0.8$). This implicates that paradigm is a moderator of the sex difference in language lateralization assessed with the dichotic listening paradigm. However, the subdivision into studies applying different paradigms largely overlaps with the division into studies that either focus on sex differences or report sex differences as a by product. None of the

studies that reported a sex difference as a by product applied the CV(C) task, while the majority of studies that focus on sex differences did apply the CV(C) task. To assess the potential influence of publication bias, studies were divided on the basis of their main topic (sex difference or otherwise). Seven studies focused on sex differences, including a total of 1076 subjects. Meta-analysis of these studies yielded a significant mean weighted effect size (Hedge's $g = 0.25$, $p = 0.01$) and heterogeneity increased ($I^2 = 39\%$). Four studies did not focus on sex differences, including 1240 subjects. Meta-analysis of these studies yielded no significant sex difference (Hedge's $g = -0.04$, $p = 0.56$), while these studies were homogeneous ($I^2 = 15\%$). It appears that the main topic of a study (focus on sex differences or not) is a confounder for paradigm, which also is a significant moderator. To assess the potential influence of publication bias, we compared the sub-analysis of the published studies applying the CV(C) task to a large database (Hugdahl, unpublished data) consisting of 1506 subjects that also performed the CV(C) task. The effect size of the sex difference in this database was 0.07 ($p = 0.17$), indicating no significant sex difference in asymmetry. See Fig. 7.3.

Sex differences in language lateralization measured with functional imaging

Twenty-six functional imaging studies could be included that provided data on language lateralization from males and females separately. A total of 2151 subjects could be included in the meta-analysis. All studies included only right-handed subjects, both children and adults. The difference in language lateralization between males and females was not significant (Hedge's $g = 0.09$, $p = 0.24$) and there was heterogeneity among studies ($I^2 = 44\%$). We assessed several potential moderators. First, we compared sex differences in lateralization between children and adults. Twenty studies assessed language lateralization in 1098 adult subjects. Meta-analysis of these studies yielded no sex difference (Hedge's $g = 0.12$, $p = 0.24$) and heterogeneity remained ($I^2 = 40\%$). Five studies assessed language lateralization in children. Again, no significant sex difference emerged (Hedge's $g = 0.01$, $p = 0.96$), but these studies were homogeneous ($I^2 = 0\%$).

To assess the possible influence of the applied language paradigm on sex differences in lateralization, separate analyses were performed for word generation tasks, such as verbal fluency and verb generation, for semantic decision tasks and for listening tasks (either to speech, stories, or single words). Twelve studies applied a word generation task and included a total of 1075 subjects. No sex difference was found in this analysis (Hedge's $g = -0.12$, $p = 0.15$) and studies were homogeneous ($I^2 = 0$). Eight studies on 510 subjects applied a semantic decision task. Again, no sex difference emerged (Hedge's $g = 0.01$, $p < 0.95$) and studies were homogeneous ($I^2 = 0$). Five studies applied a listening task and included 293 subjects in total. Analysis of these studies retrieved no sex difference (Hedge's $g = 0.24$, $p = 0.36$), but these studies were heterogeneous ($I^2 = 82\%$).

Finally, we compared studies that focused on sex differences to studies that reported sex differences as a by product. Sixteen studies including a total of 1036 subjects had a different main topic and reported sex differences as a by product. Meta-analysis of these studies yielded no sex difference (Hedge's $g = 0.06$, $p = 0.37$) and these studies were homogeneous ($I^2 = 0\%$). Ten studies did focus on sex differences and included 1115

subjects. Analysis of these studies found no sex difference (Hedge's $g = -0.02$, $p = 0.69$), but these studies remained heterogeneous ($I^2 = 76\%$). See Fig. 7.4.

Discussion

This study aimed to provide an overview of possible sex differences in relation to cerebral language lateralization. Meta-analyses were performed of studies on handedness, asymmetry of the PT, dichotic listening tests, and functional imaging paradigms.

A significant sex difference was observed for handedness, with more right-handedness in females. We observed no sex difference in PT asymmetry, language lateralization as measured with dichotic listening, or language lateralization as assessed with functional imaging. Sub-analyses of dichotic listening studies applying a CV(C) task did reveal a significant sex difference with lower degrees of language lateralization in females. This sex difference could not be replicated in a large unpublished database applying the same task and could be the result of publication bias.

Handedness

Males were found to have a 25% higher prevalence of non-right-handedness than females. Though the higher prevalence of non-right-handedness in males was a rather consistent finding, there was considerable variation in the extent of the sex difference, producing heterogeneous results. Heterogeneity may in part be caused by the variety in culture, or possibly in race, of the included subjects. The sex difference in non-Western samples was higher than in Western studies, indicating that cultural (or possibly racial) differences are a moderator of the sex difference in handedness.

Planum temporale asymmetry

Males, having a higher prevalence of non-right handedness, may be expected to have a lower degree of asymmetry of the PT as well, since non-right-handedness is associated with decreased PT asymmetry (Herve *et al.*, 2006). This expectation was not met, since no sex

Sex difference in language lateralization measured with functional imaging

Study name	Hedges's g	p-value	Total	Hedges's g and 95% CI
Binder *et al.* 1995	−0.12	0.85	5	
Shaywitz *et al.* 1995	1.19	0.00	38	
vd Kallen *et al.* 1998	0.40	0.35	20	
Xiong *et al.* 1998	0.80	0.20	9	
Pujol *et al.* 1999	0.10	0.62	100	
Springer *et al.* 1999	−0.15	0.45	100	
Gur *et al.* 2000	0.03	0.94	27	
Kansaku *et al.* 2000	0.98	0.01	30	
Knecht *et al.* 2000	0.14	0.22	326	
Phillips *et al.* 2000	1.69	0.00	20	
Vikingstad *et al.* 2000	0.01	0.98	36	
Gaillard *et al.* 2001	0.64	0.30	9	
Sommer *et al.* 2001	−0.73	0.07	24	
Hund-Geogiadis *et al.* 2002	−0.27	0.43	34	
Szaflarski *et al.* 2002	0.07	0.80	50	
Ahmad *et al.* 2003	−0.63	0.24	13	
Gaillard *et al.* 2003	0.30	0.53	16	
Weiss *et al.* 2003	0.16	0.70	20	
Schirmer *et al.* 2004	−0.65	0.10	25	
Balsamo *et al.* 2006	0.25	0.60	17	
Clements *et al.* 2006	0.15	0.67	30	
Eckert *et al.* 2006	0.00	1.00	99	
Haut and Bach 2006	−0.17	0.51	61	
Plante *et al.* 2006 I	−0.09	0.52	205	
Plante *et al.* 2006 II	−0.12	0.39	205	
Plante *et al.* 2006 III	−0.04	0.76	205	
Plante *et al.* 2006 IV	−0.22	0.12	205	
Szaflarski *et al.* 2006	0.11	0.46	178	
Kaiser *et al.* 2007	−0.14	0.62	44	
	0.01	0.73	2151	

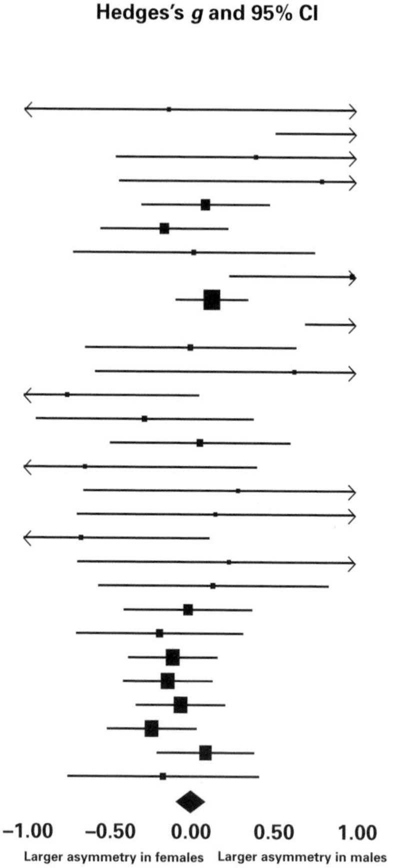

−1.00   −0.50   0.00   0.50   1.00

Larger asymmetry in females   Larger asymmetry in males

Figure 7.4 Sex differences in asymmetry of language activation.

difference emerged from the meta-analysis. It remains, however, possible that a sex difference is present in other asymmetric brain structures. Since results were heterogeneous, sub-analysis of studies were performed for studies measuring surface or volume of the PT, but heterogeneity remained high in both sub-analyses. Sub-analyses were also performed on studies that focused on sex differences and studies that had another main topic. The studies differed in the direction of their mean sex difference (more asymmetry in men in studies that focused on sex differences, and more asymmetry in women in studies with another main topic) but

significance was not reached in either analysis and heterogeneity remained high in both sub-analyses. This indicates that publication bias may be a moderator of the retrieved sex differences in PT asymmetry.

Language lateralization, dichotic listening

The meta-analysis on dichotic listening studies showed that there is no sex difference in language lateralization. Handedness of the included subjects showed no correlation with the sex difference, which implies that restricting the sample to right-handed subjects has no major impact on the sex difference in lateralization. When sub-analyses were performed on basis of the paradigm applied, a significant sex difference was retrieved by studies that used the CV(C) task, while meta-analysis of studies that applied digit or word tasks yielded no sex difference. However, studies applying a CV(C) task largely overlap with studies that had a main focus on sex differences. Sub-analyses of studies that focused on sex differences yielded a significant sex difference, while studies that focused on another topic found no sex difference. To distinguish between the influence of paradigm and that of publication bias, the effect size of the sex difference in lateralization was calculated from a large data set (Bergen Dichotic Listening Database, courtesy of Professor Hugdahl; see also Hugdahl, 2003; Hugdahl *et al.*, 2001) that also applied the CV(C) task. This database has been accomplished by merging data from several studies that all applied the same paradigm. The sample size of the database was three times larger (1506 subjects) than the sample size of our sub-analysis on published studies applying the CV(C) task (506 subjects). In the Bergen Dichotic Listening Database, no sex difference was present, indicating that publication bias is probably the most powerful moderator of the results.

Earlier reviews on sex differences in dichotic listening studies came to similar conclusions. For example, Hiscock *et al.* (1994) reviewed 114 studies that reported on sex differences in dichotic listening. Of these, 49 studies (34.8%) found at least one significant effect involving the factor sex. Most of these effects, however, involved an interaction between sex and another factor, such as age or task performance. Only 11 studies (10%) reported a main effect for sex. From these, 9 studies found higher degrees of language lateralization in males and 2 studies found higher lateralization in females. Hiscock's review did not include a quantitative analysis, since many studies did not provide enough exact data. Voyer (1996) performed a meta-analysis on perceptual half field studies in the auditory, visual, and tactile domain. He concluded that there is a modest, but significant sex difference in laterality. Voyer's results were, however, not resistant to the file drawer problem, indicating that the results may have been caused by a publication bias for studies that report a positive effect for sex.

Language lateralization, functional imaging studies

In parallel to the results of the (overall) meta-analysis on dichotic listening studies, the analysis on functional imaging studies yielded no sex difference in language lateralization. Sub-analyses of studies applying word generation tasks, semantic decision tasks, and listening tasks all produced no sex difference in language lateralization. Sub-analyses of studies on language lateralization in adults versus children also produced no sex differences. Finally, sub-analyses of studies that did or did not focus on sex difference did not produce a sex difference in either of the analyses. Thus, in contrast to dichotic listening studies, publication bias favoring studies with positive findings may not be a major factor in explaining heterogeneity among functional imaging studies. These findings are in accordance with our earlier meta-analysis on 12 functional imaging studies (Sommer *et al.*, 2004).

The absence of a sex difference in PT asymmetry and language lateralization observed in all three meta-analyses appears to be a quite consistent finding. Three hypotheses may be considered in the light of these findings. First, there may be a sex difference at the population level, but it is relatively small so that it is only sporadically observed. Were this to be true, studies with larger sample sizes would be expected to report a sex difference in lateralization more frequently than studies with smaller sample sizes, since they have more power to detect subtle differences. On inspection of our data, this appears not to be the case. Furthermore, all three meta-analyses included more than 400 males and females, which makes the chance for three false negative findings very small. Thus, the hypothesis of a true, but subtle, sex difference in cerebral asymmetry and language lateralization at the population level is not supported by our data. A second hypothesis to explain the absence of a main sex difference in language lateralization is that sex differences may be task dependent. Indeed, there was significant heterogeneity among the studies in our meta-analyses on dichotic listening and functional imaging studies, which may be congruent with this hypothesis. The results of our moderator analysis on dichotic listening studies appeared to support this idea, since a significant sex effect was retrieved only in a sub-analysis of studies using the CV(C) task. However, a much larger (unpublished) database applying the same task showed no sex difference in lateralization, which weakens the argument for a task-specific sex difference. Sub-analyses of functional imaging studies according to task did not produce a sex difference in lateralization. Thus, the argument for a task-specific sex difference is not supported by our meta-analysis.

The third hypothesis is the null-hypothesis; that there is no sex difference in cerebral asymmetry and language lateralization at the population level. If this hypothesis were to be true, the sex differences reported in the small sample studies may reflect biased reporting of chance findings, i.e., the "file drawer problem" (Rosenthal, 1991). This hypothesis is consistent with the absence of a sex difference in the large unpublished database (Hugdahl). In addition, this hypothesis offers an explanation for the different results from sub-analyses on PT asymmetry and dichotic listening studies that did or did not have sex differences in lateralization as their main topic.

Our data appear to be most consistent with a sex difference in handedness without an associated sex difference in cerebral asymmetry and language lateralization. The increased prevalence of non-right-handedness in males, in the absence of sex differences in asymmetry and lateralization is not easily explained. Several differences between men and women may account for the increased non-right-handedness in males, such as genetic, hormonal, or social influences. It could reflect sex-linked inheritance of the genetic predisposition to develop right-handedness. For example, a gene associated with handedness could be located on the X-chromosome (Corballis *et al.*, 1996). Another possibility could be different imprinting in males and females of a gene related to handedness. Indeed, an imprinted gene (*LRRTM1*, on chromosome 2p12) was recently found to be associated to handedness (Francks *et al.*, 2007). The suggestion of a genetic cause for the sex difference in handedness is supported by studies that found a higher chance for non-right-handed women to have non-right-handed offspring as compared to non-right-handed men (reviewed by Annett, 1999). However, handedness is associated to brain asymmetry and to language lateralization and the genetic basis for handedness is supposed to overlap, at least in part, with the genetics of asymmetry and lateralization (McManus, 1991; Annett, 2004). A genetic cause for increased non-right-handedness in males would therefore be expected to be paired with decreased asymmetry and language lateralization in males, which is not supported by our meta-analyses.

Higher antenatal and postnatal levels of testosterone may be another factor to cause more non-right-handedness in males. Studies in patients with abnormal levels of sex hormones appear to support this hypothesis. Schachter *et al.* (1994) investigated the prevalence of non-right-handedness in a group of women whose mothers had been administered diethylstilbestrol (DES) during their pregnancies. Diethylstilbestrol is a synthetic estrogen, administered to prevent miscarriage, which affects the fetal brain in a similar fashion as testosterone. The DES-exposed women had a higher prevalence of non-right-handedness than control women. This finding was replicated by Schreirs and Vingerhoets (1995). Another example of the influence of testosterone on handedness is provided by females with the congenital adrenal hyperplasia (CAH) syndrome, whose adrenal glands produce abnormally high levels of testosterone as a byproduct of dysfunctional cortisol synthesis. Women with CAH were found to have a higher prevalence of non-right-handedness than their sisters with normal levels of testosterone (Nass *et al.*, 1987). The increased non-right-handedness in women with CAH was replicated by Smith and Hines (2000), but not by Helleday *et al.* (1994). Though inconsistent and rather anecdotal, these studies lend some support to the idea that higher prenatal testosterone could cause an increased prevalence of non-right-handedness, which may account for the higher prevalence of non-right-handedness in males as compared to females. The same argument as we made for a genetic cause can also be made against this explanation; why should differences in testosterone cause a sex difference in handedness but not in PT asymmetry or language lateralization? There is indeed some evidence that prenatal testosterone levels do affect language lateralization as well (Grimshaw *et al.*, 1995).

Social influences may be a better candidate to explain the retrieved sex difference in handedness only. It can be hypothesized that social pressure to use the right hand for unimanual tasks, such as writing and eating, is higher for females than for males. Alternatively, females may be more apt to meet social preferences for using the right hand than males. In support of this hypothesis, Porac *et al.* (1986; Porac & Coren, 1981) found that women reported significantly more frequently than men to be forced to change handedness from left to right. Porac *et al.* (1986) suggested that this could explain the overall difference in handedness between the sexes. Interestingly, Annett (2004) noted in her large samples of handedness data that right-handed females more frequently use the left hand for one or two items of a handedness scale, while right-handed males were more frequently consistent right-handed for all items. In our meta-analysis we found that the sex difference in handedness was larger in non-Western samples, which may be indicative of more sex-specific social pressure in non-Western cultures. These findings strengthen the idea that females who are innate left- or mixed-handed more frequently switch to right-hand use for social activities such as writing and eating than left- or mixed-handed males.

Conclusion

Meta-analysis of handedness studies shows that the prevalence of left-handedness is 29% higher in males than in females. This increase in left-handedness is not paired with a decrease in cerebral asymmetry or language lateralization in males. No significant sex difference could be observed for PT asymmetry or for language lateralization as measured with either dichotic listening tests or functional imaging techniques.

Several factors may play a role in the increased prevalence of left-handedness in males. There is some support for sex-linked inheritance of a gene predisposing for left-handedness, either through an X-chromosomal locus for handedness or through sex specific imprinting. Testosterone also appears to affect handedness and possibly also language lateralization. Higher levels of antenatal testosterone may predict more left-handedness, though evidence is anecdotal. Finally, social pressure to use the right hand may be different for males than for females, which could induce a sex difference in

handedness. Or perhaps, females may be more adaptive to social norms to use the right hand. This hypothesis is supported by higher frequencies of hand switching in females than in males, and by less consistent preference to use the right hand for unimanual tasks in females as compared to males. The social pressure hypothesis is the only hypothesis that can explain the increased left-handedness in men in the absence of a sex difference in PT asymmetry and language lateralization.

ACKNOWLEDGMENT

This chapter uses extracts and figures from: Sommer, I. E. C., Aleman, A., Somers, M., Boks, M. P. M. & Kahn, R. S. (2008). Sex differences in handedness, asymmetry of the Planum Temporale and functional language lateralization. *Brain Research*, **1206**, 76–88.

REFERENCES

Afifi, M. (2007). Gender differences in mental health. *Singapore Med J*, **48**(5), 385–91.

Ahmad, Z., Balsamo, L. M., Sachs, B. C., Xu, B. & Gaillard, W. D. (2003). Auditory comprehension of language in young children: neural networks identified with fMRI. *Neurology*, **60** (10), 1598–605.

Annett, M. (1973). Handedness in families. *Ann Hum Genet*, **37**, 93–105.

Annett, M. (1999). Left-handedness as a function of sex, maternal versus paternal inheritance, and report bias. *Behav Genet*, **29**(2), 103–14.

Annett, M. (2004). Hand preference observed in large healthy samples: classification, norms and interpretations of increased non-right-handedness by the right shift theory. *Br J Psychol*, **95**(3), 339–53.

Ashton, G. C. (1982). Handedness: an alternative hypothesis. *Behav Genet*, **12**, 125–47.

Balsamo, L. M., Xu, B. & Gaillard, W. D. (2006). Language lateralization and the role of the fusiform gyrus in semantic processing in young children. *Neuroimage*, **31**(3), 1306–14.

Beckman, L. & Elston, R. (1962). Data on bilateral variation in man: handedness, hand clasping and arm folding in Swedes. *Hum Biol*, **34**, 99–103.

Binder, J. R., Rao, S. M., Hammeke, T. A. *et al.* (1995). Lateralized human brain language systems demonstrated by task subtraction functional magnetic resonance imaging. *Arch Neurol*, **52**(6), 593–601.

Boles, D. B. (1984). Sex in lateralized tachistoscopic word recognition. *Brain Lang*, **23**(2), 307–17.

Bradshaw, J. L. & Sheppard, D. M. (2000). The neurodevelopmental frontostriatal disorders: evolutionary adaptiveness and anomalous lateralization. *Brain Lang*, **73**(2), 297–320.

Bryden, M. P. (1982). *Laterality: Functional Asymmetry in the Intact Brain*. New York: Academic Press.

Chance, S. A., Casanova, M. F., Switala, A. E. & Crow, T. J. (2006). Minicolumnar structure in Heschl's gyrus and planum temporale: asymmetries in relation to sex and callosal fiber number. *Neurosci*, **143**(4), 1041–50.

Chapman, J. P., Chapman, L. J. & Allen, J. A. (1987). The measurement of foot preference. *Neuropsychologia*, **25**, 579–84.

Clark, M. M. (1957). *Left-handedness: Laterality Characteristics and their Educational Implications*. London: University of London Press.

Clements, A. M., Rimrodt, S. L., Abel, J. R. *et al.* (2006). Sex differences in cerebral laterality of language and visuospatial processing. *Brain Lang*, **98**(2), 150–8.

Corballis, M. C., Lee, K., McManus, I. C. & Crow, T. J. (1996). Location of the handedness gene on the X and Y chromosomes. *Am J Med Genet*, **67**(1), 50–2.

Coren, S. & Porac, C. (1980). Birth factors and laterality: effects of birth order, parental age, and birth stress on four indices of lateral preference. *Behav Genet*, **10**, 123.

Crovitz, H. F. & Zener, K. (1962). A group test for assessing hand and eye-dominance. *Am J Psychol*, **75**, 271–6.

Dawson, J. L. M. B. (1972). Temne Arunta hand-eye dominance and cognitive style. *Int J Psychol*, **7**, 219–33.

Davis, A. & Annett, M. (1994). Handedness as a function of twinning, age and sex. *Cortex*, **30**(1), 105–11.

Demura, S., Tada, N., Matsuzawa, J. *et al.* (2006). The influence of gender, athletic events, and athletic experience on the subjective dominant hand and the determination of the dominant hand based on the laterality quotient (LQ) and the validity of the LQ. *J Physiol Anthropol*, **25**(5), 321–9.

DeLisi, L. E., Hoff, A. L., Neale, C. & Kushner, M. (1994). Asymmetries in the superior temporal lobe in male and female first-episode schizophrenic patients: measures of the planum temporale and superior temporal gyrus by MRI. *Schizophr Res*, **12**(1), 19–28.

Dos Santos Sequeira, S., Woerner, W., Walter, C. *et al.* (2006). Handedness, dichotic-listening ear advantage, and gender effects on planum temporale asymmetry – a volumetric investigation using structural magnetic resonance imaging. *Neuropsychologia*, **44**(4), 622–36.

Dusek, C. D. & Hicks, R. A. (1980). Multiple birth risk factors and handedness in elementary school children. *Cortex*, **16**, 471–8.

Elalmiş D. D. & Tan, U. (2005). Hand preference in Turkish population. *Int J Neurosci*, **115**(5), 705–12.

Ellis, S. J., Ellis, P. J. & Marshall, E. (1988). Hand preferences in a normal population. *Cortex*, **24**, 157–63.

Eckert, M. A., Leonard, C. M., Possing, E. T. & Binder, J. R. (2006). Uncoupled leftward asymmetries for planum morphology and functional language processing. *Brain Lang*, **98**(1), 102–11.

Falek, A. (1959). Handedness: a family study. *Am J Hum Genet*, **2**, 52–62.

Fairweather, H., Brizzolara, D., Tabossi, P. & Umiltà, C. (1982). Functional cerebral lateralisation: dichotomy or plurality? *Cortex*, **18**(1), 51–65.

Foundas, A. L., Leonard, C. M. & Hanna-Pladdy, B. (2002). Variability in the anatomy of the planum temporale and posterior ascending ramus:do right- and left handers differ? *Brain Lang*, **83**(3), 403–24.

Francks, C., Maegawa, S., Lauren, J. *et al.* (2007). LRRTM1 on chromosome 2p12 is a maternally suppressed gene that is associated paternally with handedness and schizophrenia. *Mol Psychiatry*, **12**(12), 1129–39.

Gaillard, W. D., Pugliese, M., Grandin, C. B. *et al.* (2001). Cortical localization of reading in normal children: an fMRI language study. *Neurology*, **57**(1), 47–54.

Gaillard, W. D., Balsamo, L. M., Ibrahim, Z., Sachs, B. C. & Xu, B. (2003). fMRI identifies regional specialization of neural networks for reading in young children. *Neurology*, **60**(1), 94–100.

Grimshaw, G. M., Sitarenios, G. & Finegan, J. A. (1995). Mental rotation at 7 years: relations with prenatal testosterone levels and spatial play experiences. *Brain Cogn*, **29**(1), 85–100.

Gur, R. E. & Gur, R. C. (1977). Sex differences in the relations among handedness, sighting-dominance and eye-acuity. *Neuropsychologia*, **15**, 585–90.

Gur, R. C., Alsop, D., Glahn, D. *et al.* (2000). An fMRI study of sex differences in regional activation to a verbal and a spatial task. *Brain Lang*, **74**(2), 157–70.

Hardyck, C., Petrinovich, L. F. & Goldman, R. D. (1976). Left-handedness and cognitive deficit. *Cortex*, **12**, 266–79.

Harris, L. J. (1980). Lateralised sex differences: substrate and significance. *Behav Brain Sci*, **3**, 236–7.

Hatta, T. & Nakatsuka, Z. (1976). Note on hand preference of Japanese people. *Percept Mot Skills*, **42**(2), 530.

Hatta, T., Ayetani, N. & Yoshizaki, K. (1984). Dichotic listening by chronic schizophrenic patients. *Int J Neurosci*, **23**(1), 75–80.

Haut, K. M. & Barch, D. M. (2006). Sex influences on material-sensitive functional lateralization in working and episodic memory: men and women are not all that different. *Neuroimage*, **32**(1), 411–22.

Hedges, L. V. & Olkin, I. (1985). *Statistical Methods for Meta-analysis*. Orlando, Florida: Academic Press.

Heim, A. W. & Watts, K. P. (1976). Handedness and cognitive bias. *Q J Exp Psychol*, **28**, 355–60.

Helleday, J., Siwers, B., Ritzen, E. M. & Hugdahl, K. (1994). Normal lateralization for handedness and ear advantage in a verbal dichotic listening task in women with congenital adrenal hyperplasia (CAH). *Neuropsychologia*, **32**(7), 875–80.

Herve, P. Y., Crivello, F., Perchey, G., Mazoyer, B. & Tzourio-Mazoyer, N. (2006). Handedness and cerebral anatomical asymmetries in young adult males. *Neuroimage*, **29**(4), 1066–79.

Higgins, J. P., Thompson, S. G., Deeks, J. J. & Altman, D. G. (2003). Measuring inconsistency in meta-analyses. *B M J*, **327**(7414), 557–60.

Hiscock, M., Inch, R., Jacek, C., Hiscock-Kalil, C. & Kalil, K. M. (1994). Is there a sex difference in human laterality? I. An exhaustive survey of auditory laterality studies from six neuropsychology journals. *J Clin Exp Neuropsychol*, **16**(3), 423–35. Review.

Hiscock, M. & Mackay, M. (1985). The sex difference in dichotic listening: multiple negative findings. *Neuropsychologia*, **23**(3), 441–4.

Holland, S. K., Plante, E., Weber Byars, A. *et al.* (2001). Normal fMRI brain activation patterns in children performing a verb generation task. *Neuroimage*, **14**(4), 837–43.

Hugdahl, K. (2003). Dichotic listening in the study of auditory laterality. In K. Hugdahl & R. J. Davidson (eds.) *The Asymmetrical Brain*. Cambridge, MA: MIT Press, pp. 441–76.

Hugdahl, K., Carlsson, G. & Eichele, T. (2001). Age effects in dichotic listening to consonant–vowel syllables: interactions with attention. *Dev Neuropsychol*, **20**, 449–57.

Hund-Georgiadis, M., Lex, U., Friederici, A. D. & von Cramon, D. Y. (2002). Non-invasive regime for language lateralization in right- and left-handers by means of functional MRI and dichotic listening. *Exp Brain Res*, **145**(2), 166–76.

Jones, B. & Bell, J. (1980). Handedness in engineering and psychology students. *Cortex*, **16**, 521–5.

Kaiser, A., Kuenzli, E., Zappatore, D. & Nitsch, C. (2007). On females' lateral and males' bilateral activation during language production: a fMRI study. *Int J Psychophysiol*, **63**(2), 192–8.

Kansaku, K., Yamaura, A. & Kitazawa, S. (2000). Sex differences in lateralization revealed in the posterior language areas. *Cereb Cortex*, **10**(9), 866–72.

Knaus, T. A., Bollich, A. M., Corey, D. M., Lemen, L. C., Foundas, A. L. (2004). Sex-linked differences in the anatomy of the perisylvian language cortex: a volumetric MRI study of gray matter volumes. *Neuropsychology*, **18**(4), 738–47.

Knecht, S., Drager, B., Deppe, M. *et al.* (2000). Handedness and hemispheric language dominance in healthy humans. *Brain*, **123**(12), 2512–18.

Komai, T. & Fukuoka, G. (1934). A study on the frequency of left-handedness and left-footedness among Japanese school children. *Hum Biol*, **6**, 33–41.

Kraft, R. H. (1982). Relationship of ear specialization to degree of task difficulty, sex, and lateral preference. *Percept Mot Skills*, **54**(3), 703–14.

Kulynych, J. J., Vladar, K., Jones, D. W. & Weinberger, D. R. (1994). Gender differences in the normal lateralization of the supra-temporal cortex: MRI surface rendering morphometry of Heschl's gyrus and the planum temporale. *Cereb Cortex*, **4**, 107–18.

Lamm, O. & Epstein, R. (1997). Dichotic listening in children: the reflection of verbal and attentional changes with age. *J Exp Child Psychol*, **65**(1), 25–42.

Lansky, L. M., Feinstein, H. & Peterson, J. M. (1988). Demography of handedness in two samples of randomly selected adults (N = 2083). *Neuropsychologia*, **26**, 465–77.

Leiber, L. & Axelrod, S. (1981). Intra-familial learning is only a minor factor in manifest handedness. *Neuropsychologia*, **19**, 273–88.

Levander, M. & Schalling, D. (1988). Hand preference in a population of Swedish college students. *Cortex*, **24**, 149–56.

Lewis, R. S., Orsini, D. L. & Satz, P. (1988). Individual differences in the cerebral organization of language using input and output interference measures of lateralization. *Arch Clin Neuropsychol*, **3**(2), 111–19.

Liederman, J., Kantrowitz, L. & Flannery, K. (2005). Male vulnerability to reading disability is not likely to be a myth: a call for new data. *J Learn Disabil*, **38**(2), 109–29.

Lipsey, M. W. & Wilson, D. B. (2001). The way in which intervention studies have "personality" and why it is important to meta-analysis. *Eval Health Prof*, **24**, 236–54.

Mathiowetz, V., Wiemer, D. M. & Federman, S. M. (1986). Grip and pinch strength: norms for 6- to 19-year-olds. *Am J Occup Ther*, **40**(10), 705–11.

Maccoby, E. E. & Konrad, K. W. (1966). Age trends in selective listening. *J Exp Child Psychol*, **3**(2), 113–22.

McFarland, K. & Anderson, J. (1980). Factor stability of the Edinburgh Handedness Inventory as a function of the test-retest performance, age and sex. *Br J Psychol*, **71**, 135–42.

McGlone, J. (1980). Sex differences in the human brain: a critical survey. *Behav Brain Sci*, **3**, 215–63.

McManus, I. C. (1991). The inheritance of left-handedness. *Ciba Found Symp*, **162**, 251–67.

McKeever, W. F. (1986). The influences of handedness, sex, familial sinistrality and androgyny on language laterality, verbal ability, and spatial ability. *Cortex*, **22**(4), 521–37.

Medland, S. E., Perelle, I., De Monte, V. & Ehrman, L. (2004). Effects of culture, sex, and age on the distribution of handedness: an evaluation of the sensitivity of three measures of handedness. *Laterality*, **9**(3), 287–97.

Michel, G. F. & Harkins, D. A. (1986). Postural and lateral asymmetries in the ontogeny of handedness during infancy. *Dev Psychobiol*, **19**(3), 247–58.

Munro, P. & Govier, E. (1993). Dynamic gender-related differences in dichotic listening performance. *Neuropsychologia*, **31**(4), 347–53.

Nachson, I., Denno, D. & Aurand, S. (1983). Lateral preferences of hand, eye and foot: relation to cerebral dominance. *Int J Neurosci*, **18**, 1–10.

Nass, R., Baker, S., Speiser, P. *et al.* (1987). Hormones and handedness: left-hand bias in female congenital adrenal hyperplasia patients. *Neurology*, **37**(4), 711–15.

Oldfield, R. C. (1971). The assessment and analysis of handedness: the Edinburgh inventory. *Neuropsychologia*, **9**(1), 97–113.

Pedersen, P. M., Jorgensen, H. S., Nakayama, H., Raaschou, H. O. & Olsen, T. S. (1995). Aphasia in acute stroke: incidence, determinants, and recovery. *Ann Neurol*, **38**(4), 659–66.

Pelecanos, M. (1969). Some Greek data on handedness, hand clasping and arm folding. *Hum Biol*, **41**, 275–8.

Peters, M. (1986). Incidence of left-handed writers and the inverted writing position in a sample of 2194 German elementary school children. *Neuropsychologia*, **24**, 429–33.

Phillips, M. D., Lowe, M. J., Lurito, J. T., Dzemidzic, M. & Mathews, V. P. (2001). Temporal lobe activation demonstrates sex-based differences during passive listening. *Radiology*, **220**, 202–7.

Plante, E., Schmithorst, V. J., Holland, S. K. & Byars, A. W. (2006). Sex differences in the activation of language cortex during childhood. *Neuropsychologia*, **44**(7), 1210–21.

Porac, C. & Coren, S. (1981). *Lateral Preferences and Hum Behaviour*. New York: Springer Verlag.

Porac, C., Coren, S. & Searleman, A. (1986). Environmental factors in hand preference formation: evidence from attempts to switch the preferred hand. *Behav Genet*, **16**(2), 251–61.

Porac, C. & Buller, T. (1990). Overt attempts to change hand preference: a study of group and individual characteristics. *Can J Psychol*, **44**(4), 512–21.

Preis, S., Jancke, L., Schmitz-Hillebrecht, J. & Steinmetz, H. (1999). Child age and planum temporale asymmetry. *Brain Cogn*, **40**(3), 441–52.

Pujol, J., Deus, J., Losilla, J. M. & Capdevila, A. (1999). Cerebral lateralization of language in normal left-handed people studied by functional MRI. *Neurology*, **52**(5), 1038–43.

Rosenthal, R. (1991). *Meta-analytic Procedures for Social Research*. London: Sage Publications.

Sakuma, M., Hoff, A. L. & DeLisi, L. E. (1996). Functional asymmetries in schizophrenia and their relationship to cognitive performance. *Psychiatry Res*, **65**(1), 1–13.

Schachter, S. C. (1994). Handedness in women with intrauterine exposure to diethyl stilbestrol. *Neuropsychologia*, **32**(5), 619–23.

Scheirs, J. G. & Vingerhoets, A. J. (1995). Handedness and other laterality indices in women prenatally exposed to DES. *J Clin Exp Neuropsychol*, **17**(5), 725–30.

Schirmer, A., Zysset, S., Kotz, S. A. & Yves von Cramon, D. (2004). Gender differences in the activation of inferior frontal cortex during emotional speech perception. *Neuroimage*, **21**(3), 1114–23.

Searleman, A., Tweedy, J. & Springer, S. (1979). Interrelationships among subject variables believed to predict cerebral organisation. *Brain Lang*, **7**, 267–76.

Shaywitz, B. A., Shaywitz, S. E., Pugh, K. R. *et al.* (1995). Sex differences in the functional organization of the brain for language. *Nature*, **373**(6515), 607–9.

Shimizu, A. & Endo, M. (1983). Handedness and familial sinistrality in a Japanese student population. *Cortex*, **19**, 265–72.

Sicotte, N. L., Woods, R. P. & Mazziotta, J. C. (1999). Handedness in twins: a meta-analysis. *Laterality*, **4**, 265–86.

Silverberg, R., Obler, L. K. & Gordon, H. W. (1979). Handedness in Israel. *Neuropsychologia*, **17**, 83–87.

Singh, M. (1990). Lateralized interference in concurrent manual activity: influence of age in children. *Int J Neurosci*, **50**(1–2), 55–8.

Singh, M. & Bryden, M. P. (1994). "The factor structure of handedness in India", *Int J Neurosci*, **74**, 33–43.

Singh, M., Manjary, M. & Dellatolas, G. (2001). Lateral preferences among indian school children. *Cortex*, **37**(2), 231–41.

Smith, L. L. & Hines, M. (2000). Language lateralization and handedness in women prenatally exposed to diethylstilbestrol (DES). *Psychoneuroendocrinology*, **25**(5), 497–512.

Sommer, I. E., Aleman, A., Bouma, A. & Kahn, R. S. (2004). Do women really have more bilateral language representation than men? A meta-analysis of functional imaging studies. *Brain*, **127**(8), 1845–52.

Sommer, I. E. C., Ramsey, N. F., Mandl, R. C. W. & Kahn, R. S. (2003). Language lateralization in women with schizophrenia. *Schizophr Res*, **60**(2–3), 183–90.

Springer, J. A., Binder, J. R., Hammeke, T. A. *et al.* (1999). Language dominance in neurologically normal and epilepsy subjects: a functional MRI study. *Brain*, **122**(11), 2033–46.

Szaflarski, J. P., Binder, J. R., Possing, E. T. *et al.* (2002). Language lateralization in left-handed and ambidextrous people: fMRI data. *Neurology*, **59**(2), 238–44.

Szaflarski, J. P., Holland, S. K., Schmithorst, V. J. & Byars, A. W. (2006). fMRI study of language lateralization in children and adults. *Hum Brain Mapp*, **27**(3), 202–12.

Takahashi, T., Suzuki, M., Zhou, S. Y. *et al.* (2006). Temporal lobe gray matter in schizophrenia spectrum: a volumetric MRI study of the fusiform gyrus, parahippocampal gyrus, and middle and inferior temporal gyri. *Schizophr Res.*, **87**(1–3), 116–26.

Teng, E. L., Lee, P. & Chang, P. C. (1976). Handedness in a Chinese population: biological, social and pathological factors. *Science*, **193**, 1148–50.

Vadlamudi, L., Hatton, R., Byth, K. *et al.* (2006). Volumetric analysis of a specific language region – the planum temporale. *J Clin Neurosci*, **13**(2), 206–13.

van der Kallen, B. F., Morris, G. L., Yetkin, F. Z. *et al.* (1998). Hemispheric language dominance studied with functional MR: preliminary study in healthy volunteers and patients with epilepsy. *AJNR Am J Neuroradiol*, **19**(1), 73–7.

Vikingstad, E. M., George, K. P., Johnson, A. F. & Cao, Y. (2000). Cortical language lateralization in right handed normal subjects using functional magnetic resonance imaging. *J Neurol Sci*, **175**: 17–27.

Voyer, D. (1996). On the magnitude of laterality effects and sex differences in functional lateralities. *Laterality*, **1**(1), 51–83.

Wada, J., Clarke, R. & Hamm, A. (1975). Cerebral asymmetry in humans. Cortical speech zones in 100 adult and 100 infant brains. *Arch Neurol*, **32**, 239–46.

Walder, D. J., Seidman, L. J., Makris, N. *et al.* (2007). Neuroanatomic substrates of sex differences in language dysfunction in schizophrenia: a pilot study. *Schizophr Res*, **90**(1–3), 295–301.

Watkins, K. E., Paus, T., Lerch, J. P. *et al.* (2001). Structural asymmetries in the human brain: a voxel-based statistical analysis of 142 MRI scans. *Cereb Cortex*, **11**(9), 868–77.

Weiss, E. M., Siedentopf, C., Hofer, A. *et al.* (2003). Brain activation pattern during a verbal fluency test in healthy male and female volunteers: a functional magnetic resonance imaging study. *Neurosci Lett*, **352**(3), 191–4.

Xiong, J., Rao, S., Gao, J. H., Woldorff, M. & Fox, P. T. (1998). Evaluation of hemispheric dominance for language using functional MRI: a comparison with positron emission tomography. *Hum Brain Mapp*, **6**(1), 42–58.

Yim, S. Y., Cho, J. R. & Lee, I. Y. (2003). Normative data and developmental characteristics of hand function for elementary school children in Suwon area of Korea: grip, pinch and dexterity study. *J Korean Med Sci*, **18**(4), 552–8.

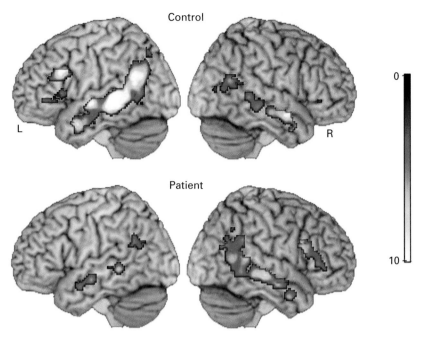

Figure 9.1 Hemispheric surface rendering of an activated LANG region of interest (ROI) is illustrated for a control (top), showing leftward asymmetry superimposed on the individual anatomic MRIs after stereotactic normalization. Hemispheric surface rendering of an activated LANG region of interest is illustrated for a schizophrenia patient (bottom), showing rightward asymmetry superimposed on the individual anatomic MRIs after stereotactic normalization. The LANG ROI corresponds to three merged regions, namely the pars triangularis of the inferior frontal gyrus, the middle temporal gyrus, and the angular gyrus.

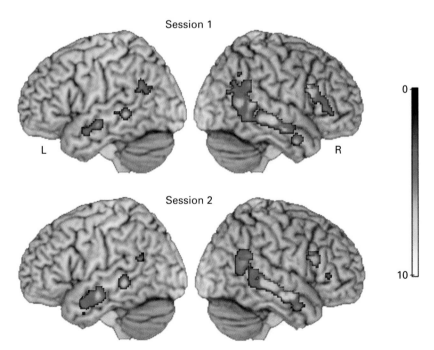

Figure 9.2 Hemispheric surface rendering of an activated LANG region of interest is illustrated for one schizophrenia patient at two test sessions (session 1 was baseline, and session 2 was 21 months after the first session); this shows a rightward asymmetry superimposed on the individual anatomic MRIs after stereotactic normalization.

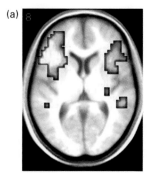

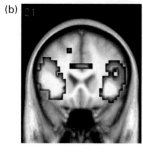

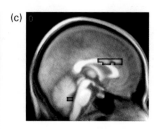

Figure 11.1 a, b, and c SPM(T)s for the group hallucination analysis.

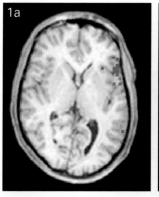

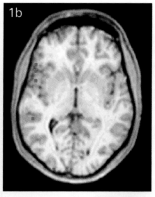

Figure 11.2 a, b, and c SPM(T)s for the group language analysis.

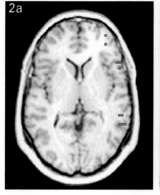

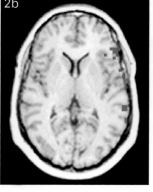

Figure 6.1 Examples of language activation patterns of a monozygotic pair consisting of (a) a left-hander and (b) a right-hander with opposite language lateralization.

Figure 6.2 Another monozygotic twin pair of unequal handedness, but with almost identical language lateralization to those shown in Fig. 6.1.

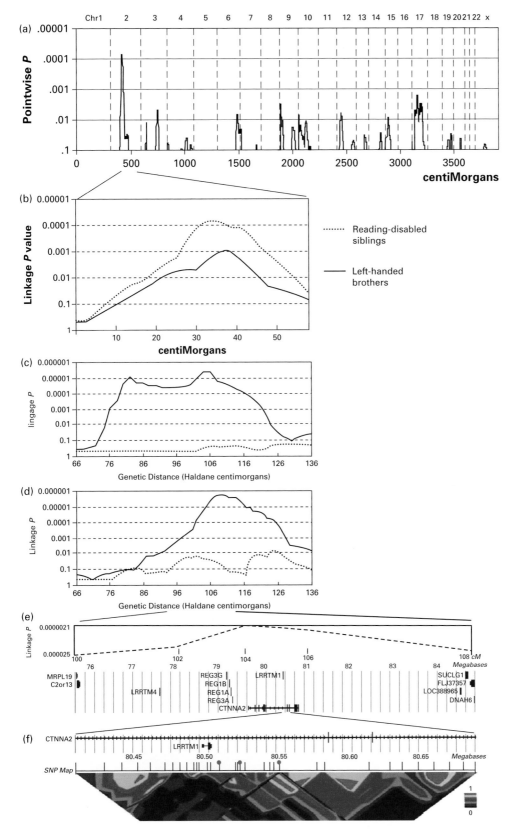

Figure 13.1 The full caption is available on page 185.

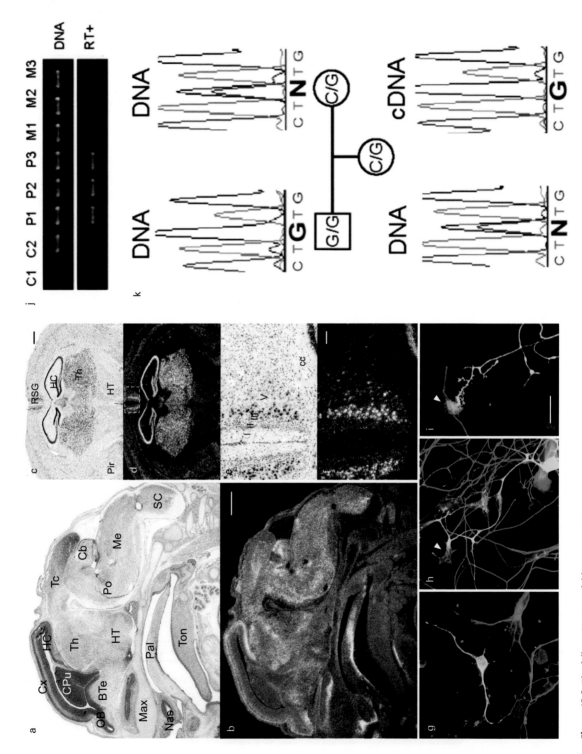

Figure 13.2 The full caption is available on page 189.

SECTION 2

Language lateralization and psychosis

8

Hand-preference and population schizotypy: A meta-analysis

Metten Somers, Iris E. C. Sommer, and René S. Kahn

Summary

Language functions in schizophrenia patients are represented more bilaterally (i.e., less lateralized) than in healthy subjects. This decreased lateralization is also observed in individuals at increased risk for schizophrenia. Language lateralization is related to handedness; in that left- and mixed-handed individuals more frequently have decreased lateralization in comparison to right-handed subjects. In line with this, population schizotypy has repeatedly, though inconsistently, been associated with left-handedness. In order to define the exact association between handedness and schizotypy, we performed meta-analyses on the available literature. We found that non-right-handed subjects, but not strong left-handers, had higher scores on schizotypy questionnaires than right-handed subjects. Mixed-handers showed a trend towards higher schizotypy in comparison to strong left-handers. It is argued that the higher schizotypy in non-right-handed individuals reflects the higher incidence of bilateral language lateralization in this group. Bilateral brain organization may underlie loosening of association, possibly leading to higher schizotypy scores. It is hypothesized that increased right-hemisphere involvement contributes to unconventional, divergent thought, of which schizotypy can be considered an extreme example.

Introduction

Non-right-handedness has been associated with schizophrenia at least since the 1950s (Straaten, 1955). Indeed, meta-analysis shows that the frequency of non-right-handedness is almost twice as high in schizophrenia patients in comparison to healthy subjects (Sommer *et al.*, 2001a). Handedness is related to cerebral lateralization, though this association is rather weak; approximately 95% of right-handed subjects have left-cerebral dominance for language function (Szaflarski *et al.*, 2006) and 5% have bilateral or right cerebral dominance. In non-right-handed subjects 70% have left cerebral dominance and 30% show a right dominant or bilateral pattern of language dominance (Pujol *et al.*, 1999). Given the ease with which handedness can be assessed, and the weak but consistent association between handedness and cerebral lateralization, hand preference seems a useful indirect reflection of cerebral dominance in larger groups. The increased frequency of non-right-handedness in schizophrenia patients has been attributed to a higher incidence of bilateral language lateralization as compared to healthy subjects. Functional imaging studies showed that this was indeed the case (Sommer *et al.*, 2001b; Li *et al.*, 2007a; Sommer *et al.*, 2004; 2003). The lower degree of language lateralization is caused by increased language activity in frontal and temporal areas of the right hemisphere (Sommer *et al.*, 2001b; 2003). Increased language activity of the right hemisphere was also present in unaffected monozygotic co-twins of schizophrenia patients (Sommer *et al.*, 2004; Spaniel *et al.*, 2007), indicating that decreased language lateralization is a genetic predisposition for schizophrenia. As such, decreased language lateralization and possibly non-right-handedness may be useful endophenotypes for psychosis. The association between decreased cerebral dominance and psychosis is not restricted to schizophrenia, but has also been shown in patients with unipolar and bipolar affective psychosis (Sommer *et al.*, 2007) and subjects at high genetic risk for psychosis (Li *et al.*, 2007b). It is hypothesized that more bilateral language representation facilitates magical and delusional ideas by means of the more diffuse semantic activation in the right hemisphere as compared to the left. These more diffuse semantic activations may also be involved in creative thinking and as such may constitute a selective evolutionary advantage (Leonhard & Brugger, 1998). Population schizotypy (i.e., non-clinical subjects with a schizotypal tendency) can be considered to be part of the schizophrenia spectrum. It can consequently be hypothesized that such subjects will also have decreased language lateralization. Whether schizotypal thinking is indeed associated with decreased language lateralization is yet elusive since no functional imaging on language lateralization has been performed in these subjects, though some support is provided by dichotic listening studies (Broks *et al.*, 1984; Rawlings & Borge, 1987; Poreh *et al.*, 1994). Hand preference in population schizotypy, however, has been investigated extensively in large samples. Several studies have assessed possible associations between mixed-, left-, and non-right-handedness and higher scores on the Schizotypal Personality Questionnaire (SPQ) (Raine, 1991; Kim *et al.*, 1992; Preti *et al.*, 2007) as well as on the Oxford–Liverpool Inventory of Feelings and Experiences (O-life) and Rust Inventory of Schizotypy Cognition (RISC) scales (Annett & Moran, 2006). Evidence is heterogeneous and at times contradictory (Dragovic *et al.*, 2005), which precludes any definite conclusions on handedness in population schizotypy. In order to elucidate the evidence for a possible association between hand preference and schizotypal tendency, we performed meta-analyses on the present literature. Primarily, we aimed to investigate whether schizotypy is elevated in non-right-handers in comparison to right-handers. Secondarily, we investigated whether there is a difference between mixed handedness (ambidexterity) in comparison to both strong right- and left- handedness.

Methods

Search criteria

Searches were performed in PubMed and Embase databases up to December 2007. In addition, reference

lists from journal articles were searched for cross-references. Combinations of the following search terms were used: "(left-)handedness", "hand preference", "magical ideation", "schizotyp(y)(al)", and "psychosis proneness". Further, we combined "schizotypal personality disorder" and "functional laterality" as MESH terms. Only journals in English were searched.

Inclusion criteria

Papers were included for meta-analysis if they met the following criteria.

(1) Subjects should be at least 11 years old, since the use of schizotypy scales has not been validated before that age (Cyhlarova & Claridge, 2005). Hand preference can reliably be investigated from that age (Bryden *et al.*, 2000). Studies of subjects with a mean age above 65 were excluded, since the effect of aging itself might blur results.

(2) Hand preference should be measured either by self-report, observation, or by a validated hand preference questionnaire such as the Edinburgh Handedness Inventory (EHI) (Oldfield, 1971) or the Annett Hand Preference Questionnaire (AHPQ) (Annett, 1970).

(3) The usage of a schizotypy scale with either the presence of (or possibility to reconstruct) mean test scores and standard deviation per hand-preference group *or* available exact F-, t-, or p- values.

(4) Investigated individuals were not selected on the basis of a special condition possibly related to language lateralization or handedness (such as dyslexia, schizophrenia, or epilepsy). Control subjects for studies investigating such subjects were allowed.

Combination of measurement methods

Handedness

As explained earlier handedness is a useful implicit measure of cerebral lateralization. However, hand preference can be dichotomously dissected in right-handedness (RH) and non-right-handedness (NRH), with non-right-handedness including left- (LH), mixed- (Mix) and even weak right-handers (McManus, 1985), or hand preference can be considered a trichotomous model comprising right-, mixed- and left-handedness (Peters, 1998). In addition, more sub-classifications are used, for example see Annett's 7 or 8-group model (Annett, 2004). In our meta-analysis we investigated associations between schizotypy and handedness using both a dichotomous and trichotomous model of handedness.

A RH/NRH dichotomy

For the analysis of right- vs. non-right-handedness we required studies to either split up subjects in an RH/NRH group, or show data that allowed for the formation of such a division. For the latter procedure we applied the following rules: when studies used a trichotomous model of hand preference left- and mixed-handed subjects were pooled into one NRH group. This required the author to explicitly define hand-preference boundaries. When an author did not explicitly define boundaries and used the AHPQ, Annett's criteria for subdivision of hand-preference were applied (1 = RH, 2–7 = Mix, 8 = LH). After pooling NRH and LH subjects, a combined test score mean, weighted for group size, was calculated.

A RH/Mix/LH trichotomy

For the analysis of the trichotomous model of hand preference we used LH, Mix and RH groups as defined by the authors of a study. If a study further sub-classified hand-preference groups, subjects were again pooled now to yield the three groups. If pooling was necessary, a combined test score mean, weighted for group size, was calculated. Apart from the analysis of LH and RH vs. Mix, we also compared LH and RH.

Schizotypy scales

For the current meta-analysis, studies were selected that primarily or secondarily investigated the association of hand preference and schizotypal traits in the population. To be considered for inclusion, schizotypal cognition had to be measured by validated tests of schizotypy for non-clinical subjects, such as the

Perceptual Abberation Scale (PAS) (Chapman *et al.*, 1978), the Magical Ideation Scale (MIS) (Eckblad & Chapman, 1983), the Schizotypy Questionnaire (STA) (Claridge & Broks, 1984), the Rust Inventory of Schizotypal Cognition (RISC) (Rust, 1988), the Peters *et al.* Delusion Inventory (PDI) (Peters *et al.*, 1999), the Schizotypal Personality Questionnaire (SPQ) (Raine, 1991) and the Oxford–Liverpool Inventory of Feelings and Experiences (O-Life) (Mason *et al.*, 1995). Most instruments are inventories of positive signs of schizotypy such as disorganization, magical ideation, paranoia and perceptual abberations. In addition, the SPQ and O-life also measure negative schizotypy items, such as social anxiety and flat affect. The O-life test consists of four scales measuring unusual experiences (UnEx) and cognitive disorganization (CogDis) as well as introvertive anhedonia (IntAn) and impulsive nonconformity (ImpCon), but these questionnaires are not designed to sum up scales to produce a single measure (Mason & Claridge, 2006). The SPQ measures all nine traits of schizotypal personality disorder as described in DSM-IIIR (Spitzer *et al.*, 1987) and can be dissected in a three-factor model consisting of cognitive/perceptual, interpersonal, and disorganized features (Raine *et al.*, 1994), although some studies also use a two-factor model. A total SPQ score can also be calculated. For our meta-analyses of the association between schizotypy and non-right-handedness vs. right-handedness as well as mixed-handedness vs. left- and right-handedness we used scores from scales of positive schizotypy. When subscores of positive schizotypy could not be obtained, we also allowed total SPQ scores of the two SPQ factors "cognitive/perceptual" and "disorganization". In addition, we also aimed to perform a meta-analysis of the association of SPQ subscales with non-right-and mixed-handedness to investigate whether a specific association between schizotypy factors and hand preference exists.

Meta-analytic techniques

Schizotypy and right-handedness vs. non-right-handedness

For the analysis of schizotypy and right- vs. non-right-handedness we used the program Comprehensive Meta-analysis (www.meta-analysis.com). Primarily, the magnitude and direction of effect for schizotypal cognition and hand preference was calculated for each individual study. When means and standard deviations were not available, effect sizes were computed from exact p-values, t-values, or F-values (cf. Lipsey & Wilson, 2001). Effect sizes for schizotypy scores in right-handers vs. non-right-handers of all studies were combined and weighted for sample size to obtain a mean weighted effect size ("Hedges's g") (Hedges & Olkin, 1985) and p-values using the random effects module of Comprehensive Meta-analysis software. Further, the homogeneity statistic (I^2) was calculated (Higgins *et al.*, 2003) to assess heterogeneity of results across studies. The homogeneity statistic, I^2, quantifies the effect of heterogeneity, providing a measure of the degree of inconsistency in the studies' results (Higgins *et al.*, 2003). Because negative values of I^2 are put equal to zero, I^2 varies between 0% and 100%; I^2 describes the percentage of total variation across studies due to heterogeneity rather than chance. A value of 0% indicates no observed heterogeneity. Larger values show increasing heterogeneity: 25% can be considered low, 50% moderate, and 75% high heterogeneity (Higgins *et al.*, 2003).

Schizotypy and mixed-handedness vs. left- and right-handedness

For the meta-analysis of schizotypy and Mix vs. RH and LH the program Comprehensive Meta-analysis was again used for statistical analysis. The direction of effect for schizotypal cognition in Mix vs. RH and Mix vs. LH was calculated as above, after which effect sizes for schizotypy scores of all studies were combined and weighted for sample size of the studies to obtain a mean weighted effect size ("Hedges's g") (Hedges & Olkin, 1985) and p-values using random effects. Further, as described earlier the homogeneity statistic (I^2) was calculated for both comparisons (Higgins *et al.*, 2003) to assess the heterogeneity of results across studies.

Schizotypal Personality Questionnaire (SPQ) factors and RH vs. NRH

For studies showing separate SPQ factor scores the direction of effect for the cognitive/perceptual,

interpersonal, and disorganization factors was calculated separately for RH vs. NRH using Comprehensive Meta-analysis software. Hereafter, effect sizes for each factor were combined and weighted for sample size of the studies to obtain a mean weighted effect size ("Hedges's g") (Hedges & Olkin, 1985) and p-values using random effects. The homogeneity statistic (I^2) was calculated for both comparisons (Higgins *et al.*, 2003) to assess heterogeneity of results across studies.

Results

Inclusion

Eighty-six journal articles were identified and screened of which twelve met all criteria for inclusion. Three studies applied the MIS (Nalcaci *et al.*, 2000; Barnett & Corballis, 2002). Of these, one study (showing a p-value and direction of effect) could only be used in the analysis of extreme hand preference (Nicholls *et al.*, 2005). One study used the PDI (Preti *et al.*, 2007) and two the STA (Claridge *et al.*, 1998; Gregory *et al.*, 2003). One study investigated two samples of subjects that were included for meta-analysis separately (Annett & Moran, 2006). In the first sample the STA as well as the UnEx scale from the O-life was used, but detailed data was only shown for the STA. For the second sample the RISC was used. The other study that used the O-life also showed data only for the Unusual Experiences (UnEx) subscale of positive schizotypy (Shaw *et al.*, 2001). One study used the SPQ as well as the PAS on a sample of adolescents and a sample of adults (Chen & Su, 2006), but only SPQ results were used for meta-analysis. The remaining studies used the SPQ only (Stefanis *et al.*, 2006; Dragovic *et al.*, 2005). Of these, one study investigated comparable subgroups, which allowed for averaging of data (Dragovic *et al.*, 2005). From one study that used a two-factor SPQ model the F-value for cognitive-perceptual dysfunction in the analysis of RH vs. Mix could be used (Kim *et al.*, 1992). Thus, the results from all but three studies that showed SPQ total scores, were scores of positive schizotypy. Since two studies described two different samples (Annett & Moran, 2006; Chen & Su, 2006), a total of fourteen samples

Schizotypy (RH vs. NRH) with outlier

Study name	Hedges's g	p-value	RH	NRH	Hedges's g and 95% CI
Claridge et al. 1998	0.25	0.001	399	282	
Nalcaci et al. 2000	−0.34	0.091	42	56	
Shaw et al. 2001	0.09	0.011	2096	1314	
Barnett et al. 2002	2.18	0.000	217	33	
Gregory et al. 2003	0.04	0.682	236	173	
Dragovic et al. 2005	−0.06	0.536	355	129	
Annett et al. 2006 1	0.16	0.029	430	303	
Annett et al. 2006 2	0.14	0.352	116	66	
Stefanis et al. 2006	0.22	0.011	974	155	
Chen et al. 2006 1	−0.16	0.130	191	151	
Chen et al. 2006 2	0.30	0.000	585	435	
Preti et al. 2007	0.20	0.095	527	77	
	0.22	0.010	6168	3174	

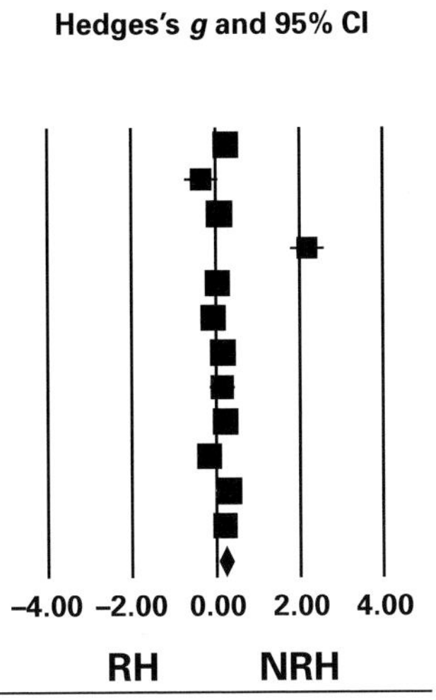

−4.00 −2.00 0.00 2.00 4.00

RH   NRH

Figure 8.1 The association between schizotypy and right handedness vs. non-right-handedness showing a significant effect for non-right-handedness with Hedges's $g = 0.22$ and $p = 0.01$, implicating higher total schizotypy scores in the non-right-handers as compared to the right-handers.

from twelve studies could be included for meta-analysis with a total of 10 058 subjects. Ten studies comprising twelve samples allowed a dichotomous division in RH and NRH, yielding 6168 right-handed and 3174 non-right-handed subjects. Using a trichotomous division yielded 5379 right-handed, 2153 mixed-handed, and 379 left-handed subjects. Nine studies (ten samples) allowed for the comparison of RH and Mix. Eight studies with a total of nine samples allowed for the comparison of LH (379 subjects) and Mix (2133 subjects). Nine studies comprising ten samples could be used for the analysis of extreme hand preference, with 5956 RH and 448 LH subjects.

Schizotypy and right-handedness vs. non-right-handedness

The overall meta-analysis investigating the association between schizotypy and right-handedness vs. non-right-handedness showed a significant effect for non-right-handedness with Hedges's $g = 0.22$ and $p = 0.01$, implicating higher total schizotypy scores in the non-right-handers as compared to the right-handers. These

findings are plotted in Fig. 8.1. Heterogeneity was high with $I^2 = 91\%$. After removing an outlier of more than two standard deviations (Barnett & Corballis, 2002), the effect of handedness on schizotypy scores remained significant, though small (Hedges's $g = 0.11$, $p = 0.015$). Heterogeneity decreased, with $I^2 = 66\%$. Removing the only study that investigated adolescents slightly lowered the effect size as well as heterogeneity (Hedges's $g = 0.09$, $p < 0.05$, $I^2 = 57\%$).

Schizotypy and mixed-handedness vs. strong left- and right-handedness

The analysis investigating the association between schizotypy and mixed handedness vs. extreme left- or right-handedness yielded a significant effect for mixed-handedness in comparison to right-handedness (Hedges's $g = 0.51$, $p = 0.0003$, Fig. 8.2). Heterogeneity was high with $I^2 = 95\%$. The difference in schizotypy score between left-handedness and mixed-handedness was also significant (Hedges's $g = 0.33$, $p = 0.026$, Fig. 8.3). Heterogeneity was again high, with $I^2 = 76\%$. The size of this effect seemed partially driven by the Barnett and

Schizotypy (RH vs. Mix) with outlier

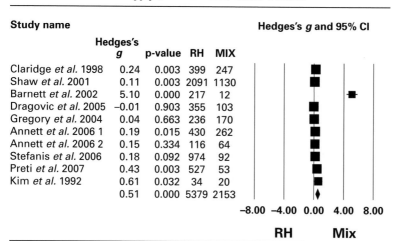

Figure 8.2 The association between schizotypy and mixed-handedness vs. extreme right-handedness showing a significant effect with Hedges's $g = 0.51$ and $p = 0.0003$, implicating higher schizotypy scores in mixed handed subjects than in strong right-handers.

Schizotypy (LH vs. Mix) with outlier

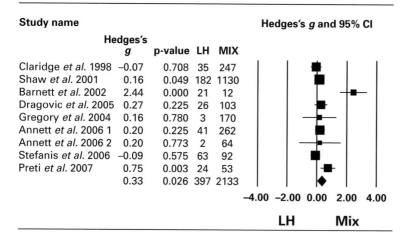

Figure 8.3 The association between schizotypy and mixed-handedness vs. extreme left-handedness showing a significant effect with Hedges's $g = 0.33$ and $p = 0.026$, implicating higher schizotypy scores in mixed handed subjects than in strong left-handers.

Corballis study, which was again an outlier of more than two standard deviations. However, after removal of this study mixed-handers still scored significantly higher then right-handers (Hedges's $g = 0.16$, $p < 0.0001$) with heterogeneity decreasing to $I^2 = 35\%$. In the comparison of mixed- and left-handers there was a comparable effect, with significance only at trend level (Hedges's $g = 0.15$, $p = 0.053$) and a low I^2 of 28%.

Meta-analysis of schizotypy in strong right- and left-handed subjects from these studies showed no difference (Hedges's $g = 0.06$, $p = 0.51$), with $I^2 = 61\%$.

Discussion

This study aimed to examine the association between schizotypy and handedness by performing a meta-analysis on the literature from 1970 until 2007 concerning population schizotypy and hand preference. We could include twelve studies, providing schizotypy scores of 10 058 subjects in total. In the main analysis we found a subtle but significant effect that remained significant after excluding a positive outlier (Hedges's $g = 0.11$), indicating higher schizotypy in non-right-handed individuals as compared to right-handed ones. In the subsequent analysis we found that mixed-handed subjects show a subtle increase in schizotypy as compared to right-handed individuals (Hedges's $g = 0.16$), a similar trend was observed for higher schizotypy in mixed-handers as compared to left-handed subjects (Hedges's $g = 0.15$). We did not find any difference in schizotypy score between strong left- and strong right-handedness. This indicates that non-right-handedness, and especially mixed-handedness is associated with schizotypy, although the effect is only small. This finding parallels observations in patients with schizophrenia (Sommer *et al.*, 2001a; Dragovic & Hammond, 2005) who also show increased prevalence of non-right-handedness. In schizophrenia as well as in population schizotypy decreased cerebral lateralization, resulting in bilateral language representation, is considered the underlying basis for the increased frequency of non-right-handedness (Crow, 1997; Shaw *et al.*, 2001). Although no functional imaging has been performed on language lateralization in population schizotypy, several dichotic listening studies found schizotypal subjects to exhibit a relatively greater left-ear preference for unilaterally presented verbal stimuli than normal controls (Broks *et al.*, 1984; Rawlings & Borge, 1987; Poreh *et al.*, 1994), which suggests increased language dominance of the right hemisphere. Indeed, a more bilateral pattern of language lateralization is likely to underlie the

association between population schizotypy and non-right-handedness observed in this meta-analysis. This is supported by the finding that relatives of schizophrenia patients, who are known to have increased schizotypy scores (Appels *et al.*, 2004), also show decreased language lateralization (Sommer *et al.*, 2004; Li *et al.*, 2007b). As such, we hypothesize that our finding of higher schizotypy in non-right-handers originates from a higher prevalence of bilateral language representation. Our results may be explained by the suggestion that the prevalence of bilateral language representation is even higher in mixed-handers than in strong left-handers. However, this remains speculative, since the accurate prevalence of bilateral language lateralization in mixed-handedness as compared to strong left-handers is presently not known. In contrast to bilateral language representation, strong right-hemispheric lateralization has not been associated with psychosis (e.g., Sommer *et al.*, 2001b). Right-hemisphere language dominance shows a linear increase with the strength of left-handedness, so that strongly left-handed subjects have higher prevalences of right cerebral dominance than mixed-handed subjects (Isaacs *et al.*, 2006; Knecht *et al.*, 2000). This may be the reason why our meta-analysis found no increase in schizotypy in left-handers as compared to right-handers.

In addition to schizophrenia, bilateral language representation, i.e., a lack of cerebral lateralization and its corresponding lack in hand dominance, has been associated with various phenomena, from autism (Annett, 1999; Herbert *et al.*, 2002), dyslexia and ADHD (Foster *et al.*, 2002; Giedd *et al.*, 2001) to cognitive skills. With regards to the latter, Crow *et al.* found that schoolchildren with equal hand skill – functioning at a "point of hemispheric indecision" – show relative cognitive dysfunction on verbal and mathematical tasks (Crow *et al.*, 1998) as compared to schoolchildren with stronger lateralized hand skill. In addition, in a large internet-based study a deficit in spatial ability was shown for adults writing with either hand (Peters *et al.*, 2006) as compared to adults who had clear right- or left-hand preferences. Another recent study showed that from a group of adults participating in a Television IQ test, adults writing with either hand performed worse on arithmetic, memory, and reasoning tasks (Corballis *et al.*, 2008). In contrast, Knecht *et al.* found no differences in cognitive achievement between left-, bilaterally, and right-lateralized subjects as measured by fTCD (Knecht *et al.*, 2001), but the sample of this study (i.e. *n* = 326) may have been too small to detect subtle differences.

Exactly how decreased cerebral lateralization predisposes to schizophrenia spectrum tendencies remains elusive. The contribution of increased right hemisphere activity might originate from the more diffuse spreading of activation that is shown in tasks of semantic priming, in contrast to the more focused spreading characteristic for the left hemisphere (Chiarello *et al.*, 1990), which could facilitate the occurrence of distant associations and thus irrational thinking. Indeed, semantic network activations have been shown to spread further within a shorter period of time in thought-disordered schizophrenia patients. Indirect semantic priming measured by event-related potentials was increased in these patients relative to non-thought-disordered and healthy controls (Kreher *et al.*, 2008). Further, fMRI studies have shown activation of the right-hemisphere homolog of Wernicke's area during speech production in (right-handed) thought-disordered schizophrenia patients (Kircher *et al.*, 2002), while controls performing the same task showed left-lateralized activity.

It has been suggested that psychosis, as well as schizotypy, is related to creativity through right-hemisphere involvement (Weinstein & Graves, 2002). This can be understood from a point of view that considers both phenomena as a different result of divergent thought, with a common neurobiological origin. Creativity can be defined as the ability to utilize non-prepotent associations of problem elements in order to discover non-obvious solutions to a problem (Mednick, 1962). Psychometric measures of creativity have been proposed to be related to diffuse rather than focused attention (Rowe *et al.*, 2007). This might be related to the diffuse processes supposedly associated with right-hemisphere function and psychosis. Indeed, right-hemisphere homologs of the language areas are shown to be involved in creative

problem solving (Jung-Beeman *et al.*, 2004). More evidence for the interrelatedness of creative capacity and psychosis proneness comes from research showing visual artists to score higher on measures of positive schizotypy as measured with the O-life (Burch *et al.*, 2006). In addition, Preti *et al.* found that creative artists have both a higher incidence of non-right-handedness as well as increased scores on the Peters *et al.* Delusion Inventory, independently from their level of psychopathology and higher use of drugs (Preti & Vellante, 2007). These findings could be understood from an evolutionary perspective, assuming that the capability of divergent thought as a result of decreased cerebral dominance constitutes a selective evolutionary advantage through creative thinking, supposedly yielding a benefit at the population level. As a trade off for such benefits, a minor group capable of divergent thought, but incapable of adequately organizing such thoughts, could be at risk for psychosis. Here, the right-hemispheric diffuse focus and more remote associations that regularly lead to creative solution, now yield paranoia or ideas of reference, by using non-obvious associations to connect unrelated common events. The resulting idiosyncratic feeling of interconnectedness of such events might predispose for magical thinking, ideas of reference, and finally delusions.

In conclusion, non-right-handed subjects had higher schizotypy levels than right-handed subjects, while there was no difference between strong right- and strong left-handed subjects. This supports the hypothesis of decreased lateralization being a vulnerability model for schizophrenia-spectrum features. It is also in line with previous studies that show specific vulnerability for ambidextrous subjects, rather than for strong left-handers in several cognitive domains (e.g., Crow *et al.*, 1998; Peters *et al.*, 2006). Our findings are in line with a possible evolutionary explanation of this vulnerability model. Herein, schizotypal and creative thought might represent variants of divergent thought, which in itself seems mediated by the right hemisphere. Further neuroimaging studies on cerebral lateralization of high schizotypy subjects are required to elucidate the origins of the relation between non-right-handedness and schizotypy.

ACKNOWLEDGMENT

This chapter uses extracts and figures from Somers, M., Sommer, I. E. & Kahn, R. S. (in press). Hand preference and population schizotypy. *Schizophrenia Research*.

REFERENCES

Annett, M. (1970). A classification of hand preference by association analysis. *Br J Psychol*, **61**, 303–21.

Annett, M. (1999). The theory of an agnosic right shift gene in schizophrenia and autism. *Schizophr Res*, **39**, 177–82.

Annett, M. (2004). Hand preference observed in large healthy samples: classification, norms and interpretations of increased non-right-handedness by the right shift theory. *Br J Psychol*, **95**, 339–53.

Annett, M. & Moran, P. (2006). Schizotypy is increased in mixed-handers, especially right-handed writers who use the left hand for primary actions. *Schizophr Res*, **81**, 239–46.

Appels, M. C., Sitskoorn, M. M., Vollema, M. G. & Kahn, R. S. (2004). Elevated levels of schizotypal features in parents of patients with a family history of schizophrenia spectrum disorders. *Schizophr Bull*, **30**, 781–90.

Barnett, K. J. & Corballis, M. C. (2002). Ambidexterity and magical ideation. *Laterality*, **7**, 75–84.

Broks, P., Claridge, G., Matheson, J. & Hargreaves, J. (1984). Schizotypy and hemisphere function-IV. Story comprehension under binaural and monaural listening conditions. *Personal Indiv Diff*, **5**(6), 665–70.

Bryden, P. J., Pryde, K. M. & Roy, E. A. (2000). A developmental analysis of the relationship between hand preference and performance: II. A performance-based method of measuring hand preference in children. *Brain Cogn*, **43**, 60–4.

Burch, G. S., Pavelis, C., Hemsley, D. R. & Corr, P. J. (2006). Schizotypy and creativity in visual artists. *Br J Psychol*, **97**, 177–90.

Chapman, L. J., Chapman, J. P. & Raulin, M. L. (1978). Body-image aberration in Schizophrenia. *J Abnorm Psychol*, **87**, 399–407.

Chen, W. J. & Su, C. H. (2006). Handedness and schizotypy in non-clinical populations: influence of handedness measures and age on the relationship. *Laterality*, **11**, 331–49.

Chiarello, C., Burgess, C., Richards, L. & Pollock, A. (1990). Semantic and associative priming in the cerebral hemispheres: some words do, some words don't ... sometimes, some places. *Brain Lang*, **38**, 75–104.

Claridge, G. & Broks, P. (1984). Schizotypy and hemisphere function: I. Theoretical considerations and the measurement of schizotypy. *Personal Indiv Diff*, **5**(6), 633–48.

Claridge, G., Clark, K., Davis, C. & Mason, O. (1998). Schizophrenia risk and handedness: a mixed picture. *Laterality*, **3**, 209–20.

Corballis, M. C., Hattie, J. & Fletcher, R. (2008). Handedness and intellectual achievement: an even-handed look. *Neuropsychologia*, **46**, 374–8.

Crow, T. J. (1997). Is schizophrenia the price that *Homo sapiens* pays for language? *Schizophr Res*, **28**, 127–41.

Crow, T. J., Crow, L. R., Done, D. J. & Leask, S. (1998). Relative hand skill predicts academic ability: global deficits at the point of hemispheric indecision. *Neuropsychologia*, **36**, 1275–82.

Cyhlarova, E. & Claridge, G. (2005). Development of a version of the Schizotypy Traits Questionnaire (STA) for screening children. *Schizophr Res*, **80**, 253–61.

Dragovic, M. & Hammond, G. (2005). Handedness in schizophrenia: a quantitative review of evidence. *Acta Psychiatr Scand*, **111**, 410–19.

Dragovic, M., Hammond, G. & Jablensky, A. (2005). Schizotypy and mixed-handedness revisited. *Psychiatry Res*, **136**, 143–52.

Eckblad, M. & Chapman, L. J. (1983). Magical ideation as an indicator of schizotypy. *J Consult Clin Psychol*, **51**, 215–25.

Foster, L. M., Hynd, G. W., Morgan, A. E. & Hugdahl, K. (2002). Planum temporale asymmetry and ear advantage in dichotic listening in Dev Dyslexia and Attention-Deficit/ Hyperactivity Disorder (ADHD). *J Int Neuropsychol Soc*, **8**, 22–36.

Giedd, J. N., Blumenthal, J., Molloy, E. & Castellanos, F. X. (2001). Brain imaging of attention deficit/hyperactivity disorder. *Ann N Y Acad Sci*, **931**, 33–49.

Gregory, A. M., Claridge, G., Clark, K. & Taylor, P. D. (2003). Handedness and schizotypy in a Japanese sample: an association masked by cultural effects on hand usage. *Schizophr Res*, **65**, 139–45.

Hedges L. V. & Olkin, I. (1985). *Statistical Methods for Meta-analysis*. Orlando, Florida: Academic Press.

Herbert, M. R., Harris, G. J., Adrien, K. T. *et al.* (2002). Abnormal asymmetry in language association cortex in autism. *Ann Neurol*, **52**, 588–96.

Higgins, J. P., Thompson, S. G., Deeks, J. J. & Altman, D. G. (2003). Measuring inconsistency in meta-analyses. *BMJ*, **327**, 557–60.

Isaacs, K. L., Barr, W. B., Nelson, P. K. & Devinsky, O. (2006). Degree of handedness and cerebral dominance. *Neurology*, **66**, 1855–8.

Jung-Beeman, M., Bowden, E. M., Haberman, J. *et al.* (2004). Neural activity when people solve verbal problems with insight. *PLoS Biol*, **2**, E97.

Kim, D., Raine, A., Triphon, N. & Green, M. F. (1992). Mixed handedness and features of schizotypal personality in a non-clinical sample. *J Nerv Ment Dis*, **180**, 133–5.

Kircher, T. T., Liddle, P. F., Brammer, M. J. *et al.* (2002). Reversed lateralization of temporal activation during speech production in thought disordered patients with schizophrenia. *Psychol Med*, **32**, 439–49.

Knecht, S., Drager, B., Deppe, M. *et al.* (2000). Handedness and hemispheric language dominance in healthy humans. *Brain*, **123**(12), 2512–18.

Knecht, S., Drager, B., Floel, A. *et al.* (2001). Behavioural relevance of atypical language lateralization in healthy subjects. *Brain*, **124**, 1657–65.

Kreher, D. A., Holcomb, P. J., Goff, D. & Kuperberg, G. R. (2008). Neural evidence for faster and further automatic spreading activation in schizophrenic thought disorder. *Schizophr Bull*, **34**(3), 473–82.

Leonhard, D. & Brugger, P. (1998). Creative, paranormal, and delusional thought: a consequence of right hemisphere semantic activation? *Neuropsychiatry Neuropsychol Behav Neurol*, **11**, 177–83.

Li, X., Branch, C. A., Ardekani, B. A. *et al.* (2007a). fMRI study of language activation in schizophrenia, schizoaffective disorder and in individuals genetically at high risk. *Schizophr Res*, **96**, 14–24.

Li, X., Branch, C. A., Bertisch, H. C. *et al.* (2007b). An fMRI study of language processing in people at high genetic risk for schizophrenia. *Schizophr Res*, **91**, 62–72.

Lipsey, M. W. & Wilson, D. B. (2001). The way in which intervention studies have "personality" and why it is important to meta-analysis. *Eval Health Prof*, **24**, 236–54.

Mason, O. & Claridge, G. (2006). The Oxford-Liverpool Inventory of Feelings and Experiences (O-LIFE): further description and extended norms. *Schizophr Res*, **82**, 203–11.

Mason, O., Claridge, G. & Jackson, M. (1995). New scales for the assessment of schizotypy. *Personal Individ Diff*, **18**(1), 7–13.

McManus, I. C. (1985). Handedness, language dominance and aphasia: a genetic model. *Psychol Med Monogr Suppl*, **8**, 1–40.

Mednick, S. A. (1962). The associative basis of the creative process. *Psychol Rev*, **69**, 220–32.

Nalcaci, E., Kalaycioglu, C., Cicek, M. & Budanur, O. E. (2000). Magical ideation and right-sided hemispatial inattention on a spatial working memory task: influences of sex and handedness. *Percept Mot Skills*, **91**, 883–92.

Nicholls, M. E., Orr, C. A. & Lindell, A. K. (2005). Magical ideation and its relation to lateral preference. *Laterality*, **10**, 503–15.

Oldfield, R. C. (1971). The assessment and analysis of handedness: the Edinburgh inventory. *Neuropsychologia*, **9**, 97–113.

Peters, E. R., Joseph, S. A. & Garety, P. A. (1999). Measurement of delusional ideation in the normal population: introducing the PDI (Peters *et al.* Delusions Inventory). *Schizophr Bull*, **25**, 553–76.

Peters, M. (1998). Description and validation of a flexible and broadly usable handedness questionnaire. *Laterality*, **3**, 77–96.

Peters, M., Reimers, S. & Manning, J. T. (2006). Hand preference for writing and associations with selected demographic and behavioral variables in 255,100 subjects: the BBC internet study. *Brain Cogn*, **62**, 177–89.

Poreh, A. M., Whitman, D. R. & Ross, T. P. (1994). Creative thinking abilities and hemispheric asymmetry in schizotypal college students. *Curr Psych*, **12**, 344–52.

Preti, A., Sardu, C. & Piga, A. (2007). Mixed-handedness is associated with the reporting of psychotic-like beliefs in a non-clinical Italian sample. *Schizophr Res*, **92**, 15–23.

Preti, A. & Vellante, M. (2007). Creativity and psychopathology: higher rates of psychosis proneness and nonright-handedness among creative artists compared to same age and gender peers. *J Nerv Ment Dis*, **195**, 837–45.

Pujol, J., Deus, J., Losilla, J. M. & Capdevila, A. (1999). Cerebral lateralization of language in normal left-handed people studied by functional MRI. *Neurology*, **52**, 1038–43.

Raine, A. (1991). The SPQ: a scale for the assessment of schizotypal personality based on DSM-III-R criteria. *Schizophr Bull*, **17**, 555–64.

Raine, A., Reynolds, C., Lencz, T. *et al.* (1994). Cognitive-perceptual, interpersonal, and disorganized features of schizotypal personality. *Schizophr Bull*, **20**, 191–201.

Rawlings, D. & Borge, A. (1987). Personality and hemisphere function: two experiments using the dichotic shadowing technique. *Personality and Individual Differences*, **8**(4), 483–8.

Rowe, G., Hirsh, J. B. & Anderson, A. K. (2007). Positive affect increases the breadth of attentional selection. *Proc Natl Acad Sci USA*, **104**, 383–8.

Rust, J. (1988). The Rust Inventory of Schizotypal Cognitions (RISC). *Schizophr Bull*, **14**, 317–22.

Shaw, J., Claridge, G. & Clark, K. (2001). Schizotypy and the shift from dextrality: a study of handedness in a large non-clinical sample. *Schizophr Res*, **50**, 181–9.

Sommer, I., Ramsey, N., Kahn, R., Aleman, A. & Bouma, A. (2001a). Handedness, language lateralisation and anatomical asymmetry in schizophrenia: meta-analysis. *Br J Psychiatry*, **178**, 344–51.

Sommer, I. E., Ramsey, N. F. & Kahn, R. S. (2001b). Language lateralization in schizophrenia, an fMRI study. *Schizophr Res*, **52**, 57–67.

Sommer, I. E., Ramsey, N. F., Mandl, R. C. & Kahn, R. S. (2003). Language lateralization in female patients with schizophrenia: an fMRI study. *Schizophr Res*, **60**, 183–90.

Sommer, I. E., Ramsey, N. F., Mandl, R. C., van Oel, C. J. & Kahn, R. S. (2004). Language activation in monozygotic twins discordant for schizophrenia. *Br J Psychiatry*, **184**, 128–35.

Sommer, I. E., Vd Veer, A. J., Wijkstra, J., Boks, M. P. & Kahn, R. S. (2007). Comparing language lateralization in psychotic mania and psychotic depression to schizophrenia; a functional MRI study. *Schizophr Res*, **89**, 364–5.

Spaniel, F., Tintera, J., Hajek, T. *et al.* (2007). Language lateralization in monozygotic twins discordant and concordant for schizophrenia. A functional MRI pilot study. *Eur Psychiatry*, **22**, 319–22.

Spitzer, R. L., Skodol, A. E., Gibbon, M. & Williams, J. B. W. (1987). *DSM-III-R:Diagnostic and Statistical Manual of Mental Disorders*, 3rd edn. Washington, DC: American Psychiatric Association.

Stefanis, N. C., Vitoratou, S., Smyrnis, N. *et al.* (2006). Mixed handedness is associated with the disorganization dimension of schizotypy in a young male population. *Schizophr Res*, **87**, 289–96.

Straaten, v. A. (1955). [Considerations on the occurrence of manifest left-handedness in schizophrenia.] *Ned Tijdschr Geneeskd*, **99**, 706–10.

Szaflarski, J. P., Holland, S. K., Schmithorst, V. J. & Byars, A. W. (2006). fMRI study of language lateralization in children and adults. *Hum Brain Mapp*, **27**, 202–12.

Weinstein, S. & Graves, R. E. (2002). Are creativity and schizotypy products of a right hemisphere bias? *Brain Cogn*, **49**, 138–51.

9

Functional imaging studies on language lateralization in schizophrenia patients

Annick Razafimandimby, Olivier Maïza, and Sonia Dollfus

Summary

Functional cerebral imaging allows us to investigate the functional dominance directly using functional laterality indices (FLI). Functional laterality indices are usually measured based on activated voxel counting or on normalized blood-oxygen-level-dependent (BOLD) signal variations in the left and right hemispheres. Functional imaging studies of language processing using FLI have supported Crow's hypothesis that schizophrenia would be a result of an anomaly in the hemispheric specialization for language. Compared to control subjects, reduced or reversed FLI have been found in schizophrenic patients during language tasks such as verb generation, verbal fluency, semantic decision-making, and listening to stories and sentences. However, confounding variables such as handedness, gender, task performance, clinical state, or antipsychotic dose has led to different interpretations of this decreased or reversed hemispheric lateralization for language observed in schizophrenia patients. Other functional imaging studies have shown that decreased language lateralization is also observed in affective disorders, in patients with a high genetic risk for schizophrenia, and in patients experiencing their first episode of schizophrenia. Taken together, these results indicate that decreased language lateralization can be considered a trait marker for psychosis. However, they must be confirmed in larger samples and further studies must determine whether there is a greater prevalence of this trait in members of the families of identified psychotic patients than in the general population, as well as whether it is associated with psychotic spectrum disorders in such families. Nevertheless, preliminary results support Crow's hypothesis that there is a continuum of psychosis between bipolar and schizophrenic disorders.

Introduction

There are three major reasons to study hemispheric specialization or dominance of language in schizophrenia. First, some key symptoms of schizophrenia, such as auditory verbal hallucinations (AVH) and formal thought disorders, are related to language functions. Second, the hemispheric specialization of language is a well known left-lateralized function in right-handed healthy subjects (Broca, 1861), and this lateralization may be determined during fetal development. For example, the leftward asymmetry of the planum temporale appears between weeks 29 and 31 of gestation, and this asymmetry could underlie the hemispheric dominance of language (Geschwind & Levitsky, 1968). The neuro-developmental hypothesis posits that a dysfunction during brain development occurs in subjects who will develop schizophrenia. Thus, the study of functional lateralization in schizophrenia is of great interest regarding this hypothesis. Third, numerous studies on handedness and on anatomical and functional cerebral imaging have supported Crow's hypothesis that a reduced hemispheric specialization for language plays a role in schizophrenia. Crow proposed that a failure to develop normal cerebral lateralization predisposes individuals to psychosis; he further suggested, "Schizophrenia is the price *Homo sapiens* pays for language" (Crow, 1997a).

Many studies on handedness have shown an increase of mixed-handedness in nearly 20% of patients with schizophrenia, compared to 3.8% of the normal population (Green *et al.*, 1989; Satz & Green, 1999). In

Language Lateralization and Psychosis, ed. Iris E. C. Sommer and René S. Kahn. Published by Cambridge University Press.
© Cambridge University Press 2009.

addition, mixed-handedness is significantly related to the severity of formal thought disorders or to auditory hallucinations (Manoach, 1994; Dollfus *et al.*, 2002). However, handedness is an indirect index of hemispheric language dominance and can also be influenced by environment and education.

To what extent does cerebral imaging contribute to the investigation of hemispheric lateralization? Anatomical cerebral MRI studies have shown a reduction or a reversal of the normal volume asymmetry of the superior temporal gyrus (Highley *et al.*, 1999), and in particular, of the planum temporale in schizophrenia (Shapleske *et al.*, 1999). However, these results are controversial due to great anatomical inter-subject variability. Anatomical asymmetry is also an indirect index of functional dominance of language. In order to directly investigate this functional dominance, the use of functional cerebral imaging with positron emission tomography (PET) or functional magnetic resonance imaging (fMRI) allows us to determine the hemispheric specialization for language (Herve *et al.*, 2006).

In this chapter, we present the different methods and language tasks that are used to evaluate functional lateralization, as well as the confounding variables that can affect the functional lateralization of language in schizophrenia. Finally, we present some studies supporting the idea that reduced language lateralization may be a marker of schizophrenia.

Methods to evaluate the functional lateralization of language

In order to evaluate the hemispheric dominance of language, functional laterality indices (FLI) need to be computed. On the basis of activation maps induced by language tasks, the dominant hemisphere displays the strongest and the most extended activation. The formulas that are usually used are:

FLI = (Left – Right)/(Left + Right) or
FLI = (Left – Right)/(Left + Right) × 100

The value that is used is the number or the t-value sum of activated voxels, i.e., values above a set statistical threshold in the left and right hemispheres (Fernandez *et al.*, 2003). The FLI can be evaluated using activated voxels in regions of interest (ROIs) that are defined anatomically or functionally in both hemispheres. Anatomical ROIs can be hemispheres, lobes, or smaller anatomical regions, and can be traced in each individual subject using either their native space or a reference stereotaxic space (Tzourio-Mazoyer *et al.*, 2002). Functional ROIs are regions significantly activated by the task in a group of subjects (Adcock *et al.*, 2003). Whatever the anatomical or functional methods used, the use of language-specific ROIs provides more consistent FLI than those computed in whole hemispheres (Rutten *et al.*, 2002).

The FLI is a normalized variable. With the formula shown above, the FLIs fall between +1 and –1 or +100 and –100; the upper and lower values correspond to complete left or right dominance with no activated voxels in the right or left side, respectively. Functional laterality indices that are mid-range (for example, from +0.2 to –0.2 or +20 to –20) correspond to an absence of dominance and are characteristic of ambilateral subjects. This voxel counting method has been used in the majority of schizophrenia studies (Koeda *et al.*, 2006; Sommer *et al.*, 2001; Sommer *et al.*, 2003; Sommer *et al.*, 2004b; Weiss *et al.*, 2004; Weiss *et al.*, 2006; Li *et al.*, 2007). However, with activated voxel counting, deactivation cannot be taken into account since only positive values are recorded. As deactivation is relevant to determining hemispheric specialization for language, the use of simple differences of normalized regional cerebral blood flow or blood-oxygen-level-dependent (BOLD) values between the left and right hemispheres (FLI = Right – Left or Left – Right) in a priori defined ROIs has been proposed (Tzourio-Mazoyer *et al.*, 2004; Dollfus *et al.*, 2005; Artiges *et al.*, 2000). Is is notable that stronger lateralization indices are obtained when deactivation occurs in only one side. Lastly, the signal intensity changes measured in the ROIs' voxels that exceeded a predefined activation level have been used to calculate FLI (Jansen *et al.*, 2006). This method is known to produce robust and reproducible laterality results in healthy subjects but has never been used in schizophrenia patients.

Language tasks and the networks involved

Auditory verbal imagery

Cognitive models propose that AVH are derived from inner speech that is mistakenly identified as external or "alien" through defective self-monitoring (Frith & Done, 1988). This suggests that the functional neuro-anatomy of monitoring inner speech may be abnormal in patients who are prone to AVH. Both covert articulation and imagining another person's speech involve the generation of inner speech, but imagining speech (auditory verbal imagery) places greater demands on verbal self-monitoring (McGuire *et al.*, 1995). Auditory verbal imagery consists of imagining another person's speech and involves both the generation and monitoring of inner speech. McGuire and collaborators showed that auditory verbal imagery was associated with reduced activation in the left middle temporal gyrus and in the supplementary motor area in schizophrenia patients prone to auditory hallucinations compared to patients with schizophrenia but no history of hallucinations and compared to healthy volunteers (McGuire *et al.*, 1996). Moreover, another study using a similar paradigm in another group of hallucination-prone patients demonstrated attenuated activation in several cerebral regions, notably in the right middle and superior temporal cortex (Shergill *et al.*, 2000). According to the authors, a predisposition to verbal hallucinations in schizophrenia could be associated with a failure to activate areas implicated in the normal monitoring of inner speech. However, these two studies did not evaluate functional lateralization of auditory verbal imagery.

Language production tasks

Verbal fluency is a widely used neuropsychological test of language production, requiring subjects to generate a word in response to a cue. This requires the retrieval of lexically associated words from long-term memory storage and involves high demands on frontally mediated strategic processes. Other derived production tasks, such as verb generation and free speech

production, have been used to investigate schizophrenia in conjunction with PET or fMRI. Previous functional cerebral imaging studies indicated that a verbal fluency task in healthy subjects is associated with activation of a distributed set of brain regions, including the left frontal cortex, that corresponds to the Broca area, the dorsolateral prefrontal cortex, the premotor cortex, and the right cerebellum (Pujol *et al.*, 1999; Frost *et al.*, 1999; Lurito *et al.*, 2000; Hubrich-Ungureanu *et al.*, 2002). When schizophrenia patients performed a verbal fluency task, researchers found that the activation network included the same regions in patients and in healthy controls, except that decreased activation was observed in the patients with negative symptoms. Moreover, the activation was primarily concentrated in the language areas of the left hemisphere in controls, while more widespread and unfocused activation was found in patients (even in those with a never-treated first episode of schizophrenia) (Boksman *et al.*, 2005).

Neuroimaging studies using verbal fluency tasks in schizophrenia patients have produced controversial findings concerning the involvement of the frontal cortex. There are some reports of reduced prefrontal activity in patients (Yurgelun-Todd *et al.*, 1996; Curtis *et al.*, 1998; Kircher *et al.*, 2002; Boksman *et al.*, 2005; Fu *et al.*, 2005b), while one study found that patients and controls showed similar patterns of prefrontal activation (Spence *et al.*, 2000). It has also been noted that the cognitive demands of the specific experimental task and the resulting test performance can be confounding factors that lead to reduced brain activation in poorly performing patients (Callicott *et al.*, 2003; Curtis *et al.*, 1999). This is supported by a study that found that patients, who were matched with controls for the task performance levels, did not exhibit reduced leftward frontal activity (Frith *et al.*, 1995).

Moreover, in a recent study using a paced letter verbal fluency task, acutely psychotic schizophrenia patients showed less activation than the healthy controls; however, these differences were less marked than the differences between the patients in remission and the healthy comparison subjects (Fu *et al.*, 2005b). Indeed, direct group comparison revealed that while the patients in remission showed less activation in the right middle and bilateral inferior frontal cortex than the controls, no significant difference was observed in the prefrontal cortex between the acute psychosis patients and the healthy subjects. These observations seemed counter-intuitive in light of the evidence that prefrontal function in schizophrenia was more impaired in patients with positive psychotic symptoms than those in remission (Spence *et al.*, 1998). However, compromised prefrontal function in schizophrenia may be manifested as increased activation during cognitive processing. For example, Fu *et al.* have found that healthy volunteers with positive psychotic symptoms induced by ketamine showed greater engagement of prefrontal areas during verbal fluency than when performing the task while taking placebo (Fu *et al.*, 2005a). Moreover, during a verbal fluency task in first-episode schizophrenia, Jones *et al.* reported significantly increased activation in the left prefrontal cortex in the quetiapine-treated patients and the healthy control sample compared with the drug-naïve sample (Jones *et al.*, 2004). Another report (Schaufelberger *et al.*, 2005) showed lower activation in the right prefrontal cortex in patients with first episode psychosis compared to healthy volunteers, which was consistent with previous studies (Curtis *et al.*, 1998; Ashton *et al.*, 2000; Fu *et al.*, 2005b). This report regarding a phonological verbal fluency task also showed greater activation in a more superior portion of the right prefrontal cortex but no difference between subjects in terms of task performance. All these observations are consistent with the notion that schizophrenia patients have alterations in the prefrontal cortex, i.e., either increased or decreased neural recruitment. Such alterations could depend on the level of task difficulty or the severity of the psychotic symptoms; the changes could also be related to a compensatory response that is required to maintain normal task performance.

There are also differential patterns of temporal lobe activation during the performance of verbal fluency tasks. Deactivation of the left temporal lobe is observed both in healthy controls and patients while performing a language production task, and individual analysis showed that deactivation was localized to the left Heschl gyrus (Dollfus & Brazo, 2003). This area is considered the primary auditory cortex and has been implicated in auditory verbal hallucinations (Lennox

et al., 2000). According to the studies of Frith *et al.* (1995) and Yurgelun-Todd *et al.* (1996), patients performing a fluency task failed to deactivate the left Heschl gyrus. However, two other studies employing a silent fluency task did not find any difference in deactivation in the same region between patients and healthy controls (Dye *et al.*, 1999; Spence *et al.*, 2000). These conflicting results can be explained by the variability of the chronicity and the severity of the psychosis reported in these studies. Indeed, the patients included in the report by Frith *et al.* (1995) had severe and chronic symptoms, while those included in the studies of Dye *et al.* (1999) and Spence *et al.* (2000) were either in complete remission or were stabilized with few symptoms respectively. Another factor, medication, cannot fully explain this discrepancy since the patients included in the study of Spence *et al.* (2000) as well as those in the study of Frith *et al.* (1995) and Yurgelun-Todd *et al.* (1996) were all receiving antipsychotic medication. However, we cannot completely exclude the possibility that psychotropic drugs influence cerebral activity. Indeed, one report has shown that D-cycloserine, a partial agonist at the glycine recognition site of the N-methyl-D-aspartate receptor, in addition to conventional antipsychotic medication, increases temporal activation associated with improvement of negative symptoms in schizophrenic patients performing a word fluency task (Yurgelun-Todd *et al.*, 2005).

Taken together, these results provide evidence of modified activation in both the frontal and temporal cortex during verbal fluency tasks in schizophrenia patients compared to healthy volunteers. This reduced recruitment may depend on the psychotic state and the level of task difficulty. However, these reports did not specifically evaluate the functional lateralization of language, and in fact few studies have evaluated functional lateralization using a production task in patients with schizophrenia. One study used a vocalized verbal fluency task and a spontaneous word production task in patients with prominent negative symptoms and moderate doses of antipsychotics (Artiges *et al.*, 2000). This study found that there was lower activation in the left frontal regions associated with increased activity of the right frontal and prefrontal cortex in schizophrenia patients compared to healthy controls. Functional laterality indices were also evaluated based on normalized cerebral blood flow in both hemispheres, and a decreased leftward asymmetry was observed in patients compared to controls. Other reports, using a letter verbal fluency task, found the same results in high-functioning schizophrenia patients and in unmedicated patients during an acute episode of schizophrenia (Weiss *et al.*, 2004; Weiss *et al.*, 2006).

Semantic decision tasks

Functional lateralization for language was also assessed through the combination of two language tasks: a paced verb generation task and a semantic decision task (Sommer *et al.*, 2001; Sommer *et al.*, 2003). This task combination induced bilateral activation in the frontal, temporal, and temporo-parietal language areas. Functional laterality indices were computed with the method of voxel counting in a language-specific ROI defined as the union of the inferior frontal gyrus, the superior and middle temporal gyri, and the supramarginal and angular gyri, regions known to be involved in language processing. Compared to controls, schizophrenia patients showed normal activity of the left ROI but increased activations in the right ROI. The FLI analysis indicated that cerebral dominance for language was significantly reduced in patients compared to controls. The authors concluded that decreased language lateralization observed in schizophrenia patients resulted from increased right hemispheric language activation, which might suggest a failure to inhibit non-dominant language areas in schizophrenia.

Language comprehension tasks

Linguistic research has demonstrated that there are multiple levels of representation in mapping sound to meaning. The implicit goal of speech perception studies is to understand sub-lexical stages in the process of speech recognition (i.e., auditory comprehension).

Functional imaging data are consistent with the bilateral organization of speech comprehension processes. A consistent and uncontroversial finding is that,

compared to a resting baseline, listening to speech activates the superior temporal gyrus bilaterally: the posterior part of the superior temporal gyrus and the superior temporal sulcus, both implicated in the phonological-level processes (Hickok & Poeppel, 2007). Moreover, most studies dealing with language comprehension have documented the role of the pars triangularis of the inferior frontal gyrus in semantic processing during speech listening (Gabrieli *et al.*, 1998; Mazoyer *et al.*, 1993), with co-activation of the middle temporal gyrus extending posteriorly to the angular gyrus or the inferior parietal lobe (Binder *et al.*, 1997; Crinion *et al.*, 2003; Papathanassiou *et al.*, 2000; Tzourio *et al.*, 1998; Schlosser *et al.*, 1998; Perani *et al.*, 1996). These regions belong to the heteromodal associative cortex, which might be involved in the pathophysiology of schizophrenia, according to Pearlson *et al.* (1996).

Verbal auditory stimulation without visual stimulation, consisting of a story presented binaurally through earphones, was used to study 15 schizophrenia patients (Woodruff *et al.*, 1997). In a first analysis, the authors compared schizophrenia patients with a history of auditory hallucinations (trait-positive), to schizophrenia patients without a history of auditory hallucinations (trait-negative) and to healthy volunteers. During the auditory stimulation (i.e., the story listening), the comparison of the trait-positive and trait-negative patients revealed no clear difference in temporal activation. However, the schizophrenia patients (trait-positive and trait-negative combined), showed significantly less activation in the left superior temporal gyrus but more activation in the right middle temporal gyrus relative to the healthy controls. In a second analysis, the same authors (Woodruff *et al.*, 1997) examined seven schizophrenic patients while they were actually experiencing severe auditory verbal hallucinations (hallucinatory-state positive) and again after their hallucinations had diminished (hallucinatory-state negative). The temporal cortex (right middle and left superior temporal gyri) was significantly less activated during the auditory speech listening in the hallucinatory-state positive condition than in the hallucinatory-state negative condition. However, in that study the authors did not evaluate functional lateralization by calculating

FLI. They suggested that the auditory hallucinations might compete with external speech for processing sites within the temporal cortex. This notion of competition is consistent with the patients' practice of listening to music or to speech as a means of alleviating auditory hallucinations (Nayani & David, 1996; Gallagher *et al.*, 1994).

The generative mechanism of functional auditory hallucinations is known to be closely associated with human voice perception. Consequently, investigating the cerebral response to the human voice is relevant to schizophrenia. In healthy subjects, functional MRI studies have shown that the human voice-specific area is located in the superior temporal sulcus with right hemisphere dominance (Belin & Zatorre, 2003; Belin *et al.*, 2000). A recent functional study scanned 14 schizophrenia patients and 14 controls while they listened to reverse sentences and identifiable non-vocal sounds (Koeda *et al.*, 2006). This comparison allowed the authors to investigate the neural bases of human voice perception without semantic processing, and demonstrated that the patients presented less activation than controls in the right superior temporal sulcus, the right middle temporal gyrus, and the bilateral posterior cingulated gyrus. This indicated that the voice-specific network in the right hemisphere was disrupted in the schizophrenia patients. Moreover, they also calculated FLI based on the activated voxel numbers in the anterior part of the middle temporal gyrus in both hemispheres. However, there was no significant difference in the functional lateralization between schizophrenia patients and controls.

Other language tasks can also be used to investigate cerebral activation during language comprehension processing in schizophrenia patients versus healthy controls. One study used a story comprehension task that compared activation while listening to a French story to listening to the same story in Tamil (a language unknown to the subjects) in order to focus on the semantic network. Functional laterality indices were computed as the difference of the BOLD signal variations in the right and left ROIs (Dollfus *et al.*, 2005). A similar study also used a comprehension task, which consisted of listening to sentences, or listening to reverse sentences, or identifiable non-vocal sounds

(Koeda *et al.*, 2006). Both studies showed reduced recruitment in the left ROIs. These ROIs corresponded on the one hand to the pars triangularis of the inferior frontal gyrus, the middle temporal, and the angular gyri (Dollfus *et al.*, 2005), and on the other hand to the pars triangularis of the inferior frontal gyrus, the posterior part of the superior temporal gyrus, and the inferior parietal gyrus (Koeda *et al.*, 2006). The authors of both studies concluded that there was decreased activation in regions related to the language semantic network. Both reports also calculated FLI and demonstrated significantly lower FLI in patients than in controls. This finding supports a decreased leftward lateralization in schizophrenia.

We wish to note that interpretations of average results can be misleading when they involve a dichotomous group of individuals with disparate results. For example, detecting an average reduction in left hemisphere recruitment during a language task can be either due to a small decrease in activity in most subjects, or to the presence of a subgroup of rightward asymmetrical subjects. Each scenario leads to strikingly different interpretations from the perspective of hemispheric specialization (Herve *et al.*, 2006). In our study (Dollfus *et al.*, 2005), each schizophrenic patient was compared one by one to a healthy subject matched for gender, age, education level, and handedness. We found that patients had reduced FLI as compared to matched controls in 16 of 21 pairs (76%), while 28.6% of the schizophrenic patients and 9.5% of healthy subjects showed an atypical (rightward) hemispheric specialization for language (Fig. 9.1). These observations raise the question of whether the inclusion of patients with atypical lateralization for language might have skewed the average results of the cohort. To address this question, we included schizophrenia patients with similar typical (leftward) functional lateralization as controls in using the same language task (Dollfus *et al.*, 2008). Consequently, no difference in functional lateralization was observed between patients and controls, as assessed by FLI in areas involved in language semantic processing. However, the results showed a significant functional deficit in the medial part of the left superior frontal gyrus in patients compared to controls; this region is considered a core region for theory of mind processing.

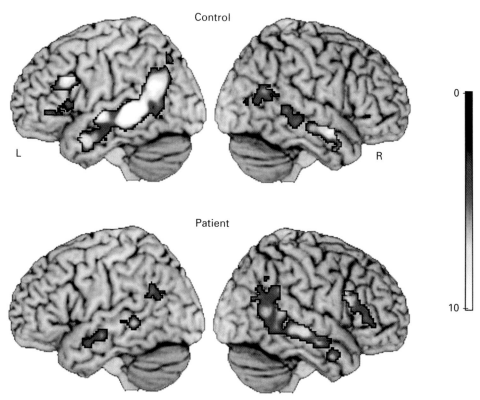

Figure 9.1 Hemispheric surface rendering of an activated LANG region of interest (ROI) is illustrated for a control (top), showing leftward asymmetry superimposed on the individual anatomic MRIs after stereotactic normalization. Hemispheric surface rendering of an activated LANG region of interest is illustrated for a schizophrenia patient (bottom), showing rightward asymmetry superimposed on the individual anatomic MRIs after stereotactic normalization. The LANG ROI corresponds to three merged regions, namely the pars triangularis of the inferior frontal gyrus, the middle temporal gyrus, and the angular gyrus. (See color plate section.)

Moreover, this deficit was also observed in patients experiencing a first episode of schizophrenia and in patients with bipolar disorder (Maiza *et al.*, 2008). In all of these studies, the language task was the same: it consisted of listening to a story that involved social interactions, leading the subjects to infer the characters' mental states in order to understand the story. Consequently, we assumed that this major functional deficit in patients could be the result of a defect in the core region of the theory of mind neural network. This functional defect was not the result of reverse hemispheric lateralization for language, and was found in chronic schizophrenic patients as well as in first-

episode schizophrenics and in patients with bipolar disorders. Consequently, this functional deficit may be considered a functional abnormality of psychosis. This functional defect, present at the beginning of schizophrenia, may persist throughout the course of the illness and may not be specific to schizophrenia.

Confounding variables for hemispheric lateralization for language

Potential confounding factors, such as handedness, gender, severity of the psychotic symptoms, task performances, or medication have to be considered in interpreting the results of functional imaging studies.

Concerning handedness, only one study used functional imaging to test possible associations between schizophrenia and handedness in terms of language lateralization (Razafimandimby *et al.*, 2006). Compared to controls, the authors reported decreased leftward asymmetry in the semantic integration areas in patients, irrespective of their handedness. Consequently, the reduced leftward language lateralization can be considered a characteristic of schizophrenia that is independent of handedness.

Although gender effects have been reported on hemispheric specialization for language in healthy subjects, no association between gender and illness has been reported (Sommer *et al.*, 2003).

Other factors linked to schizophrenia, such as impaired task performance or clinical state, could be expected to correlate with reduced FLI. With regard to task performance, Artiges *et al.* showed that right-hemisphere activity was negatively correlated to the number of words produced during the generation task (Artiges *et al.*, 2000). These authors suggested that the origin of this increased right frontal activation, observed in patients, could represent a functional brain adaptation to cognitive impairments. However, no link between comprehension scores and FLI was reported by Sommer *et al.* (2001) or by Dollfus *et al.* (2005). It can be concluded that lower performance levels in patients might have an effect on the language area activity, depending on the task, but this cannot explain the reduced functional cerebral asymmetry observed in schizophrenia patients.

Few investigators have studied whether antipsychotic medication has an impact on hemispheric dominance. Overall studies have reported decreased language lateralization including schizophrenia patients treated with antipsychotic medication. To date, we cannot exclude the role of these drugs on the modification of functional asymmetries during the language tasks, although one study found decreased lateralization of language in unmedicated patients (Weiss *et al.*, 2006).

There are few reports in the literature addressing the issue of whether clinical symptoms can confound language lateralization results. A longitudinal functional imaging study showed that auditory hallucinations decrease bilateral activity in the temporal cortex during the presentation of speech (Woodruff *et al.*, 1997), but functional asymmetries were not evaluated. Another group reported a negative correlation between the severity of auditory hallucinations and FLI in a population in which patients with rightward language lateralization had been excluded (Sommer *et al.*, 2001). Thus, patients with severe hallucinations were the least leftward lateralized. However, other studies did not find any relationship between decreased leftward FLI in patients and the severity of language disorders (such as auditory hallucinations and conceptual disorganization) as assessed with PANSS (Weiss *et al.*, 2004; Dollfus *et al.*, 2005) and BPRS (Koeda *et al.*, 2006). In fact, reduced language lateralization was found in patients regardless of whether the prevalent symptoms were negative symptoms (Artiges *et al.*, 2000), auditory hallucinations (Sommer *et al.*, 2001; Sommer *et al.*, 2003), or formal thought disorders (Kircher *et al.*, 2002).

Taken together, these functional cerebral imaging studies provided direct evidence of an anomaly of language hemispheric specialization in schizophrenic patients. Further, given that this anomaly might not be the consequence of language disorders, the questions can be raised whether this reduced language lateralization is stable over time, is observed in other psychoses, is observed in the first episode of psychosis, and is observed in relatives of schizophrenia patients.

Longitudinal studies on language lateralization in schizophrenic patients

To date, only one study has investigated the time course of functional lateralization of language in schizophrenia (Razafimandimby *et al.*, 2007). Out of 21 pairs of schizophrenic patients and matched controls that were included in a previous study (Dollfus *et al.*, 2005), 10 pairs underwent a second fMRI session 21 months after the first session. All of the patients were stabilized outpatients without any hospitalization or any psychotic exacerbation during the follow-up period. The mean illness duration at the first session

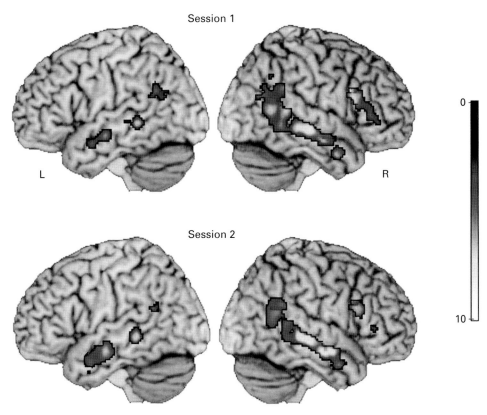

Figure 9.2 Hemispheric surface rendering of an activated LANG region of interest is illustrated for one schizophrenia patient at two test sessions (session 1 was baseline, and session 2 was 21 months after the first session); this shows a rightward asymmetry superimposed on the individual anatomic MRIs after stereotactic normalization. (See color plate section.)

was 12.1 ± 8.6 years. This study showed that in both healthy controls and patients, the indices of lateralization did not differ between the first and the second session and were strongly correlated across both sessions. Moreover, FLI correlated neither with task performance assessed through a comprehension questionnaire nor with the severity of the psychotic symptoms. These results suggest that reduced leftward lateralization for language is stable over time and may correspond to an abnormality of language-related brain organization in schizophrenic patients (Fig. 9.2). However, this study involved patients at an advanced stage of the disease. Thus, in order to determine whether reduced hemispheric lateralization is a core feature of schizophrenia, further investigation of

functional language lateralization in patients experiencing a first episode of schizophrenia is needed. Even so, structural studies have provided evidence for an evolutionary process targeting brain regions underlying language functions in first-episode patients (Kasai et al., 2003; Whitford et al., 2006): this process may influence language lateralization.

Language lateralization in first-episode schizophrenia

No study has focused on functional language lateralization in first-episode schizophrenia. However, Weiss et al. conducted an fMRI study that included seven unmedicated schizophrenic patients, five of whom were experiencing their first episode of the illness (Weiss *et al.*, 2006). A covert verbal fluency task was used to assess functional language lateralization through FLI computed using the classical method of voxel counting. In this study, schizophrenic patients were less left lateralized than controls. This result confirms that the decrease of hemispheric specialization is not relative to antipsychotic exposure, since no patient had been treated. It also indicates that this anomaly might be present at the beginning of the illness. Although the sample was heterogeneous as to illness duration (five were first-episode and two were chronic patients), the individual data showed that five out of seven patients displayed a lower degree of left lateralization than the controls, and that three of these five patients were rightward lateralized. Although further studies are needed to clarify the time course of this change in the brain's organization of language processing in schizophrenic patients, the results of this study support the hypothesis that schizophrenics have decreased functional lateralization for language since the beginning of the disease.

Functional lateralization in subjects at high risk of schizophrenia

Functional cerebral studies in subjects at high risk for schizophrenia can provide better understanding of the pathophysiology of schizophrenia in terms of identifying abnormalities that exist prior to the onset of the disease and, hence, that may not be related to symptoms or medication. Such abnormalities might reflect a predisposition to develop schizophrenia, and might have a clinical utility if they could be used to predict which high-risk individuals will go on to develop schizophrenia (Whalley *et al.*, 2006).

Li *et al.* investigated language processing in three groups: 21 subjects at high genetic risk for schizophrenia, 20 patients suffering from schizophrenia or schizoaffective disorder, and 36 control subjects at low risk for schizophrenia (Li *et al.*, 2007). All subjects were scanned while performing a visual word/pseudoword discrimination task. Functional laterality indices were computed for different ROIs with the following formula:

$FLI = (L - R)/(L + R)$, where L and R were the t-value sum of activated voxels in the left and right hemispheres, respectively. In the control subjects, activation during the task was left-lateralized in the Broca area, whereas in both patients and high-risk subjects, activation was more bilateral in the same area. Surprisingly, the reasons for this loss of leftward lateralization were different in the two groups. In schizophrenic patients, it corresponded to increased activations in the right hemisphere while, for high-risk subjects, it was due to decreased activation in the left hemisphere. The authors concluded that there was a lesser degree of hemispheric specialization for language present in patients before the beginning of the illness.

Language lateralization in the relatives of schizophrenic patients

The only fMRI study that investigated healthy relatives of patients included 12 monozygotic twin pairs discordant for schizophrenia and 12 monozygotic healthy twin pairs (Sommer *et al.*, 2004b). In the pairs discordant for schizophrenia, the twins affected by the disease had been ill for an average of 17 years. It was therefore very unlikely that their co-twins would develop the disease later on. Compared to controls, schizophrenic patients and their healthy co-twins were less leftward lateralized. In both the well and the ill twins decreased lateralization was caused by increased language activity in the right hemisphere areas. Moreover, schizophrenic patients and their co-twins did not differ significantly in regards to language lateralization. The authors concluded that the decreased language lateralization may be genetically, rather than environmentally determined. Moreover, since this anomaly was found in healthy relatives of patients, it might be considered as a marker of a predisposition to develop schizophrenia.

Language lateralization in other psychoses

To address the question of specificity of decreased language lateralization, Sommer *et al.* conducted an fMRI study of 14 patients with psychotic unipolar depression, 13 patients with psychotic mania, 14 patients with schizophrenia, and 14 healthy controls (Sommer *et al.*, 2007). Functional lateralization of the subjects was assessed using the same task and methods as in their study on monozygotic twins (Sommer *et al.*, 2004a). Patients from the three affected groups had a lower degree of functional lateralization of language than did healthy controls. Therefore, according to the authors, the anomaly of functional lateralization for language may not be specific to schizophrenia, but may be a general characteristic of psychosis.

In conclusion, all functional imaging studies (Artiges *et al.*, 2000; Dollfus *et al.*, 2005; Koeda *et al.*, 2006; Sommer *et al.*, 2001; Sommer *et al.*, 2003; Weiss *et al.*, 2004; Sommer *et al.*, 2004b; Weiss *et al.*, 2006) using FLI to study language lateralization support Crow's hypothesis that schizophrenia is associated with anomalies in the hemispheric specialization for language (Crow, 1997b). Schizophrenia patients had reduced or reversed FLI compared to control subjects during language tasks such as verb generation, verbal fluency, semantic decision making, and story and sentence listening. However, confounding variables can lead to different interpretations of the significance of the observed reduced hemispheric lateralization in schizophrenia.

Taken together, these studies support the point of view that a lower degree of language lateralization can be considered a trait marker for schizophrenia, according to the criteria of Szymanski (Szymanski *et al.*, 1994). Indeed, this decreased language lateralization:

- is distributed differently in psychotic individuals than in controls
- correlates with the subsequent development of psychotic spectrum illness in high-risk subjects
- is found in family members of psychotic patients
- is a reliable and stable trait over time.

However, studies have to demonstrate whether it occurs preceding the development of clinical manifestation of psychotic spectrum disease. The absence of specificity of this decreased language lateralization also needs to be confirmed in larger samples. However, these reports of decreased hemispheric lateralization in bipolar disorders support Crow's hypothesis of a continuum of psychosis between bipolar and schizophrenic disorders.

REFERENCES

Adcock, J. E., Wise, R. G., Oxbury, J. M., Oxbury, S. M. & Matthews, P. M. (2003). Quantitative fMRI assessment of the differences in lateralization of language-related brain activation in patients with temporal lobe epilepsy. *Neuroimage*, **18**, 423–38.

Artiges, E., Martinot, J. L., Verdys, M. *et al.* (2000). Altered hemispheric functional dominance during word generation in negative schizophrenia. *Schizophr Bull*, **26**, 709–21.

Ashton, L., Barnes, A., Livingston, M. & Wyper, D. (2000). Cingulate abnormalities associated with PANSS negative scores in first episode schizophrenia. *Behav Neurol*, **12**, 93–101.

Belin, P. & Zatorre, R. J. (2003). Adaptation to speaker's voice in right anterior temporal lobe. *Neuroreport*, **14**, 2105–9.

Belin, P., Zatorre, R. J., Lafaille, P., Ahad, P. & Pike, B. (2000). Voice-selective areas in human auditory cortex. *Nature*, **403**, 309–12.

Binder, J. R., Frost, J. A., Hammeke, T. A. *et al.* (1997). Human brain language areas identified by functional magnetic resonance imaging. *J Neurosci*, **17**, 353–62.

Boksman, K., Theberge, J., Williamson, P. *et al.* (2005). A 4.0-T fMRI study of brain connectivity during word fluency in first-episode schizophrenia. *Schizophr Res*, **75**, 247–63.

Broca, P. (1861). Perte de la parole, ramollissement chronique et destruction partielle du lobe antérieur gauche du cerveau. *Bull Soc Anthropol Paris*, **2**, 235–8.

Callicott, J. H., Mattay, V. S., Verchinski, B. A. *et al.* (2003). Complexity of prefrontal cortical dysfunction in schizophrenia: more than up or down. *Am J Psychiatry*, **160**, 2209–15.

Crinion, J. T., Lambon-Ralph, M. A., Warburton, E. A., Howard, D. & Wise, R. J. (2003). Temporal lobe regions engaged during normal speech comprehension. *Brain*, **126**, 1193–201.

Crow, T. J. (1997a). Is schizophrenia the price that *Homo sapiens* pays for language? *Schizophr Res*, **28**, 127–41.

Crow, T. J. (1997b). Schizophrenia as failure of hemispheric dominance for language. *Trends Neurosci*, **20**, 339–43.

Curtis, V. A., Bullmore, E. T., Brammer, M. J. *et al.* (1998). Attenuated frontal activation during a verbal fluency task in patients with schizophrenia. *Am J Psychiatry*, **155**, 1056–63.

Curtis, V. A., Bullmore, E. T., Morris, R. G. *et al.* (1999). Attenuated frontal activation in schizophrenia may be task dependent. *Schizophr Res*, **37**, 35–44.

Dollfus, S. & Brazo, P. (2003). Bases neurales des troubles du langage dans la schizophrénie. Cerveau et langage, Traité des sciences cognitives, Hermès Science Publications, Caen et Paris, **5**, 249–74.

Dollfus, S., Buijsrogge, J. A., Benali, K., Delamillieure, P. & Brazo, P. (2002). Sinistrality in subtypes of schizophrenia. *Eur Psychiatry*, **17**, 272–7.

Dollfus, S., Razafimandimby, A., Delamillieure, P. *et al.* (2005). Atypical hemispheric specialization for language in right-handed schizophrenia patients. *Biol Psychiatry*, **57**, 1020–8.

Dollfus, S., Razafimandimby, A., Maiza, O. *et al.* (2008). Functional deficit in the medial prefrontal cortex during a language comprehension task in patients with schizophrenia. *Schizophr Res*, **99**(1–3), 304–11.

Dye, S. M., Spence, S. A., Bench, C. J. *et al.* (1999). No evidence for left superior temporal dysfunction in asymptomatic schizophrenia and bipolar disorder. PET study of verbal fluency. *Br J Psychiatry*, **175**, 367–74.

Fernandez, G., Specht, K., Weis, S. *et al.* (2003). Intrasubject reproducibility of presurgical language lateralization and mapping using fMRI. *Neurology*, **60**, 969–75.

Frith, C. D. & Done, D. J. (1988). Towards a neuropsychology of schizophrenia. *Br J Psychiatry*, **153**, 437–43.

Frith, C. D., Friston, K. J., Herold, S. *et al.* (1995). Regional brain activity in chronic schizophrenic patients during the performance of a verbal fluency task. *Br J Psychiatry*, **167**, 343–9.

Frost, J. A., Binder, J. R., Springer, J. A. *et al.* (1999). Language processing is strongly left lateralized in both sexes. Evidence from functional MRI. *Brain*, **122**(Pt 2), 199–208.

Fu, C. H., Abel, K. M., Allin, M. P. *et al.* (2005a). Effects of ketamine on prefrontal and striatal regions in an overt verbal fluency task: a functional magnetic resonance imaging study. *Psychopharmacology*, **183**, 92–102.

Fu, C. H., Suckling, J., Williams, S. C. *et al.* (2005b). Effects of psychotic state and task demand on prefrontal function in schizophrenia: an fMRI study of overt verbal fluency. *Am J Psychiatry*, **162**, 485–94.

Gabrieli, J. D., Poldrack, R. A. & Desmond, J. E. (1998). The role of left prefrontal cortex in language and memory. *Proc Natl Acad Sci USA*, **95**, 906–13.

Gallagher, A. G., Dinan, T. G. & Baker, L. J. (1994). The effects of varying auditory input on schizophrenic hallucinations: a replication. *Br J Med Psychol*, **67**(Pt 1), 67–75.

Geschwind, N. & Levitsky, W. (1968). Human brain: left-right asymmetries in temporal speech region. *Science*, **161**, 186–7.

Green, M. F., Satz, P., Smith, C. & Nelson, L. (1989). Is there atypical handedness in schizophrenia? *J Abnorm Psychol*, **98**, 57–61.

Herve, P. Y., Razafimandimby, A., Dollfus S. & Tzourio-Mazoyer, N. (2006). Functional laterality imaged. *Neurosci Imag*, **1**(3), 183–205.

Hickok, G. & Poeppel, D. (2007). The cortical organization of speech processing. *Nat Rev Neurosci*, **8**, 393–402.

Highley, J. R., McDonald, B., Walker, M. A., Esiri, M. M. & Crow, T. J. (1999). Schizophrenia and temporal lobe asymmetry. A post-mortem stereological study of tissue volume. *Br J Psychiatry*, **175**, 127–34.

Hubrich-Ungureanu, P., Kaemmerer, N., Henn, F. A. & Braus, D. F. (2002). Lateralized organization of the cerebellum in a silent verbal fluency task: a functional magnetic resonance imaging study in healthy volunteers. *Neurosci Lett*, **319**, 91–4.

Jansen, A., Menke, R., Sommer, J. *et al.* (2006). The assessment of hemispheric lateralization in functional MRI - robustness and reproducibility. *Neuroimage*, **33**, 204–17.

Jones, H. M., Brammer, M. J., O'Toole, M. *et al.* (2004). Cortical effects of quetiapine in first-episode schizophrenia: a preliminary functional magnetic resonance imaging study. *Biol Psychiatry*, **56**, 938–42.

Kasai, K., Shenton, M. E., Salisbury, D. F. *et al.* (2003). Progressive decrease of left superior temporal gyrus gray matter volume in patients with first-episode schizophrenia. *Am J Psychiatry*, **160**, 156–64.

Kircher, T. T., Liddle, P. F., Brammer, M. J. *et al.* (2002). Reversed lateralization of temporal activation during speech production in thought disordered patients with schizophrenia. *Psychol Med*, **32**, 439–49.

Koeda, M., Takahashi, H., Yahata, N. *et al.* (2006). Language processing and human voice perception in schizophrenia: a functional magnetic resonance imaging study. *Biol Psychiatry*, **59**, 948–57.

Lennox, B. R., Park, S. B., Medley, I., Morris, P. G. & Jones, P. B. (2000). The functional anatomy of auditory hallucinations in schizophrenia. *Psychiatry Res*, **100**, 13–20.

Li, X., Branch, C. A., Ardekani, B. A. *et al.* (2007). fMRI study of language activation in schizophrenia, schizoaffective disorder and in individuals genetically at high risk. *Schizophr Res*, **96**, 14–24.

Lurito, J. T., Kareken, D. A., Lowe, M. J., Chen, S. H. & Mathews, V. P. (2000). Comparison of rhyming and word generation with FMRI. *Hum Brain Mapp*, **10**, 99–106.

Maiza, O., Razafimandimby, P., Delamillieure, P. *et al.* (2008). Functional deficit in medial prefrontal cortex: a common neural basis for impaired communication in chronic schizophrenia and bipolar disorders. *Schizophr Res*, **98**(1), 39.

Manoach, D. S. (1994). Handedness is related to formal thought disorder and language dysfunction in schizophrenia. *J Clin Exp Neuropsychol*, **16**, 2–14.

Mazoyer, B., Tzourio-Mazoyer, N., Frak, V. *et al.* (1993). The cortical representation of speech. *J Cogn Neurosci*, **5**, 467–79.

McGuire, P. K., Silbersweig, D. A., Murray, R. M. *et al.* (1996). Functional anatomy of inner speech and auditory verbal imagery. *Psychol Med*, **26**, 29–38.

McGuire, P. K., Silbersweig, D. A., Wright, I. (1995). Abnormal monitoring of inner speech: a physiological basis for auditory hallucinations. *Lancet*, **346**, 596–600.

Nayani, T. H. & David, A. S. (1996). The auditory hallucination: a phenomenological survey. *Psychol Med*, **26**, 177–89.

Papathanassiou, D., Etard, O., Mellet, E. *et al.* (2000). A common language network for comprehension and production: a contribution to the definition of language epicenters with PET. *Neuroimage*, **11**, 347–57.

Pearlson, G. D., Petty, R. G., Ross, C. A. & Tien, A. Y. (1996). Schizophrenia: a disease of heteromodal association cortex? *Neuropsychopharmacology*, **14**, 1–17.

Perani, D., Dehaene, S., Grassi, F. *et al.* (1996). Brain processing of native and foreign languages. *Neuroreport*, **7**, 2439–44.

Pujol, J., Deus, J., Losilla, J. M. & Capdevila, A. (1999). Cerebral lateralization of language in normal left-handed people studied by functional MRI. *Neurology*, **52**, 1038–43.

Razafimandimby, A., Maiza, O., Herve, P. Y. *et al.* (2007). Stability of functional language lateralization over time in schizophrenia patients. *Schizophr Res*, **94**, 197–206.

Razafimandimby, A., Tzourio-Mazoyer, N., Herve, P. Y. *et al.* (2006). Handedness and hemispheric specialization for language in schizophrenic patients. *Schizophr Res*, Supplement **1**, 33–4.

Rutten, G. J., Ramsey, N. F., van Rijen, P. C. & van Veelen, C. W. (2002). Reproducibility of fMRI-determined language lateralization in individual subjects. *Brain Lang*, **80**, 421–37.

Satz, P. & Green, M. F. (1999). Atypical handedness in schizophrenia: some methodological and theoretical issues. *Schizophr Bull*, **25**, 63–78.

Schaufelberger, M., Senhorini, M. C., Barreiros, M. A. (2005). Frontal and anterior cingulate activation during overt verbal fluency in patients with first episode psychosis. *Rev Bras Psiquiatr*, **27**, 228–32.

Schlosser, M. J., Aoyagi, N., Fulbright, R. K., Gore, J. C. & McCarthy, G. (1998). Functional MRI studies of auditory comprehension. *Hum Brain Mapp*, **6**, 1–13.

Shapleske, J., Rossell, S. L., Woodruff, P. W. & David, A. S. (1999). The planum temporale: a systematic, quantitative review of its structural, functional and clinical significance. *Brain Res Brain Res Rev*, **29**, 26–49.

Shergill, S. S., Bullmore, E., Simmons, A., Murray, R. & McGuire, P. (2000). Functional anatomy of auditory verbal imagery in schizophrenic patients with auditory hallucinations. *Am J Psychiatry*, **157**, 1691–3.

Sommer, I. E., Ramsey, N. F. & Kahn, R. S. (2001). Language lateralization in schizophrenia, an fMRI study. *Schizophr Res*, **52**, 57–67.

Sommer, I. E., Ramsey, N. F., Mandl, R. C. & Kahn, R. S. (2003). Language lateralization in female patients with schizophrenia: an fMRI study. *Schizophr Res*, **60**, 183–90.

Sommer, I. E., Ramsey, N. F., Mandl, R. C., van Oel, C. J. & Kahn, R. S. (2004b). Language activation in monozygotic twins discordant for schizophrenia. *Br J Psychiatry*, **184**, 128–35.

Sommer, I. E., Ramsey, N. F., Mandl, R. C., van Oel, C. J. & Kahn, R. S. (2004a). Language activation in monozygotic twins discordant for schizophrenia. *Br J Psychiatry*, **184**, 128–35.

Sommer, I. E., Vd Veer, A. J., Wijkstra, J., Boks, M. P. & Kahn, R. S. (2007). Comparing language lateralization in psychotic mania and psychotic depression to schizophrenia: a functional MRI study. *Schizophr Res*, **89**, 364–5.

Spence, S. A., Hirsch, S. R., Brooks, D. J. & Grasby, P. M. (1998). Prefrontal cortex activity in people with schizophrenia and control subjects. Evidence from positron emission tomography for remission of "hypofrontality" with recovery from acute schizophrenia. *Br J Psychiatry*, **172**, 316–23.

Spence, S. A., Liddle, P. F., Stefan, M. D. (2000). Functional anatomy of verbal fluency in people with schizophrenia and those at genetic risk. Focal dysfunction and distributed disconnectivity reappraised. *Br J Psychiatry*, **176**, 52–60.

Szymanski, S., Kane, J. & Lieberman, J. (1994). *Trait Markers in Schizophrenia: Are They Diagnostic?* DSM-IV Source Book, Washington DC, pp. 477–92.

Tzourio, N., Crivello, F., Mellet, E., Nkanga-Ngila, B. & Mazoyer, B. (1998). Functional dominance for speech comprehension in left handers vs right handers. *Neuroimage*, **8**, 1–16.

Tzourio-Mazoyer, N., Josse, G., Crivello, F. & Mazoyer, B. (2004). Interindividual variability in the hemispheric organization for speech. *Neuroimage*, **21**, 422–35.

Tzourio-Mazoyer, N., Landeau, B., Papathanassiou, D. (2002). Automated anatomical labeling of activations in SPM using a macroscopic anatomical parcellation of the MNI MRI single-subject brain. *Neuroimage*, **15**, 273–89.

Weiss, E. M., Hofer, A., Golaszewski, S. (2004). Brain activation patterns during a verbal fluency test-a functional MRI study in healthy volunteers and patients with schizophrenia. *Schizophr Res*, **70**, 287–91.

Weiss, E. M., Hofer, A., Golaszewski, S. *et al.* (2006). Language lateralization in unmedicated patients during an acute episode of schizophrenia: a functional MRI study. *Psychiatry Res*, **146**, 185–90.

Whalley, H. C., Simonotto, E., Moorhead, W. (2006). Functional imaging as a predictor of schizophrenia. *Biol Psychiatry*, **60**, 454–62.

Whitford, T. J., Grieve, S. M., Farrow, T. F. (2006). Progressive grey matter atrophy over the first 2–3 years of illness in first-episode schizophrenia: a tensor-based morphometry study. *Neuroimage*, **32**, 511–19.

Woodruff, P. W., Wright, I. C., Bullmore, E. T. (1997). Auditory hallucinations and the temporal cortical response to speech in schizophrenia: a functional magnetic resonance imaging study. *Am J Psychiatry*, **154**, 1676–82.

Yurgelun-Todd, D. A., Coyle, J. T., Gruber, S. A. *et al.* (2005). Functional magnetic resonance imaging studies of schizophrenic patients during word production: effects of D-cycloserine. *Psychiatry Res*, **138**, 23–31.

Yurgelun-Todd, D. A., Waternaux, C. M., Cohen, B. M. *et al.* (1996). Functional magnetic resonance imaging of schizophrenic patients and comparison subjects during word production. *Am J Psychiatry*, **153**, 200–5.

10

The role of the right hemisphere for language in schizophrenia

Alexander Rapp

Summary

Although there is no question that the left hemisphere is the superior language processor, a growing body of research proves the "non-verbal" right hemisphere is as well involved in the language comprehension process on higher linguistic levels. Traditionally, especially the processing of non-literal and figurative expressions is attributed to the right cerebral hemisphere. This chapter will review the lateralization of non-literal language in healthy individuals and schizophrenia.

Non-literal language is a heterogeneous linguistic entity of speech forms that go beyond the literal meaning of the words and require the ability to process more than the literal meaning of an utterance in order to grasp the speaker's intention. It includes metaphors, proverbs, idioms, irony, sarcasm, and metonymy.

There is good evidence in the literature that schizophrenic patients are impaired in understanding various types of non-literal expressions, although not all schizophrenia patients have problems in understanding non-literal language. The general consensus used to be that non-literal language represents a "right hemisphere language function" and that thereby these deficits are evidence for a right hemisphere deficit in schizophrenia. However, recent research on the functional neuroanatomy of non-literal language suggests that both hemispheres significantly contribute to non-literal language processing with marked differences between different types of non-literal language. Task instructions and linguistic properties of the non-literal utterances significantly alter hemispheric lateralization. These factors limit the conclusions that can be drawn from behavioral studies on non-literal language comprehension in schizophrenia. Some evidence comes from recent research with functional magnetic resonance imaging in schizophrenia, in which altered right hemisphere activation in schizophrenia could be demonstrated during metaphor comprehension. In addition, evidence for reversed lateralization comes from an imaging study investigating emotional prosody in schizophrenia.

Taken together, the evidence about lateralization processes of higher order language functions in psychosis is less clear than for lower level semantics such as processing of single words or literal sentences.

Left lateralization of language is among the most well established findings in research on cerebral lateralization. Although there is no question that the left hemisphere is the superior language processor, a growing body of research has demonstrated significant linguistic abilities in the "non-verbal" right hemisphere (Lindell, 2006). Traditionally, especially the processing of non-literal and figurative expressions is attributed to the right cerebral hemisphere (Burgess & Chiarello, 1996; Bookheimer, 2002). Non-literal language is a heterogeneous linguistic entity of speech forms that go beyond the literal meaning of the words and require the ability to process more than the literal meaning of an utterance in order to grasp the speaker's intention in a given context. Non-literal language includes metaphors, proverbs, idioms, irony, sarcasm, and metonymy. Research on these types of language has attracted a lot of interest in schizophrenia research mainly for two reasons. First, deficits in understanding non-literal expressions are long-known to be important symptoms of schizophrenia (Gorham, 1956). In addition, right hemisphere language functions may provide important insights into language lateralization processes in this disorder. Among others, Crow (Crow, 2004; Mitchell & Crow, 2005) suggested that reduced cerebral lateralization could affect language functions normally located in

Language Lateralization and Psychosis, ed. Iris E. C. Sommer and René S. Kahn. Published by Cambridge University Press.
© Cambridge University Press 2009.

the right hemisphere. He hypothesized that reversed left-lateralization effects for right hemisphere language functions might occur. Such reversed lateralization effects have indeed been demonstrated for emotional prosody (Mitchell *et al.*, 2004) and formal thought disorder (Kircher *et al.*, 2002) in schizophrenia.

This chapter will review lateralization processes for non-literal language in healthy subjects, brain lesioned patients, and schizophrenia patients with special focus on metaphor, proverbs, idioms, irony, and sarcasm.

Metaphors (such as "hard work is a ladder" or "life is a journey") are used for conceptualizing and making expressible relevant parts of our lives that are otherwise difficult to explain. Taken literally, metaphoric statements are mostly wrong (Carroll, 1999). The meaning of a metaphor is implied through association and comparison of similarities between different expressions that are not stated explicitly. Beyond semantic and word-by-word analysis, understanding the figurative meaning of a metaphor requires mental linkage of different category domains normally not related to each other (Gibbs, 1990; Glucksberg, 2003). In linguistics, metaphors are often divided into salient and non-salient metaphors (Giora, 2003). Salient metaphors (such as "broken heart") are frequently used in everyday language. They are sometimes called "dead" metaphors. In contrast, non-salient metaphors are not conventional in everyday language.

A metonymy is a trope in which one entity is used to stand for another associated entity (for example "Kremlin" for "the Russian government"). Metonymies are often used in newspaper headlines. In contrast to metaphors, metonymy works more by contiguity between two concepts, whereas metaphors work more by the similarity between them (Lakoff & Johnson, 1980). Proverbs are simple, popularly known sayings based on a common sense or practical experience. Proverbs are often – but not always – metaphorical. Idioms are structurally "frozen", which means they are fixed expressions. Idioms form a large group both in terms of syntactic and semantic characteristics. Some idioms – like metaphors – can be understood by comparison of the semantic entities within, whereas others can not (like "kick the bucket", which in English language is an idiomatic expression for "to die").

In verbal irony the speaker uses words that express something other – in most cases the opposite – of what he literally says. Detecting irony involves rather complex mental representations, as the listener needs to understand not only that the speaker does not mean exactly what she/he said, but also that she/he does not expect to be taken literally. Irony comprehension deserves intact "theory of mind" processing (Brune, 2005). Sarcasm is mostly defined as a severe form of irony often intended to insult or wound. In sarcastic expressions the speaker says the opposite of what he means (for example "this is just great" after something bad happens). Sarcasm can be difficult to grasp in written form and is easily misinterpreted.

Although all these language forms are usually mentioned together in the psychiatric literature on hemispheric lateralization, the various different forms of non-literal language differ in their structure, communicative function, and processing demands (Winner & Gardner, 1993; Zaidel *et al.*, 2002; Giora, 2007). For example, metaphor describes or shows something in a different way, while irony reveals something about the speaker. (Some forms of humor and processing indirect requests and faux pas can as well be seen as non-literal expressions. However, this chapter will focus on the above-mentioned language forms, because most studies have been carried out with these types of non-literal language. See Lindell, 2006; Mitchell & Crow, 2005; and Champagne-Lavau *et al.*, 2006 for comprehensive review of other types of non-literal language.)

Hemispheric lateralization of non-literal language has been of interest in the literature for some time. There are studies in patients with brain lesions, as well as research using functional magnetic resonance imaging, repetitive transcranial magnetic stimulation (rTMS), and hemifield investigations.

Metaphor comprehension has been investigated in a number of studies with heterogeneous results. Most studies in patients with brain lesions used picture matching tasks, where patients with a lesion in either hemisphere had to match orally presented metaphors with an appropriate picture (Hillekamp *et al.*, 1996; MacKenzie, 1997; Winner & Gardner, 1997; Gagnon *et al.*, 2003). In this task, patients with left hemisphere damage performed well (Winner & Garner, 1977), whereas right hemisphere-lesioned patients often choose pictures with a literal interpretation of the metaphor (Winner & Gardner, 1977; Hillekamp *et al.*, 1996). However, results from these tests poorly correlate with other tests of metaphor comprehension (Zaidel *et al.*, 2002; Rinaldi *et al.*, 2004; Papagno *et al.*, 2006). For example in a study by Rinaldi *et al.* (2004), right hemisphere-damaged patients performed much better when matching the meaning of metaphors with sentences than with pictures. Other studies assessed brain-lesioned patients' ability to give short verbal explanations of metaphoric expressions. Patients with right hemisphere lesions gave adequate descriptions of metaphors (Giora *et al.*, 2000; Winner & Gardner, 1977); however, it has been hypothesized that this may be only the case for short, highly conventional metaphors (Giora *et al.*, 2000). In contrast, left hemisphere-damaged patients often offer "concrete" or "literal" verbal explanations of the metaphors (Winner & Gardner, 1977), despite that some authors reported an antithetical tendency of left hemisphere-damaged patients towards metaphoric interpretations (McIntyre, 1976; Burgess & Chiarello, 1996). Results from lesion studies on phrasal metaphors are not fully compatible with studies investigating single metaphoric words either (see Gagnon *et al.*, 2003; Faust & Weisper, 2000). Besides these lesion studies, a number of brain imaging studies have investigated the functional neuroanatomy of metaphor comprehension. As in the lesion studies, results are heterogeneous concerning cerebral lateralization. Whereas some studies reported differences between metaphoric phrases (Rapp *et al.*, 2004, 2007) or words (Lee & Dapretto, 2006) relative to literal expressions only in the left cerebral hemisphere, other studies reported differences in both hemispheres (Ahrens *et al.*, 2007; Stringaris *et al.*, 2006, 2007; Eviatar & Just, 2006; Mashal *et al.*, 2005, 2007). Importantly, none of these studies has replicated a finding from a 1994 positron emission tomography study, which found differences between metaphoric and literal sentences only in the right hemisphere (Bottini *et al.*, 1994). Taken together, data from both lesion and fMRI studies suggest that (1) both hemispheres contribute to metaphor comprehension and

that (2) there are moderators that can affect the extent to which the right cerebral hemisphere is involved in comprehending metaphoric expressions. However, there is no general consensus about these moderators (Giora, 2007). Some authors suggested that linguistic properties of the metaphors modulate right hemisphere involvement. For example, the "graded salience hypothesis" postulates that only "non-salient" metaphors, but not commonly used figurative expressions, are processed in the right cerebral hemisphere (Giora, 1997). This theory is supported by some (Ahrens *et al.*, 2007; Giora *et al.*, 2000) but not all (Rapp *et al.*, 2004, 2007; Lee & Dapretto, 2006) investigations. In addition, task differences within the studies significantly modulated right hemisphere involvement (Winner & Gardner, 1977; Rinaldi *et al.*, 2004; Kacinik & Chiarello, 2007). Based on these findings it has been concluded that other factors than metaphoricity per se are crucial for the extent that the right hemisphere is needed for metaphor comprehension (Rapp *et al.*, 2004; Giora, 2007). This conclusion is of importance for studies in clinical populations, because a deficit in metaphor comprehension does not necessarily imply a right hemisphere deficit (Rapp *et al.*, 2007; Champagne-Lavau *et al.*, 2007).

As in the case of metaphors, research on the functional neuroanatomy of idioms yielded heterogeneous results. Zempleni and colleagues (2007) investigated comprehension of Dutch idioms in 15 healthy subjects and found differential activation in both cerebral hemispheres for understanding idioms relative to matched literal expressions. In line with this result, Lauro and colleagues found differences for Italian idioms relative to literal expressions in both cerebral hemispheres when subjects were judging whether a sentence (either proverb or literal) is congruent with a picture (Lauro *et al.*, 2007).

Rizzo and colleagues (Rizzo *et al.*, 2007) used repetitive transcranial magnetic stimulation (rTMS) to investigate the neuroanatomy of idiom comprehension. In their study, 14 healthy subjects were treated with rTMS while they were matching the meaning of Italian idioms with one out of four pictures that showed the figurative meaning of the idiom. Repetitive transcranial magnetic stimulation to the left inferior frontal region attenuated the accuracy of idiom comprehension in both hemi-spheres. They concluded that the prefrontal cortex of both cerebral hemispheres is involved in idiom com-prehension. However, bilateral comprehension pro-cesses may not occur in all types of idiomatic expressions. In an investigation from the same work-group, rTMS over the right cerebral hemisphere failed to influence idiom comprehension when opaque idi-oms were used as stimuli. As in metaphors, laterality of idioms is significantly affected by the type of task and type of idiom used in brain lesion studies (Olivieri *et al.*, 2004; Papagno & Caporali, 2007).

In contrast to the findings in metaphor and idioms, all brain lesion studies on irony and sarcasm compre-hension consistently showed a significant role of the right cerebral hemisphere (Bihrle *et al.*, 1986; McDonald, 2000; Giora *et al.*, 2000; Zaidel *et al.*, 2002; Shamay-Tsoory *et al.*, 2005), although different tasks and stimulus types were used in these studies. Right hemisphere involvement in irony comprehension is further supported by two recent fMRI investigations. Eviatar and Just (2006) used fMRI to examine brain activation patterns while 16 healthy participants read brief three-sentence stories that concluded with either a literal, metaphoric, or ironic sentence. The fMRI images acquired during the reading of the critical sen-tence revealed a selective response of the brain to the two types of non-literal utterances. Ironic statements resulted in significantly higher activation levels than literal statements in the right superior and middle tem-poral gyri, with metaphoric statements resulting in intermediate levels in these regions. In addition, Wang *et al.* (2006) demonstrated right hemisphere fMRI activation during irony comprehension in children.

Laterality in metonymy comprehension is largely unknown. However, preliminary fMRI results from our workgroup suggest that phrasal metonymies – like metaphors – activate the left inferior frontal gyrus in contrast to literal sentences (Rapp *et al.*, unpublished manuscript).

Besides patients with brain lesions, subjects with schizophrenia exhibit difficulties in understanding non-literal language. Language comprehension def-icits in general represent a hallmark symptom of schiz-ophrenia (Crow, 1997, 2000). However, it has been noted early on that schizophrenic patients are exceedingly impaired in the use of non-literal language. Anecdotal reports of inability to understand non-literal language ("schizophrenic concretism") date back to the beginning of the last century (Finckh, 1906; Vigotsky, 1934; Gorham, 1956). The characteristic problems of schizophrenic patients in understanding non-literal language have been shown in numerous studies and clinical reports (see Thoma & Daum, 2006 and Champagne-Lavau *et al.*, 2006 for comprehensive reviews). They are included in established psycho-pathology rating scales. For example the positive and negative syndrome scale (PANSS) (Kay *et al.*, 1987), includes an item in which the patient is asked to give a verbal explanation of a proverb. The answer is then rated in terms of concreteness. Following a discussion in the middle of the last century, it is now clear that non-literal language comprehension deficits are not a specific symptom of schizophrenia (Andreasen, 1977), but can be present in many psychiatric disorders including autism (Dennis *et al.*, 2001) and Alzheimer's disease (Papagno, 2001).

Impaired non-literal language comprehension skills in schizophrenia have been demonstrated for all types of non-literal language. Schizophrenic patients exhibit severe difficulties interpreting metaphors and prov-erbs, with an impaired interpretation of non-literal utterances including a preference for the literal rather than figurative interpretation of metaphors (Chapman, 1960; Cutting & Murphy, 1990; Drury *et al.*, 1998). They have difficulties in selecting appropriate pictures to match the figurative meaning of metaphors, and this deficit is present early in the course of the illness (Anand *et al.*, 1994). It has been suggested that non-literal language comprehension deficits might be a potential endophenotypical marker of schizophre-nia (Allen & Schuldberg, 1989; Langdon & Coltheart, 2004; Nunn & Peters, 2001; Thoma & Daum, 2006). De-Bonis *et al.* (1997) demonstrated that schizophrenia patients are impaired in matching metaphors and prov-erbs that are similar in meaning at a figurative level. Patients also have deficits in detecting and compre-hending irony (Langdon *et al.*, 2002; Drury *et al.*, 1998; Mitchley *et al.*, 1998; Herold *et al.*, 2002; Hensler *et al.*, 2007) and sarcasm (Leitman *et al.*, 2006).

Furthermore, deficits have been demonstrated in the comprehension and use of indirect speech (Mitchell & Crow, 2005), metonymy (Rhodes & Jakes, 2004; Hensler et al., 2007) and humor (Drury et al., 1998; Mitchell & Crow, 2005; Falkenberg et al., 2007). Non-literal language deficits seem to have significant impact on social interaction (Brune, 2005; Langdon et al., 2002) and are associated with impaired psychosocial functioning (Rapp et al., 2007b).

Disruptions of non-literal language comprehension are clinically tested routinely by asking the patient to interpret metaphorical proverbs (Finckh, 1906; Kay et al., 1987; Vigotsky, 1934). Typically, only the literal but not the metaphoric meaning is realized (Gorham, 1956; Iakimova et al., 2005; Watson et al., 1979), although not all patients exhibit this deficit (Titone et al., 2002; Iakimova et al., 2005; Thoma & Daum, 2005).

Few studies have investigated the relationship between non-literal language comprehension and psychopathology in schizophrenia. Langdon et al. (2002) demonstrated an association between poor appreciation of irony and positive formal thought disorder in the PANSS. Negative formal thought disorder was associated with impaired metaphor comprehension. In the context of laterality research, these issues are of importance since formal thought disorder itself is likewise associated with laterality (see Chapter 12). Yet, it has been criticized that most studies used inconsistent diagnostic tools and investigated moderately ill patients (Thoma & Daum, 2006). Several models have been proposed for non-literal language comprehension deficits in schizophrenia including impairment in theory of mind functions (Corcoran et al., 1995; Mitchley et al., 1998; Janssen et al., 2003; Brune, 2005), deficits in context processing (Besche et al., 1996) or executive functions (Brune & Bodenstein, 2005; Sponheim et al., 2003; Janssen et al., 2003) (see Champagne-Lavau et al., 2006 for review).

Laterality of non-literal language comprehension in schizophrenia has been of scientific interest for some time. Impaired non-literal language comprehension skills have been seen as an argument for right hemisphere involvement in the pathophysiology of the disorder (e.g., Kircher et al., 2001; Langdon et al., 2002; Langdon & Coultheart, 2004; Mitchell & Crow, 2005).

However, so far only few studies have investigated laterality of non-literal language in psychosis directly. Because of the marked differences in the studies mentioned above, this is a crucial point.

Champagne-Lavau and colleagues (2007) investigated idiom comprehension in both right hemisphere damaged patients and subjects with DSM-IV schizophrenia. The result showed differences between the two groups: whereas right hemisphere damaged patients were impaired only in understanding non-idiomatic metaphors, schizophrenia patients had difficulties in understanding both idiomatic and non-idiomatic metaphors. The authors concluded that different cognitive deficits may account for the difficulties of the two groups (Champagne-Lavan et al., 2006, 2007). In other words, many different cognitive dysfunctions may result in an impairment of non-literal utterances.

Functional imaging studies may help to clarify the question whether a right or left hemisphere deficit is crucial for non-literal language comprehension deficits in schizophrenia. Kircher et al. (2007) investigated comprehension of metaphoric sentences in patients with schizophrenia and healthy control subjects. Twelve subacute in- and outpatients with schizophrenia (DSM-IV) and a control group of twelve healthy volunteers matched for sex, age, and demographic variables participated in this event-related fMRI experiment. All subjects were carefully selected right-handers (Annett, 1970). The control group did not significantly differ in verbal IQ (Lehrl & Triebig, 1995) and Digit span. The mean duration of illness in the patients was nine years and all were on stable doses of atypical antipsychotic medication.

A set of 60 sentences (30 metaphors with their literal counterparts) were chosen as stimuli for the fMRI experiment. The sentences were matched for syntax structure, number of words, word frequency, content, and tense. The metaphors were non-salient, which means they were created de novo for the experiment and are not listed in the German Duden dictionary for idioms (Duden, 1998). To avoid effects of complex syntax processing, all stimulus sentences were simple statements (like: an "a" is a "b"). Sentence pairs differed only in their last one to three words and had a metaphoric (e.g., "the lover's words are harp sounds") or a literal ("the lover's words are lies") meaning. During the fMRI scan, the task

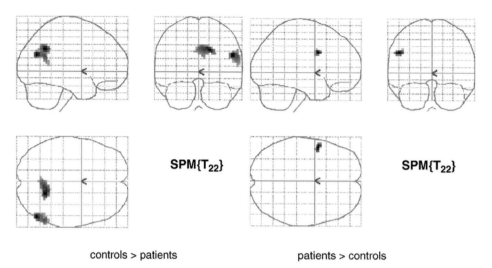

controls > patients   patients > controls

Figure 10.1 Brain activation during reading of non-salient metaphoric sentences (Kircher *et al.*, 2007). Comparison between 12 patients with DSM IV schizophrenia and healthy control subjects. Left: areas in which control subjects showed significantly greater activation compared to patients during processing of metaphors vs. baseline. Two clusters emerged, the right precuneus and the right middle/superior temporal gyrus. Right: areas in which patients showed significantly greater activation compared to controls during processing of metaphors vs. baseline: the left inferior frontal gyrus. (Kircher *et al.*, 2007, with permission from Elsevier.)

for the subjects was to read sentences silently and then to respond by pressing one of two buttons with the right index finger to indicate whether the sentence had a positive or negative connotation. Stimuli were presented in a pseudorandomized order and counterbalanced across subjects, so that subjects saw only one version of each sentence pair (metaphor or literal sentence) during the experiment. See Figure 10.1.

Compared with the patient group, the healthy subjects showed stronger signal changes for the contrast metaphors vs. low level baseline in the right superior/middle temporal gyrus (BA 39). This difference was not present during reading of literal sentences. In contrast, the patient group activated more the left inferior frontal gyrus. To test the hypothesis that the differential signal between patients and control subjects may be related to concretism, a simple regression analysis was applied. This type of analysis reveals in which brain areas the fMRI BOLD-contrast (functional magnetic resonance imaging, blood-oxygen-level-dependent) difference between the participants is explained by a covariate. The PANSS item N5 "abstract thinking difficulties" (concretism) was used as covariate. To judge this

PANSS item, the patient is asked to give a verbal explanation of a proverb and the answer is rated in terms of concreteness. A significant negative correlation with brain activation during reading metaphors was present only in the left hemisphere inferior frontal gyrus (BA 45), an area crucially involved in the comprehension of metaphors (Rapp *et al.*, 2004) and idioms (Zempleni *et al.*, 2007; Lauro *et al.*, 2007).

In another study, Zempleni (2006) investigated comprehension of familiar Dutch idioms in patients with DSM-IV schizophrenia. In healthy subjects, the task used by Zempleni induced tendentially more right hemisphere activation than the non-salient metaphors used in the Kircher *et al.* investigation (Zempleni *et al.*, 2007 in contrast to Rapp *et al.*, 2004). As in the Kircher *et al.* investigation, there was no evidence for increased right hemisphere involvement in the patient group. Instead, schizophrenic patients showed a different pattern of activation mainly in the left prefrontal cortex. However, this study has the severe limitation that only five schizophrenic patients were investigated.

Taken together, the two investigations suggest that both cerebral hemispheres contribute to metaphor comprehension, while severity of concretism in schizophrenia may be related to left hemisphere rather than right hemisphere function.

This is compatible with research on prosody, which also represents a right hemisphere language function, although recent research suggests that some prosody comprehension tasks might measure left hemisphere functions (see Wildgruber *et al.*, 2006, for this topic). Mitchell and colleagues (2004) investigated neural correlates of prosody in schizophrenia using fMRI. Twelve patients with ICD-10 schizophrenia and thirteen matched healthy controls passively listened or attended to sentences that differed in emotional prosody. Patients with schizophrenia exhibited normal right-lateralization of the passive response to "pure" emotional prosody and relative left-lateralization of the response to unfiltered emotional prosody. When attending to emotional prosody, patients with schizophrenia activated the left insula more than healthy controls. The authors concluded that schizophrenia patients show some reversal of the normal right-lateralized temporal lobe response to emotional prosody.

Other non-literal language functions such as metonymy and irony/sarcasm comprehension have not yet been investigated with functional imaging in schizophrenia. Such studies would be interesting, because of the better evidence for right hemisphere involvement in irony comprehension relative to metaphor, and the findings that suggest that irony and metaphor comprehension skills are only fairly correlated in schizophrenia (Brune, 2005) and in functional imaging studies of healthy subjects (Eviatar & Just, 2006).

In conclusion, there is good evidence in the literature that schizophrenic patients are impaired in understanding various types of non-literal expressions including metaphors, proverbs, and irony/ sarcasm, although not all schizophrenia patients have problems in understanding non-literal language. The general consensus used to be that non-literal language represents a "right hemisphere language function" and that thereby these deficits are an evidence for a right hemisphere deficit in schizophrenia (Mitchell & Crow, 2005). However, recent research on the functional neuroanatomy of non-literal language suggests that both hemispheres significantly contribute to non-literal language processing with marked differences between different types of non-literal language. Task instructions and linguistic properties of the non-literal utterances significantly alter hemispheric lateralization (Giora, 2007). These factors limit the conclusions that can be drawn from behavioral studies on non-literal language comprehension in schizophrenia. One functional imaging study demonstrated altered right hemisphere activation during non-literal language tasks in schizophrenia (Kircher *et al.*, 2007). In addition, evidence for reversed lateralization was present in a study investigating emotional prosody in schizophrenia (Mitchell *et al.*, 2004). These findings need to be replicated for other types of non-literal language.

Taken together, the evidence about lateralization processes of higher order language functions in psychosis is less clear than for lower level semantics such as processing of single words or literal sentences. The following chapters will demonstrate that symptomatology in schizophrenia, especially hallucinations and formal thought disorder, can interact or correlate with language lateralization in schizophrenia subjects. How these factors interact with laterality of non-literal language comprehension processes is not yet clear. Further research is needed to disentangle laterality of non-literal language in schizophrenia. These studies should recommend effects of task instructions and linguistic properties of non-literal expressions.

REFERENCES

Ahrens, K., Liu, H. L., Lee, C. Y. *et al.* (2007). Functional MRI of conventional and anomalous metaphors in Mandarin Chinese. *Brain Lang.*, **100**(2), 163–71.

Allen, J. & Schuldberg, D. (1989). Positive thought disorder in a hypothetically psychosis-prone population. *J. Abnorm. Psychol.*, **98**, 491.

Anand, A., Wales, R. J., Jackson, H. J. & Copolov, D. L. (1994). Linguistic impairment in early psychosis. *J. Nerv. Ment. Dis.*, **182**(9), 488–93.

Andreasen, N. C. (1977). Reliability and validity of proverb interpretation to assess mental status. *Compr. Psychiatry*, **18**(5), 465–72.

Annett, M. (1970). A classification of hand preference by association analysis. *Br. J. Psychol.*, **61**, 303–21.

Besche, C., Passerieux, C., Segui, J., Mesure, G. & Hardy-Baylé, M. C. (1996). Processing of contextual syntactic information in a decision making task in schizophrenic subjects. *Can. J. Psychiatry*, **41**(9), 587–94.

Bihrle, A. M., Brownell, H. H., Powelson, J. A. & Gardner, H. (1986). Comprehension of humorous and nonhumorous materials by left and right brain-damaged patients. *Brain Cogn.*, **5**, 399–412.

Bookheimer, S. (2002). Functional MRI of language: new approaches to understanding the cortical organization of semantic processing. *Annu. Rev. Neurosci.*, **25**, 151–88.

Bottini, G., Corcoran, R., Sterzi, R. *et al.* (1994). The role of the right hemisphere in the interpretation of figurative aspects of language. A positron emission tomography activation study. *Brain*, **117**, 1241–53.

Burgess, C. & Chiarello, C. (1996). Neurocognitive mechanisms underlying metaphor comprehension and other figurative language. *Metaphor. Symb. Act.*, **11**, 67–84.

Brune, M. (2005). "Theory of mind" in schizophrenia: a review of the literature. *Schizophr. Bull.*, **31**(1), 21–42.

Brune, M. & Bodenstein, L. (2005). Proverb comprehension reconsidered – "theory of mind" and the pragmatic use of language in schizophrenia. *Schizophr. Res.*, **75**, 233.

Carroll, D. (1999). *Psychology of Language*, 3rd edn, Pacific Grove: Brooks/Cole, pp. 142–6.

Champagne-Lavau, M., Stip, E. & Joanette, Y. (2006). Social cognition deficits in schizophrenia: accounting for pragmatic deficits in communication abilities? *Curr. Psychiatry Reviews*, **2**(3), 309–15.

Champagne-Lavau, M., Stip, E. & Joanette, Y. (2007). Language functions in right-hemisphere damage and schizophrenia: apparently similar pragmatic deficits may hide profound differences. *Brain*, **130**(2), e67.

Chapman, L. J. (1960). Confusion of figurative and literal usages of words by schizophrenics and brain damaged patients. *J. Abnorm. Soc. Psychol.*, **60**, 412–16.

Corcoran, R., Mercer, G. & Frith, C. D. (1995). Schizophrenia, symptomatology and social inference: investigating "theory of mind" in people with schizophrenia. *Schizophr. Res.*, **17**, 5–13.

Crow, T. J. (1997). Schizophrenia as failure of hemispheric dominance for language. *Trends Neurosci.*, **29**, 339–43.

Crow, T. J. (2000). Schizophrenia as the price that *Homo sapiens* pays for language: a resolution of the central paradox in the origin of the species. *Brain Res. Rev.*, **31**, 118–29.

Crow, T. J. (2004). Auditory hallucinations as primary disorders of syntax: an evolutionary theory of the origins of language. *Cogn. Neuropsychiatry*, **9**(1–2), 125–45.

Cutting, J. & Murphy, D. (1990). Preference for denotative as opposed to connotative meanings in schizophrenics. *Brain Lang.*, **39**, 459–68.

De-Bonis, M., Epelbaum, C., DeVez, V. & Feline, A. (1997). The comprehension of metaphors in schizophrenia. *Psychopathology*, **30**, 149–54.

Dennis, M., Lazenby, A. L. & Lockyer, L. (2001). Inferential language in high-function children with autism. *J. Autism Dev. Disord.*, **31**, 47–54.

Drury, V. M., Robinson, E. J. & Birchwood, M. (1998). "Theory of mind" skills during an acute episode of psychosis and following recovery. *Psychol. Med.*, **28**, 1101–2.

Duden, D. (1998). *Duden, Redewendungen und sprichwörtliche Redensarten: Wörterbuch der deutschen Idiomatik.* Dudenverlag, Mannheim, Leipzig, Wien, Zürich.

Eviatar, Z. & Just, M. A. (2006). Brain correlates of discourse processing: an fMRI investigation of irony and conventional metaphor comprehension. *Neuropsychologia*, **44**(12), 2348–59.

Falkenberg, I., Kluegel, K., Bartels, M. & Wild, B. (2007). Sense of humor in patients with schizophrenia. *Schizophr. Res.*, **95**(1–3), 259–61.

Faust, M. & Weisper, S. (2000). Understanding metaphoric sentences in the two cerebral hemispheres. *Brain Cogn.*, **43**, 186–91.

Finckh, J. (1906). Zur Frage der Intelligenzprüfung. *Zentralbl. Nervenheilkd. Psychiatr.*, **29**, 945–57.

Gagnon, L., Goulet, P., Giroux, F. & Joanette, Y. (2003). Processing of metaphoric and non-metaphoric alternative meanings of words after right- and left-hemispheric lesion. *Brain Lang.*, **87**, 217–26.

Gibbs Jr., R. W. (1990). Comprehending figurative referential descriptions. *J. Exp. Psychol.: Learn., Mem., Cogn.*, **16**, 56–66.

Giora, R. (1997). Understanding figurative and literal language: the graded salience hypothesis. *Cogn. Linguist.*, **8**, 183–206.

Giora, R. (2003). *On Our Mind: Salience, Context, and Figurative Language.* New York: Oxford University Press.

Giora, R. (2007). Is metaphor special? *Brain Lang.*, **100**(2), 111–14.

Giora, R., Zaidel, E., Soroker, N., Batori, G. & Kasher, A. (2000). Differential effects of right- and left-hemisphere damage on understanding sarcasm and metaphor. *Metaphor Symbol*, **1**(1/2), 63–83.

Glucksberg, S. (2003). The psycholinguistics of metaphor. *Trends Cogn. Sci.*, **7**(2), 92–6.

Gorham, D. R. (1956). Use of the proverbs test for differentiating schizophrenics from normals. *J. Consult. Psychol.*, **20**, 435–40.

Hensler, M., Markert, K., Saur, R., Bartels, M. & Rapp, A. M. (2007). *Sind konkretistische Denkstoerungen eine homogene Entitaet? Studie zum Verständnis verschiedener Arten nichtwörtlicher Sprache bei schizophrenen Patienten.* Paper presented at "Jahrestagung der Deutschen Gesellschaft für Psychiatrie, Psychotherapie und Nervenheilkunde", Berlin, Germany, 21–24 November 2007.

Herold, R., Tenyi, T., Lenard, K. & Trixler, M. (2002). Theory of mind deficit in people with schizophrenia during remission. *Psychol. Med.*, **32**, 1125.

Hillekamp, U., Knobloch, J. & Buelau, P. (1996). Metaphorische Sprachverarbeitung bei Hirngeschädigten: Anwendung und Analyse eines Metapherntests. *Neurol. Rehabil.*, **4**, 232–36.

Iakimova, G., Passerieux, C., Laurent, J. P. & Hardy-Bayle, M. C. (2005). ERPs of metaphoric, literal, and incongruous semantic processing in schizophrenia. *Psychophysiology*, **42**, 380–90.

Janssen, I., Krabbendam, L., Jolles, J. & Van Os, J. (2003). Alterations in theory of mind in patients with shizophrenia and non-psychotic relatives. *Acta Psychiatr. Scand.*, **108**, 110–17.

Kacinik, N. A. & Chiarello, C. (2007). Understanding metaphoric language: is the right hemisphere uniquely involved? *Brain Lang.*, **100**, 188–207.

Kay, S. R., Fiszbein, A. & Opler, L. A. (1987). The positive and negative syndrome scale (PANSS) for schizophrenia. *Schizophr. Bull.*, **13**(2), 261–76.

Kircher, T. T., Bullmore, E. T., Brammer, M. J. *et al.* (2001). Differential activation of temporal cortex during sentence completion in schizophrenic patients with and without formal thought disorder. *Schizophr. Res.*, **50**, 27–40.

Kircher, T. T., Liddle, P. F., Brammer, M. J. *et al.* (2002). Reversed lateralization of temporal activation during speech production in thought disordered patients with schizophrenia. *Psychol. Med.*, **32**(3), 439–49.

Kircher, T. T., Leube, D. T., Erb, M., Grodd, W. & Rapp, A. M. (2007). Neural correlates of metaphor processing in schizophrenia. *Neuroimage*, **34**(1), 281–9.

Lakoff, G. & Johnson, M. (1980). *Metaphors We Live By.* Chicago: University of Chicago Press.

Langdon, R. & Coltheart, M. (2004). Recognition of metaphor and irony in young adults: the impact of schizotypal personality traits. *Psychiatry Res.*, **125**, 9–20.

Langdon, R., Coltheart, M., Ward, P. B. & Catts, S. V. (2002). Disturbed communication in schizophrenia: the role of poor pragmatics and poor mind-reading. *Psychol. Med.*, **32**, 1273–84.

Lauro, L. J., Tettamanti, M., Cappa, S. F. & Papagno, C. (2007). Idiom comprehension: a prefrontal task? *Cereb. Cortex.*, **18** (1), 162–70.

Lee, S. S. & Dapretto, M. (2006). Metaphorical versus literal word meanings: fMRI evidence against a selective role of the right hemisphere. *Neuroimage*, **29**, 536–44.

Lehrl, S., Triebig, G. & Fischer, B. (1995). Multiple choice vocabulary test MWT as a valid and short test to estimate premorbid intelligence. *Acta Neurol. Scand.*, **91**, 335–45.

Leitman, D. I., Ziwich, R., Pasternak, R. & Javitt, D. C. (2006). Theory of mind (ToM) and counterfactuality deficits in schizophrenia: misperception or misinterpretation? *Psychol. Med.*, **36**(8), 1075–83.

Lindell, A. K. (2006). In your right mind: right hemisphere contributions to language processing and production. *Neuropsychol. Rev.*, **16**(3), 131–48.

MacKenzie, C., Begg, T., Brady, M. & Lees, K. R. (1997). The effects on verbal communication skills of right hemisphere stroke in middle age. *Aphasiology*, **11**, 929–45.

Mashal, N., Faust, M. & Hendler, T. (2005). The role of the right hemisphere in processing nonsalient metaphorical meanings: application of principal components analysis to fMRI data. *Neuropsychologia*, **43**(14), 2084–100.

Mashal, N., Faust, M., Hendler, T. & Jung-Beeman, M. (2007). An fMRI investigation of the neural correlates underlying the processing of novel metaphoric expressions. *Brain Lang.*, **100**(2), 115–26.

McDonald, S. (2000). Neuropsychological studies of sarcasm. *Metaphor Symbol*, **15**(1/2), 85–98.

McIntyre, M., Pritchard, P. B. & Lombroso, C. T. (1976). Left and right temporal lobe epileptics: a controlled investigation of some psychological differences. *Epilepsia*, **17**, 377–86.

Mitchell, R. L. & Crow, T. J. (2005). Right hemisphere language functions and schizophrenia: the forgotten hemisphere? *Brain*, **128**(5), 963–78.

Mitchell, R. L., Elliott, R., Barry, M., Cruttenden, A. & Woodruff, P. W. (2004). Neural response to emotional prosody in schizophrenia and in bipolar affective disorder. *Br. J. Psychiatry*, **184**, 223–30.

Mitchley, N. J., Barber, J., Gray, J. M., Brooks, N. & Livingston, M. G. (1998). Comprehension of irony in schizophrenia. *Cogn. Neuropsychiatry*, **3**, 127.

Nunn, J. & Peters, E. (2001). Schizotypy and patterns of lateral asymmetry on hemisphere-specific language tasks. *Psychiatry Res.*, **103**, 179–92.

Oliveri, M., Romero, L., Papagno, C. (2004). Left but not right temporal involvement in opaque idiom comprehension: a repetitive transcranial magnetic stimulation study. *J. Cogn. Neurosci*, **16** (5) 848–855.

Papagno, C. (2001). Comprehension of metaphors and idioms in patients with Alzheimer's disease: a longitudinal study. *Brain*, **124**, 1450–60.

Papagno, C. & Caporali, A. (2007). Testing idiom comprehension in aphasic patients: the effects of task and idiom type. *Brain Lang.*, **100**(2), 208–20.

Papagno, C., Curti, R., Rizzo, S., Crippa, F. & Colombo, M. R. (2006). Is the right hemisphere involved in idiom comprehension? A neuropsychological study. *Neuropsychology*, **20** (5), 598–606.

Rapp, A. M., Leube, D. T., Erb, M., Grodd, W. & Kircher, T. T. (2004). Neural correlates of metaphor processing. *Cogn. Brain Res.*, **20**, 395–402.

Rapp, A. M., Leube, D. T., Erb, M., Grodd, W. & Kircher, T. T. (2007a). Laterality in metaphor processing: lack of evidence from functional magnetic resonance imaging for the right hemisphere theory. *Brain Lang.*, **100**(2), 142–9.

Rapp, A. M., Bayer, W. & Langle, G. (2007b). Is language-related psychopathology a predictor of psychosocial functioning in schizophrenia? Results from a 4 year follow up study. *Schizophrenia Bulletin*, **33**, 602.

Rhodes, J. E. & Jakes, S. (2004). The contribution of metaphor and metonymy to delusions. *Psychology and Psychotherapy*, **77**, 1–17.

Rinaldi, M. C., Marangolo, P. & Baldassarri, F. (2004). Metaphor comprehension in right brain-damaged patients with visuo-verbal and verbal material: a dissociation (re) considered. *Cortex*, **40**, 479–90.

Rizzo, S., Sandrini, M. & Papagno, C. (2007). The dorsolateral prefrontal cortex in idiom interpretation: an rTMS study. *Brain Res. Bull.*, **71**(5), 523–8.

Shamay-Tsoory, S. G., Tomer, R. & Aharon-Peretz, J. (2005). The neuroanatomical basis of understanding sarcasm and its relationship to social cognition. *Neuropsychology*, **19**(3), 288–300.

Sponheim, S. R., Surerus-Johnson, C., Leskela, J. & Dieperink, M. E. (2003). Proverb interpretation in schizophrenia: the significance of symptomatology and cognitive processes. *Schizophr. Res.*, **65**, 117.

Stringaris, A. K., Medford, N., Giora, R. *et al.* (2006). How metaphors influence semantic relatedness judgments: the role of the right frontal cortex. *Neuroimage*, **33**(2), 784–93.

Stringaris, A. K., Medford, N. C., Giampietra, V., Brammer, M. J. & David, A. S. (2007). Deriving meaning: distinct neural mechanisms for metaphoric, literal, and non-meaningful sentences. *Brain Lang.*, **100**(2), 150–62.

Thoma, P. & Daum, I. (2006). Neurocognitive mechanisms of figurative language processing-evidence from clinical dysfunctions. *Neurosci. Biobehav. Rev.*, **30**(8), 1182–205.

Titone, D., Holzman, P. S. & Levy, D. L. (2002). Idiom processing in schizophrenia: literal implausibility saves the day for idiom priming. *J. Abnorm. Psychol.*, **111**, 313–20.

Vigotsky, L. S. (1934). Thought in schizophrenia. *Arch. Neurol. Psychiatry*, **31**, 1063–77.

Wang, A. T., Lee, S. S., Sigman, M. & Dapretto, M. (2006). Neural basis of irony comprehension in children with autism: the role of prosody and context. *Brain*, **129**(4), 932–43.

Watson, C. G., Plemel, D. & Burke, M. (1979). Proverb test deficit in schizophrenic and brain-damaged patients. *J. Nerv. Ment. Dis.*, **167**, 561–5.

Wildgruber, D., Ackermann, H., Kreifelts, B. & Ethofer, T. (2006). Cerebral processing of linguistic and emotional prosody: fMRI studies. *Prog. Brain Res.*, **156**, 249–68.

Winner, E. & Gardner, H. (1977). The comprehension of metaphor in brain damaged patients. *Brain.*, **100**, 717–29.

Winner, E. & Gardner, H. (1993). Metaphor and irony: two levels of understanding. In: Ortony, A. (ed.) *Metaphor and Thought*. Cambridge: Cambridge University Press, pp. 425–46.

Zaidel, E., Kasher, A., Soroker, N. & Batori, G. (2002). Effects of right and left hemisphere damage on performance of the "Right Hemisphere Communication Battery". *Brain Lang.*, **80**(3), 510–35.

Zempleni, M. Z. (2006). *Functional imaging of the hemispheric contribution to language processing*. Doctoral Dissertation, Rijksuniversiteit Groningen, Netherlands, pp. 84–108.

Zempleni, M. Z., Haverkort, M., Renken, R. A. & Stowe, L. (2007). Evidence for bilateral involvement in idiom comprehension: an fMRI study. *Neuroimage*, **34**(3), 1280–91.

11

Auditory verbal hallucinations and language lateralization

Kelly Diederen and Iris E. C. Sommer

Summary

The pathophysiology of auditory verbal hallucinations (AVH) is largely unknown. Several functional imaging studies have measured cerebral activation during AVH, but sample sizes were relatively small (1–8 subjects) and findings were inconsistent.

In this chapter we describe cerebral activation during AVH in a relatively large sample to enable group-wise analysis and obtain a representative view of the biological substrate of hallucinations. Activity during AVH is compared to activity during normal language production in the same patients.

We measured cerebral activation with fMRI in 24 psychotic patients while they experienced AVH in the scanner, and also while they silently generated words (verbal fluency). Patients indicated the presence of AVH by squeezing a balloon with their right hand. Patients were right-handed and diagnosed with schizophrenia, schizo-affective disorder, or psychosis NOS (not otherwise specified). Despite adequate pharmacotherapy, patients experienced AVH frequently. Group-wise analysis was performed on 24 fMRI scans during AVH and during word generation. Lateralization indices of both conditions were compared.

Group analysis for AVH revealed activation in the right homolog of Broca's area, bilateral insula, bilateral supramarginal gyri, right superior temporal gyrus, and in motor related areas (associated with squeezing the balloon). Broca's area and left superior temporal gyrus were not activated during AVH, nor were the hippocampi. Group analysis for word generation yielded activation in Broca's and Wernicke's area and to a lesser degree their right-sided homologs, bilateral insula, and anterior cingulate gyrus. The mean lateralization index during hallucinations (-0.11, SD $= 0.41$) was significantly lower than during word generation ($+0.14$, SD $= 0.34$) ($T(23) = -2.4$, $p < 0.02$). Lateralization of activity during AVH was not correlated with language lateralization, but rather with the degree to which the content of the AVH had a negative emotional valence.

The main difference between cerebral activity during AVH and activity during normal inner speech appears to be the lateralization. The predominant engagement of the right inferior frontal area during AVH may be related to the typical low semantic complexity and negative emotional content of AVH.

Introduction

The ancient man, who had no concept of self-fulfilment, was virtually autonomous. He heard voices inside his head and called them gods. These gods told him what to do and how to act. Their minds were divided into two parts: an executive part called "god" and a follower part called "man". When writing and other complex language activity started weakening the authority of the auditory hallucinations, this "bicameral mind" slowly broke down. The voices of the gods fell silent, and what we call consciousness was born. (Jaynes, 1976)

At the time Jaynes formulated his ideas about cerebral lateralization of language, it was not possible to study the representation of cerebral functions in vivo. Thirty years later, functional magnetic resonance imaging (fMRI) has become widely available to study cerebral functions and clinical symptoms in healthy and diseased subjects. In this chapter, fMRI is applied to study the neural substrate of auditory verbal hallucinations.

Hallucinations are among the most intriguing and characteristic symptoms of schizophrenia. In 65% hallucinations are auditory verbal in nature, i.e., "hearing voices" (Slade & Bentall, 1988). Thus, most hallucinations in schizophrenia may reflect an abnormality of

Language Lateralization and Psychosis, ed. Iris E. C. Sommer and René S. Kahn. Published by Cambridge University Press.
© Cambridge University Press 2009.

language activity. Other psychotic symptoms in schizophrenia, such as thought insertion and formal thought disorder, can also be considered a disorder of language functioning. There are several theories that try to explain auditory verbal hallucinations (AVH) and the three most dominant theories will shortly be addressed here. First, the mental imagery hypothesis states that pronounced linguistic expectations can generate a perceptual experience (David, 1999). In other words, hallucinations are thought to arise from abnormally vivid mental imagery. Probably the most influential model has been proposed by Frith (1992). According to this theory, hallucinations arise from a failure in the self-monitoring of own intentions during inner speech. In healthy subjects, language reception areas are thought to be inhibited to respond to language that is derived from covert inner speech by means of a corollary discharge system (Ford *et al.*, 2007). In this model, the corollary discharge functions as an efferent copy of the formed speech, which is sent to the auditory cortex preparing it for perceiving speech as self-generated (Creutzfeldt *et al.*, 1989). This inhibitory system may be malfunctioning in schizophrenia. A third model has been suggested by Nasrallah (1985), who hypothesized that verbal hallucinations and other language-related positive symptoms arise from inappropriate language activity of the non-dominant hemisphere. The malfunctioning inhibition system proposed by Frith may coexist with the increased right hemispheric language activity proposed by Nasrallah. Considering these three models of hallucinations, this chapter will test the theory of Nasrallah, since it proposes a central role for language processing in the etiology of hallucinations. This central position appears to be justified since the great majority of hallucinations in schizophrenia are auditory verbal in nature. Furthermore, it is a very testable model, especially when applying fMRI. The model can be tested by measuring cerebral activation in schizophrenia patients at the time they are actually experiencing auditory hallucinations.

Several previous functional imaging studies have assessed cerebral activation during AVH in an attempt to unravel its biological substrate (Silbersweig *et al.*, 1995; Lennox *et al.*, 1999; Dierks *et al.*, 1999; Shergill *et al.*, 2000; Shergill *et al.*, 2001; Copolov *et al.*, 2003; Hoffman *et al.*, 2007). Results of these studies are quite heterogeneous (reviewed by Stephane *et al.*, 2001 and Allen *et al.*, 2008). For example, Silbersweig *et al.* (1995) observed activation during hallucinations predominantly in subcortical structures in five patients and therefore stressed the role of the thalamus and limbic structures in hallucinations. In contrast, Shergill *et al.* (2000) investigated six patients and found activation of Broca's area and bilateral temporal cortices, which was used to support the model of Frith (1992). Dierks *et al.* (1999) found hallucinatory activity in the primary auditory cortex in three patients. Copolov *et al.* (2003) could not replicate primary auditory cortex activity in their sample of six patients, but found prominent activity in the parahippocampal gyrus, imposing an important role in AVH for verbal memory. Some of these studies found prominent activation in the right hemisphere (Shergill *et al.*, 2000; Lennox *et al.*, 1999), while others mainly reported activation of left hemisphere areas (Lennox *et al.*, 2000; Dierks *et al.*, 1999). The largest sample of patients hallucinating during fMRI recordings to date was recently reported by Hoffman *et al.* (2007) who found activity during AVH in temporal and frontal areas of both hemispheres in eight patients.

Inconsistency between the findings of these studies may result from the large variation in cerebral activation during hallucinations between individual patients (Hoffman *et al.*, 2007) and small samples sizes (ranging between one and eight patients). These relatively small sample sizes have limited the interpretation of the data and precluded adequately powered group-wise analyses. These limited sample sizes may be the result of the fact that acquiring functional images of patients while they are actually hallucinating is demanding: the patients need to experience AVH on several occasions (approximately >25% of the scan time) during the scan session in order to generate enough power for a meaningful comparison between hallucinations and the absence of hallucinations. Moreover, patients who hallucinate continuously have to be excluded, since adequate resting state scans are needed as comparison (again, at least 25% of the scan time should be without AVH).

In this chapter results are presented of 24 psychotic patients who actually experienced AVH in the scanner. We hypothesized that the group-wise analysis would reveal activity in language-related structures, such as Broca's and Wernicke's areas, since the percept of these hallucinations consists of words or sentences. Apart from these classical language areas, AVH may also activate other areas that are not part of the normal language system, which could be specific for hallucinations. In order to assess whether, and if so how, activation during AVH differs from normal language activity, the same patients also performed a silent word generation task while fMRI scans were acquired. Silent word generation was chosen since overt speech induces large movement artifacts.

Table 11.1 Clinical description of the participants

Mean age	37 years (SD = 10)
Mean age at onset of AVH	22 years (SD = 12)
Diagnosis	18 schizophrenia
	3 schizo-affective disorder
	3 psychosis not otherwise specified
Medication	13 clozapine, mean dose 316 mg
	4 flupentixol depot, mean dose 16 mg/week
	1 haloperidol depot 50 mg/week
	1 chlorprotixen 200 mg
	1 olanzapine 30 mg
	2 risperidone, mean dose 4 mg
	2 quetiapine, mean dose 600 mg
Sex	17 male
	7 female

Measuring the neurological substrate of auditory verbal hallucinations

Subjects

Twenty-four patients with a diagnosis of schizophrenia-spectrum disorder participated in this study. Patients were diagnosed using the Comprehensive Assessment of Symptoms and History (CASH) (Andreasen *et al.*, 1992) according to DSM-IV criteria by an independent psychiatrist. All subjects were strongly right-handed as assessed by the Edinburgh Handedness Inventory (Oldfield, 1971). All subjects were using antipsychotic medication, specified in Table 11.1, but continued to experience AVH frequently. In all patients, AVH were refractory to treatment with at least two types of antipsychotic medication.

Experimental design

Activation during hallucinations was measured over eight minutes, during which functional scans were made continuously. Patients were instructed to squeeze a balloon when they experienced AVH, and to release it when the hallucinations subsided (adapted from Hoffman *et al.*, 2007). Language activation was also measured over eight minutes during which a paced letter fluency task was presented. Letter fluency is a classical neuropsychological task of language production, which involves the generation of words beginning with a specified letter.

Patients were asked to silently generate a word starting with the letter displayed on a screen placed in front of them. Letters were presented in eight activation blocks, each block lasting 30 seconds. In each activation block ten letters were displayed at a rate of one every three seconds. As a reference condition, a crosshair was projected on the screen in order to correct for visual input.

Data acquisition

Activation maps were obtained using a Philips Achieva 3 Tesla Clinical MRI scanner. Eight-hundred 3D-PRESTO sensitivity encoding (SENSE) images depicting BOLD (blood-oxygen-level-dependent) contrast, were acquired with the following parameter settings: 40 (coronal) slices, TR/TE 21.75/32.4 ms, flip angle 10°, FOV 224 × 256 × 160, matrix 64 × 64 × 40, voxel size 4 mm isotropic. This scan sequence achieves full brain coverage within 609 ms by combining a 3D-PRESTO pulse sequence with a commercial eight-channel SENSE headcoil and in two directions (Neggers *et al.*, 2008). After completion of the functional scans, a high resolution anatomical scan, with the following parameters: TR/TE: 9.86/4.6 ms, 1 × 1 × 1 voxels, flip angle 8°, was acquired to improve localization of the functional data.

Data analysis

Functional MRI data were analyzed using statistical parametric mapping (SPM2; Welcome Department of Cognitive Neurology, London, UK). Preprocessing included reorientation and within-subject image realignment with rigid-body transformations using the fa27 as the reference, to correct for the effects of head motion.

For the hallucination paradigm a model was created using balloon squeezes as the hallucination onsets, and the time between squeezes and releases as the duration of the AVH. These hallucination periods were then compared to non-hallucinating (resting) scans.

For the letter fluency paradigm a model was created to contrast activity during presentation of the letters versus rest blocks. Functional images were analyzed on a voxel by voxel basis using multiple regression analysis (Worsley & Friston, 1995) with one factor coding for activation (task versus rest). Following the first-level analyses, second-level random-effects analyses were conducted for both the hallucination and the letter fluency paradigm to determine activation on a group-level (one sample t-tests). All thresholds corresponded to a p-value of $p < 0.05$ corrected for all voxels in the brain by the false discovery rate (FDR) (Benjamini & Hochberg, 1995).

Finally, lateralization indices were calculated on individual T-tests for both the letter fluency and the hallucination paradigm. For this purpose, a mask was created using the Anatomical Automatic Labeling (AAL) atlas (Tzourio-Mazoyer *et al.*, 2002) comprising the main areas where language processing is thought to be mediated and their contralateral homologs (Springer *et al.*, 1999). Language areas consisted of the inferior frontal triangle, the insula, the middle temporal gyrus, the superior temporal gyrus, the supramarginal gyrus, and the angular gyrus. Lateralization indices were defined as the difference in "thresholded" signal intensity changes in the left versus the right hemisphere (within the selected language regions) divided by the total sum

Table 11.2 Specific aspects of the AVH

Item of the PSYRATS	Mean (standard deviation)
Frequency (0–4)	3.5 (0.9)
Duration (0–4)	2 (1)
Location (0–4)	1.9 (1)
Loudness (0–4)	1.8 (0.9)
Beliefs about source (0–3)	2.8 (1.1)
Negative content (0–4)	3 (1)
Severity of negativity (0–4)	2.6 (0.8)
Distress (0–4)	3 (1.2)
Intensity of distress (0–4)	2.7 (0.9)
Control over AVH (0–4)	3.3 (1.1)
Number of voices (0–...)	13.1 (11.5)

of "thresholded" signal intensity changes. Differences in lateralization indices between the hallucination and the letter fluency activation were compared by means of a paired samples t-test. Pearson's correlation was used to assess an association between lateralization of AVH and lateralization of language production, and between the lateralization of hallucinatory activity and the degree to which the AVH had a negative emotional content.

Results

Clinical evaluation

Clinical symptoms of the patients were rated on the day of the fMRI scan, using the PANSS and PSYRATS interview. The mean total PANSS score was 73 (SD = 13). The mean score on the positive subscale was 19 (SD = 4), as was the mean score on the negative subscale (19, SD = 4). Details about the AVH, as rated with the PSYRATS interview are listed in Table 11.2.

Performance during the functional scans

During the eight-minute hallucination scans, the mean number of hallucinations of all subjects was 18 (SD = 13). The mean duration of a hallucination was

(a)

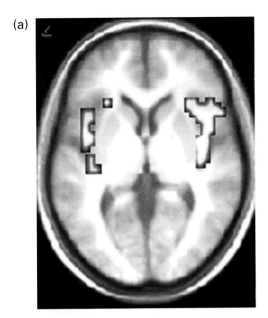

(c)

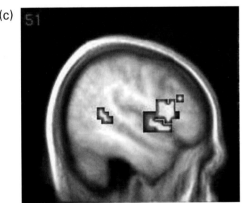

Figure 11.1 a, b, and c SPM(T)s for the group hallucination analysis. (See color plate section.)

20 (SD = 36) seconds, adding up to a mean total duration of the hallucinations of 162 (SD = 144) seconds.

For the letter fluency task, the patients showed a mean accuracy of 19.2 (SD = 1.4) words, which is a 96% (SD = 7) correct performance. Eight of the participants reported AVH also during the language task. All eight patients indicated that the hallucinations were present during the language blocks as well as in the rest condition.

(b)

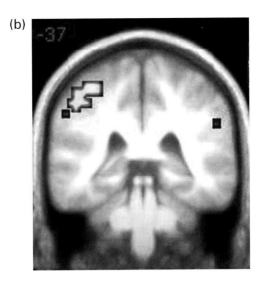

Group analysis AVH

The group analysis for AVH revealed activation in multiple brain regions. These regions included the right inferior frontal gyrus, including Broca's homolog (Figures 11.1a&c), the bilateral insula (Figure 11.1a), the bilateral supramarginal gyri (Figure 11.1b) and the right superior temporal gyrus (Figure 11.1c). Broca's area and the left superior temporal gyrus were not significantly activated. There was also significant activation in the left motor cortex and the right cerebellum, most likely as a result of the balloon squeezes. Table 11.3 shows the coordinates of all local maxima significantly activated in the group analysis.

Group analysis language task

The group analysis for the language task revealed extensive activation of multiple brain regions. These regions included Broca's area and to a lesser degree its contralateral homolog, both extending into the insula (Figure 11.2a), the bilateral temporal area (superior and middle gyri), left more than right (Figure 11.2b), and the anterior cingulate gyrus (Figure 11.2c). Table 11.4 shows the coordinates of all local maxima significantly activated in the group analysis.

Table 11.3 Z-scores, cluster size, and locations of local maxima active in the group hallucination analysis

Lobe	Area	Coordinates			Z score	Cluster size
		X	Y	Z		
R sub-lobar	Insula, ba 13	40	−4	4	5.13	466
R frontal lobe	Middle frontal gyrus, ba 9 DLPFC	48	21	28	3.55	
R frontal lobe	Inferior frontal gyrus, ba 47	28	27	−5	2.78	
R frontal lobe	Inferior frontal gyrus, ba 44	44	16	10	3.24	
R temporal lobe	Superior temporal gyrus, ba 22	51	11	−4	3.02	
L frontal lobe	Postcentral gyrus	−44	−17	45	4.64	227
L frontal lobe	Superior frontal gyrus, ba 6	−20	−8	67	3.10	
L parietal lobe	Inferior parietal lobule, ba 40 SMG	−55	−37	39	3.07	
L sub-lobar	Insula, ba 13	−44	0	4	3.47	79
L sub-lobar	Lentiform nucleus	−32	−4	0	3.70	
L frontal lobe	Precentral gyrus	−55	4	11	3.04	
L limbic lobe	Cingulate gyrus	−12	2	44	3.89	165
R frontal lobe	Medial frontal gyrus, ba 6	8	3	62	3.69	
L frontal lobe	Medial frontal gyrus, ba 6	−4	−9	48	3.49	
R cerebellum	Anterior lobe, culmen	24	−52	−21	3.87	126
R cerebellum	Posterior lobe, pyramis	20	−64	−30	3.14	
L parietal lobe	Postcentral gyrus	−55	−19	16	3.19	10
L cerebellum	Anterior lobe, dentate	−20	−59	−24	3.31	60
R temporal lobe	Superior temporal gyrus	48	−46	13	3.06	11
R parietal lobe	Supramarginal gyrus, ba 40	51	−37	30	3.02	12
L frontal lobe	Inferior frontal gyrus, ba 9	−51	6	33	3.33	9

Lateralization

The mean lateralization index was −0.11 (SD = 0.41) for the hallucination paradigm and + 0.14 (SD = 0.34) for the word generation task. The paired samples t-test revealed significantly lower lateralization during AVH as compared to covert word generation ($T(23) = -2.4$, $p < 0.02$).

The individual lateralization indices of hallucinatory activation were not correlated to the lateralization indices of word generation (Pearson's rho = 0.11, $p = 0.63$).

The negative emotional content of the AVH, as rated on item 6 of the PSYRATS, correlated with the lateralization index of the AVH (Pearson's rho = −0.5, $p = 0.01$), with a more negative emotional content of voices associated with lateralization of hallucinatory activation to the right hemisphere (Figure 11.3).

Discussion

This chapter investigated the biological substrate of AVH in 24 psychotic, mostly schizophrenic, patients. Cerebral activity was assessed while patients were actively hallucinating in the scanner. In the same patients, activity was also assessed during silent word generation. Group-wise analysis of the hallucination scans yielded the highest activation in the right inferior frontal gyrus (the homolog of Broca's area) extending into the right insula. Other areas with significant activation included the bilateral supramarginal gyri, the left insula, and the right superior temporal gyrus. Broca's area and the left superior temporal gyrus were not significantly activated during AVH. Although all patients were strongly right-handed and all hallucinations consisted of words or sentences, activation during AVH was lateralized to the right hemisphere, with a

Table 11.4 Z-scores, cluster size, and locations of local maxima active in the group letter fluency analysis

Lobe	Area	X	Y	Z	Z score
		Coordinates			
R fontal lobe	Inferior frontal gyrus	36	23	−5	6.63
L sub-lobar	Extra-nuclear, insula	−36	19	−1	6.33
L frontal lobe	Inferior frontal gyrus, ba 44	−55	12	14	6.31
R occipital lobe	Middle occipital gyrus	28	−89	4	6.23
R frontal lobe	Inferior frontal gyrus, ba 9	48	5	29	6.03
R limbic lobe	Cingulate gyrus, ba 32	4	29	32	5.94
L frontal lobe	Medial frontal gyrus, ba 8	−4	29	39	5.90
L frontal lobe	Inferior frontal gyrus, ba 9	−48	5	29	5.69
L sub-lobar	Lentiform nucleus, putamen	−24	12	3	5.65
L temporal lobe	Superior temporal gyrus, ba area 38	−48	15	−7	5.48
L frontal lobe	Precentral gyrus, ba 8	−55	2	33	5.42
L frontal lobe	Middle frontal gyrus, ba 6	−44	2	44	5.40
L parietal lobe	Superior parietal lobule	−28	−52	43	5.36
R cerebellum	Posterior lobe, declive	32	−75	−16	5.36
L temporal lobe	Middle temporal gyrus	−44	−52	7	5.34
R frontal lobe	Middle frontal gyrus, ba 6	36	−1	55	5.08
R temporal lobe	Fusiform gyrus	44	−55	−14	4.77
R limbic lobe	Anterior cingulate	4	9	25	4.72
R cerebellum	Anterior lobe, cerebellar lingual	4	−48	−18	4.72
R parietal lobe	Inferior parietal lobule	48	−40	50	4.71
L parietal lobe	Inferior parietal lobule	−48	−37	42	4.65
R cerebellum	Posterior lobe, declive	28	−63	−20	4.64
L sub-lobar	Extra-nuclear	−28	−1	−10	4.63
R sub-lobar	Lentiform nucleus	32	−20	−2	3.03

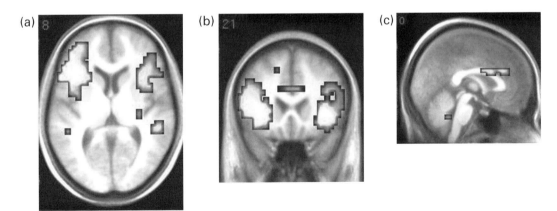

Figure 11.2 a, b, and c SPM(T)s for the group language analysis. (See color plate section.)

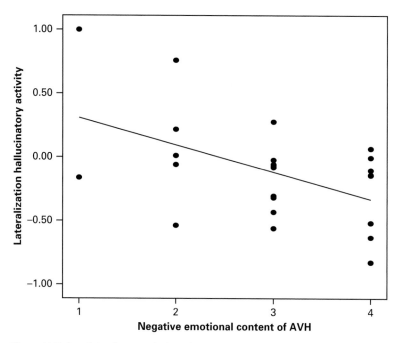

Figure 11.3 Correlation between the lateralization index of hallucinatory activation and the degree to which the emotional content of AVH is negative, as scored on item 6 of the PSYRATS.

mean lateralization index of −0.11. The lateralization index of hallucinatory activity was lower (i.e., more negative) in patients with a strong negative emotional content of AVH.

As expected, analysis of the language task, i.e., silent word generation, yielded most pronounced activity in the left inferior frontal gyrus (Broca's area), left insula, left superior temporal gyrus, and anterior cingulate gyrus. The right-sided homologs of these areas were also activated, but to a smaller degree, resulting in a mean lateralization index of +0.14. Language lateralization was not correlated to lateralization of hallucinatory activity.

The group-wise analysis showed most prominent activity during AVH in the right-sided homolog of Broca's area, while silent word generation mainly engaged Broca's area. It could be hypothesized that language activity arising from the homolog of Broca's area is more prone to become misattributed and lead to hallucinations, while speech originating from the usual

speech production area (i.e., Broca's area) is less liable to misattribution.

A similar mechanism of a right hemispheric area generating "ectopic speech" has been described in aphasia patients (Winhuizen et al., 2005; Thiel et al., 2005). Patients with severe aphasia are frequently observed to emit repetitive simple, but fully intact, utterances classified as "automatic speech" (Van Lancker & Cummings, 1999). These utterances show little variation, generally repetitions of the same word or sentence, and frequently consist of terms of abuse or swear words. As Jackson (1931–1932) already noted: "The speechless patient may occasionally swear" (cited in Van Lancker & Cummings, 1999). This observation is striking in global aphasia where speech is almost non-existent, yet the terms of abuse flow fluently and effortlessly with normal articulation and prosody (Van Lancker, 1997). Most aphasic patients are, however, not able to produce these utterances on command. Other examples of automatic speech are found in patients with left hemispherectomy at adult age (Zangwill, 1967; Burklund & Smith 1977). The negative emotional content and repetitive nature of these automatic utterances in aphasia patients, as well as the lack of voluntary control over the utterances, bears resemblance to AVH in schizophrenia patients. An obvious difference is that automatic utterances are spoken, while AVH are heard. However, before being heard, the AVH are probably generated in speech production areas that may coincide with the source of automatic speech in aphasia. Several groups have studied cerebral activation patterns of automatic speech. Functional imaging studies by Noppeney *et al.* (2005), Thivard *et al.* (2005), and Thiel *et al.* (2001) identified the right inferior frontal area as a language resource following damage or surgery to left hemisphere language areas. Interestingly, patients with prominent language activity in the right frontal areas had worse residual language function than patients whose residual language activity was restricted to remaining left areas, independent of the size of the left hemisphere lesion (Winhuizen *et al.*, 2005). This indicates that the "compensatory" language capacity of the right hemisphere is rather low and implies that destruction of eloquent language areas in the left hemisphere may reduce transcallosal inhibition, leading to "release" language activity in the right frontal areas, rather than active recruitment of a valid compensatory language system (Winhuizen *et al.*, 2005). Voets *et al.* (2006) used high-field fMRI to demonstrate that "release" language activation in subjects with left hemisphere damage is not restricted to the homolog of Broca's area, but extends further posterior to encompass the right insula. These regions (Broca's homolog and the right insula) coincide with the areas that showed greatest hallucinatory activation in the current analysis. It could therefore be hypothesized that AVH results from release language activity in the right hemisphere that is inhibited in the healthy brain.

During normal language functions, such as speaking, listening to speech, and reading, the dominant frontal language area inhibits its contralateral homolog through reciprocal callosal connections (Thiel *et al.*, 2006; Bloom & Hynd, 2005). Activity of the right homolog of Broca's area during AVH may result from insufficient inhibition of these non-dominant language areas.

Indeed, in schizophrenia patients, who frequently experience AVH, lateralization of productive and receptive language functions is decreased (Artiges *et al.*, 2000; Sommer *et al.*, 2001, 2003, 2004; Dollfus *et al.*, 2005; Weiss *et al.*, 2006; Razafimandimby *et al.*, 2007). The lower degree of language lateralization is caused by increased language activity in frontal and temporal areas of the right hemisphere (Sommer *et al.*, 2001, 2003; Dollfus *et al.*, 2005). Increased language activity of the right hemisphere is also present in unaffected monozygotic co-twins of schizophrenia patients (Sommer *et al.*, 2004; Spaniel *et al.*, 2007), indicating that decreased language lateralization is a genetic predisposition for schizophrenia. Exactly how decreased lateralization can facilitate the development of the schizophrenia phenotype remains an open question. Decreased cerebral dominance is not specific for schizophrenia since it is also observed in affective psychosis (Sommer *et al.*, 2007). This suggests that decreased lateralization is associated with psychosis, rather than with negative or cognitive symptoms. Decreased cerebral dominance may predispose for insufficient inhibition of right hemisphere language areas, which facilitates inappropriate activity of these areas. Inappropriate language activity of Broca's homolog may engender AVH.

The present finding that the right inferior frontal area is active during AVH, but much less during normal language, offers new possibilities for focal treatment of chronic AVH. For example, activity in the right inferior frontal cortex could be focally reduced by applying low frequency rTMS to this area. Repetitive transcranial magnetic stimulation is a safe and non-invasive technique that can effectively reduce AVH severity (Aleman *et al.*, 2007). Hoffman *et al.* (2007) compared the effect of rTMS applied to several stimulation sites based on hallucinatory activation maps acquired with fMRI. The right homolog of Broca's area, which showed clear hallucinatory activation in our study, also activated during AVH in their sample. This was one of the experimental sites to which they applied rTMS, together with left frontal, left and right temporal, and left and right parietal sites. Repetitive transcranial magnetic stimulation applied to frontal language areas (both right and left) was less effective than rTMS applied to temporo-parietal areas (Hoffman *et al.*, 2007). Increased distance between the coil and the brain area could explain this difference, since the frontal areas are stimulated over the musculus temporalis, which increases the distance between the TMS coil and the skull surface. The effective field strength induced by standard TMS coils decreases exponentially when distance to the coil increases, which renders the treatment less effective (Hoffman *et al.*, 2007). However, non-standard TMS coils, as the one described by Roth *et al.* (2002; 2007), have a markedly slower decrease in electrical field when distance to the coil increases, which can reach a cortical depth of up to 5.5 cm (Zangen *et al.* 2007). Application of such TMS coils may effectively reduce AVH activity in the right inferior frontal region, which could be an effective treatment for medication-resistant AVH.

In summary, group-wise analysis of 24 psychotic patients showed activation during AVH in the right homolog of Broca's area, right superior temporal gyrus, and additional bilateral gyri, but not in Broca's area nor in the left superior temporal gyrus. In contrast, silent word production in the same patients *did* engage Broca's area and the left superior temporal gyrus, among other areas. This may indicate that language produced in the homolog of Broca's area is more liable to become misattributed and lead to the experience of AVH than language generated in Broca's area. Insufficient cerebral dominance may therefore be a predisposing factor for auditory verbal hallucinations.

ACKNOWLEDGMENT

Extracts and figures in this chapter are selected from Sommer, I. E. C., Diedeven, K. M., Blom, J. D. *et al.* (2008). Auditory verbal hallucinations predominantly activate the right inferior frontal area. *Brain*, October 13.

REFERENCES

Aleman, A., Sommer, I. E. & Kahn, R. S. (2007). Efficacy of slow repetitive transcranial magnetic stimulation in the treatment of resistant auditory hallucinations in schizophrenia: a meta-analysis. *J Clin Psychiatry*, **68**(3), 416–21.

Allen, P., Larøi, F., McGuire, P. K. & Aleman, A. (2008). The hallucinating brain: a review of structural and functional neuroimaging studies of hallucinations. *Neurosci Biobehav Rev*, **32**(1), 175–91.

Andreasen, N C., Flaum. M. & Arndt, S. (1992). The comprehensive assessment of symptoms and history (CASH): an instrument for assessing psychopathology and diagnosis. *Arch Gen Psychiatry*, **49**, 615–23.

Artiges, E., Martinot, J. L., Verdys, M. *et al.* (2000). Altered hemispheric functional dominance during word generation in negative schizophrenia. *Schizophr Bull*, **26**(3), 709–21.

Benjamini, Y. & Hochberg, Y. (1995). Controlling the false discovery rate: a practical and powerful approach to multiple testing. *J R Statist Soc, Ser B (Methodol)*, **57**(1), 289–300.

Bloom, J. S. & Hynd, G. W. (2005). The role of the corpus callosum in interhemispheric transfer of information: excitation or inhibition? *Neuropsychol Rev*, **15**(2), 59–71.

Burklund, C. W. & Smith, A. (1977). Language and the cerebral hemispheres. Observations of verbal and nonverbal responses during 18 months following left ("dominant") hemispherectomy. *Neurology*, **27**(7), 627–33.

Copolov, D. L., Seal, M. L., Maruff, P. *et al.* (2003). Cortical activation associated with the experience of auditory hallucinations and perception of human speech in schizophrenia: a PET correlation study. *Psychiatry Res*, **122**(3), 139–52.

Creutzfeldt, O., Ojemann, G. & Lettich, E. (1989). Neuronal activity in the human lateral temporal lobe. II. Responses to the subject's own voice. *Exp Brain Res*, **77**(3), 476–89.

David, A. S. (1999). Auditory hallucinations: phenomenology, neuropsychology and neuroimaging update. *Acta Psychiatr Scand*, **99**(suppl 394), 95–104.

Dierks, T., Linden, D. J. E., Jandl, M. *et al.* (1999). Activation of Heschl's gyrus during auditory hallucinations. *Neuron*, **22**, 615–21.

Dollfus, S., Razafimandimby, A., Delamillieure, P. *et al.* (2005). Atypical hemispheric specialization for language in right-handed schizophrenia. *Biol Psychiatry*, **57**(9), 1020–8.

Ford, J. M., Roach, B. J., Faustman, W. O. & Mathalon, D. H. (2007). Synch before you speak: auditory hallucinations in schizophrenia. *Am J Psychiatry*, **164**(3), 458–66.

Frith, C. D. (1992). *The Cognitive Neuropsychology of Schizophrenia*. Hove: Erlbaum.

Hoffman, R. E., Hampson, M., Wu, K. *et al.* (2007). Probing the pathophysiology of auditory/verbal hallucinations by combining functional magnetic resonance imaging and transcranial magnetic stimulation. *Cereb Cortex*, **7**(11), 2733–43.

Jackson, J. H. (1931–1932). *Selected Writings of John Hughlings Jackson.* Vols I, II. Taylor, J. (ed.). London: Hodder.

Jaynes, J. (1976). *On the Origin of Consciousness in the Breakdown of the Bicameral Mind.* Boston: Houghton Mifflin Company.

Lennox, B. R., Park, S. B., Jones, P. B. & Morris, P. G. (1999). Spatial and temporal mapping of neural activity associated with auditory hallucinations. *Lancet*, **353**(9153), 644.

Lennox, B. R., Park, S. B. G., Medley, I. *et al.* (2000). The functional anatomy of auditory hallucinations in schizophrenia. *Psychiatry Res Neuroimag*, **100**, 13–20.

Nasrallah, H. A. (1985). The unintegrated right cerebral hemispheric consciousness as alien intruder: a possible mechanism for Schneiderian delusions in schizophrenia. *Compr Psychiatry*, **26**(3), 273–82.

Neggers, S. F. W., Hermans, E. J. & Ramsey, N. F. (2008). Enhanced sensitivity with fast three-dimensional BOLD fMRI: comparison of SENSE-PRESTO and 2D-EPI at 3 T. *NMR in Biomed*, **21**(7), 663–76.

Noppeney, U., Price, C. J., Duncan, J. S. & Koepp, M. J. (2005). Reading skills after left anterior temporal lobe resection: an fMRI study. *Brain*, **128**(6), 1377–85.

Oldfield, R. C. (1971). The assessment and analysis of handedness: the Edinburgh inventory. *Neuropsychologia*, **9**(1), 97–113.

Razafimandimby, A., Maiza, O., Herve, P. Y. *et al.* (2007). Stability of functional language lateralization over time in schizophrenia patients. *Schizophr Res*, **94**(1–3), 197–206.

Roth, Y., Amir, A., Levkovitz, Y. & Zangen, A. (2007). Three-dimensional distribution of the electric field induced in the brain by transcranial magnetic stimulation using figure-8 and deep H-coils. *J Clin Neurophysiol*, **24**(1), 31–8.

Roth, Y., Zangen, A. & Hallett, M. (2002). A coil design for transcranial magnetic stimulation of deep brain regions. *J Clin Neurophysiol*, **19**(4), 361–70.

Shergill, S. S., Brammer, M. J., Williams, S. C. R. *et al.* (2000). Mapping auditory hallucinations in schizophrenia using functional magnetic resonance imaging. *Arch Gen Psychiatry*, **57**, 1033–8.

Shergill, S. S., Cameron, L. A., Brammer, M. J. *et al.* (2001). Modality specific neural correlates of auditory and somatic hallucinations. *J Neurol Neurosurg Psychiatry*, **71**(5), 688–90.

Silbersweig, D. A., Stern, E., Frith, C. *et al.* (1995). A functional neuroanatomy of hallucinations in schizophrenia. *Nature*, **378**, 176–9.

Slade, P. D. & Bentall, R. P. (1988). *Sensory Deception: A Scientific Analysis of Hallucinations.* Baltimore: Johns Hopkins University Press.

Sommer, I. E. C., Ramsey, N. F. & Kahn, R. S. (2001). Lateralization in schizophrenia: an fMRI study. *Schizophr Res*, **52**, 57–67.

Sommer, I. E. C., Ramsey, N. F., Mandl, R. C. W. & Kahn, R. S. (2003). Language lateralization in women with schizophrenia. *Schizophr Res*, **60**(2–3), 183–90.

Sommer, I. E., Ramsey, N. F., Mandl, R. C., van Oel, C. J. & Kahn, R. S. (2004). Language activation in monozygotic twins discordant for schizophrenia. *Br J Psychiatry*, **184**, 128–35.

Sommer, I. E., Vd Veer, A. J., Wijkstra, J., Boks, M. P. & Kahn, R. S. (2007). Comparing language lateralization in psychotic mania and psychotic depression to schizophrenia: a functional MRI study. *Schizophr Res*, **89**(1–3), 364–5.

Spaniel, F., Tintera, J., Hajek, T. *et al.* (2007). Language lateralization in monozygotic twins discordant and concordant for schizophrenia. A functional MRI pilot study. *Eur Psychiatry*, **22**(5), 319–22.

Springer, J., Binder, J., Hammeke, T. *et al.* (1999). Language dominance in neurologically normal and epilepsy subjects: a functional MRI study. *Brain*, **122**, 2033–46.

Stephane, M., Barton, S. & Boutros, N. N. (2001). Auditory verbal hallucinations and dysfunction of the neural substrates of speech. *Schizophr Res*, **50**(1–2), 61–78.

Thiel, A., Habedank, B., Herholz, K. *et al.* (2005). From the left to the right: how the brain compensates progressive loss of language function. *Brain Lang*, **98**(1), 57–65.

Thiel, A., Herholz, K., Koyuncu, A. *et al.* (2001). Plasticity of language networks in patients with brain tumors: a positron emission tomography activation study. *Ann Neurol*, **50**(5), 620–9.

Thiel, A., Schumacher, B., Wienhard, K. *et al.* (2006). Direct demonstration of transcallosal disinhibition in language networks. *J Cereb Blood Flow Metab*, **26**(9), 1122–7.

Thivard, L., Hombrouck, J., du Montcel, S. T. *et al.* (2005). Productive and perceptive language reorganization in temporal lobe epilepsy. *Neuroimage*, **24**(3), 841–51.

Tzourio-Mazoyer, N., Landeau, B., Papathanassiou, D. *et al.* (2002). Automated anatomical labeling of activations in SPM using a macroscopic anatomical parcellation of the MNI MRI single-subject brain. *Neuroimage*, **15**(1), 273–89.

Van Lancker, D. & Cummings, J. L. (1999). Expletives: neurolinguistic and neurobehavioral perspectives on swearing. *Brain Res Brain Res Rev*, **31**(1), 83–104.

Van Lancker, D. (1997). Rags to riches: our increasing appreciation of cognitive and communicative abilities of the human right cerebral hemisphere. *Brain Lang*, **57**(1), 1–11.

Voets, N. L., Adcock, J. E., Flitney, D. E. *et al.* (2006). Distinct right frontal lobe activation in language processing following left hemisphere injury. *Brain*, **129**(3), 754–66.

Weiss, E. M., Hofer, A., Golaszewski, S. *et al.* (2006). Language lateralization in unmedicated patients during an acute episode of schizophrenia: a functional MRI study. *Psychiatry Res*, **146**(2), 185–90.

Winhuisen, L., Thiel, A., Schumacher, B. *et al.* (2005). Role of the contralateral inferior frontal gyrus in recovery of language function in poststroke aphasia: a combined repetitive transcranial magnetic stimulation and positron emission tomography study. *Stroke*, **36**(8), 1759–63.

Worsley, K. J. & Friston, K. J. (1995). Analysis of fMRI time-series revisited – again. *Neuroimage*, **2**(3), 173–81.

Zangen, A., Roth, Y., Voller, B. & Hallett, M. (2007). Transcranial magnetic stimulation of deep brain regions: evidence for efficacy of the H-coil. *Clin Neurophysiol*, **116**(4), 775–9.

Zangwill, O. L. (1967). Speech and the minor hemisphere. *Acta Neurol Psychiatr Belg*, **67**(11), 1013–20.

12

Language lateralization in patients with formal thought disorder

Carin Whitney and Tilo Kircher

Summary

Formal thought disorder (FTD) denotes language dysfunctions observed in schizophrenia that can be separated into positive and negative features. Whereas positive FTD is mainly characterized by peculiar word usage, peculiar sentence constructions, tangentiality, and loosening of associations, negative FTD manifests, among others, as impoverished speech. Patients with FTD are compromised in both their language production (FTD) and comprehension (e.g., "concretism") skills.

On the neurobiological level, brain areas relevant for linguistic processing, particularly the lateral temporal lobes but also the anterior cingulate, the lateral frontal, and medial temporal lobes have been implicated in the pathophysiology of FTD, depending on the task and the symptomatology of the patient group investigated.

Reductions in gray matter volume of the superior temporal gyrus (STG) and parts of it, specifically the Heschl gyrus (HG) and the posteriorly adjacent planum temporale (PT), have consistently been reported to be in an attenuated, diminished, or even inverse structural left–right asymmetry (L > R) in patients with FTD compared to healthy control subjects.

Functionally, the severity of FTD is associated with decreased or reversed lateralization of brain activity in the temporal lobes and STG specifically during numerous aspects of language processing, including simple auditory and higher-order semantic functions. Hereby, aberrant BOLD-signals in the left and right lateral temporal cortices have been observed in patients with positive FTD compared to healthy control subjects during language production and comprehension tasks using functional magnetic resonance imaging (fMRI). Measuring electrophysiological brain responses, recordings of event-related potentials (ERP) during perceptive linguistic performance showed decreases in components related to semantic anomalies (N400) or context updating (P300).

Since language is probably the most complex cognitive-motor task humans perform, the brain is the most complex organ and schizophrenia a complex disorder, entangling the relationship between these three entities remains a scientific challenge.

Introduction

Language dysfunctions are a key feature in schizophrenia, which clinically manifests as formal thought disorder (FTD) (Liddle *et al.*, 2002). Whereas poverty of speech and weakening of goal are referred to as negative FTD, looseness, peculiar word usage, peculiar sentence constructions, and peculiar logic, on the other hand, are subsumed under the category of disorganized speech or positive FTD. Finally, unspecific impairments of speech and thought include perseveration and distractibility. Most impressively, FTD surfaces during speech production in terms of disorganized or unintelligible utterances. The underlying cognitive impairments are complex and can be divided into "core" disturbances such as impairments involving the semantic system (Goldberg *et al.*, 1998; Goldberg & Weinberger, 2000; Kuperberg & Caplan, 2003), executive function, self-monitoring, and a number of "modulating factors" such as working memory, affective state, pragmatic and theory of mind faculties, attention and IQ (e.g., Barrera *et al.*, 2005; Kerns & Berenbaum, 2002; Landre & Taylor, 1995; Leeson *et al.*, 2005; Stirling *et al.*, 2006).

Dysfunctions within the semantic system are expressed in aberrant activation, inhibition, or selection processes within the semantic network (Kuperberg &

Caplan, 2003). As a consequence of these limitations, speech production but also specific aspects of language comprehension are compromised in patients with FTD. For example, schizophrenia patients show a deficit in their paralinguistic or pragmatic abilities including the interpretation of metaphors, understanding of jokes, sarcasm, or emotional prosody, which are all functions mainly subserved by the right hemisphere (Mitchell & Crow, 2005).

On the neurobiological level, the results of functional neuroimaging and electrophysiological studies imply a dysfunction of (1) the fronto-temporal language network and (2) disturbances in hemispheric interaction (between the left and right language homolog areas) in patients with FTD (Mitchell & Crow, 2005). With respect to FTD, the superior temporal gyrus (STG) seems to be the key component in the disrupted language network. It comprises the Heschl gyrus (HG) and the planum temporale (PT), which are the two most relevant brain regions in auditory and language processing, respectively. In schizophrenia, impairments from the early stages of auditory perception up to aberrant higher-order expressive and receptive language skills characterize findings in patients with FTD. Neuroanatomically, most of the reported structural lateralization abnormalities are observed in the STG. Lately, some studies even link the anatomical and functional changes observed in the temporal cortices and correlate them with the specific language impairments seen in patients with FTD (McCarley et al., 2002; Meisenzahl et al., 2004; Weinstein et al., 2007).

In the following three sections we will present morphological analyses, earlier metabolic investigations with positron emission tomography (PET) and functional imaging studies during language tasks, which strengthen the role of the STG in the pathogenesis of FTD. As we go along, we will embed anatomical and functional deficits of this structure into the framework of lateralization anomalies in patients with FTD. In the final section, approaches are discussed which integrate structure (i.e., reduced STG volume), function (i.e., aberrant temporal activation patterns), and symptom (i.e., FTD) relations. We have restricted our review to studies where patients with positive FTD or the disorganization syndrome were explicitly investigated or

where the severity of this syndrome has been correlated with the independent experimental measure. Only this approach allows for the reduction of the symptomatological heterogeneity of the disorder and a potential advancement in establishing a brain–symptom relationship. Deviations from this approach will be mentioned explicitly, "FTD" will be used synonymously with "positive FTD" in the following.

Formal though disorder and anatomical lateralization anomalies of the STG

The STG is a complex structure covering the HG (i.e., primary auditory cortex) and the PT, whereas the posterior section of the PT spans the classic Wernicke area. Compared to its right homologs, HG and PT volumes are larger on the left hemisphere, which is taken as an indication for the functional specialization of this hemisphere in language processing. More precisely, the PT is the most pronounced asymmetric region in the human brain (L > R) reflecting its high relevance in language functions and importance for FTD research.

Volumetric anomalies of the STG are a consistent finding in patients with schizophrenia (for reviews see Pearlson & Marsh, 1999; Shenton et al., 2001). It is not surprising that in patients suffering from FTD, such anomalies are dependent on the severity of the patient's language dysfunctions, too. Shenton and colleagues (1992) were the first to report a negative correlation between the extent of FTD and gray matter volume in the left posterior STG. In contrast to healthy controls, the posterior STG volume was decreased up to 15% in patients with FTD despite comparable whole brain volume between the two groups. Since then, most of the studies investigating FTD replicated reductions in L > R asymmetry for the STG or specific parts of this structure, e.g., the PT (Menon et al., 1995, Rajarethinam et al., 2001; Rossi et al., 1994; Shapleske et al., 1999; Subotnik et al., 2003; Weinstein et al., 2007; for negative outcomes see, e.g., DeLisi et al., 1994). Representative for a number of volumetric studies, Vita and collaborators (1995) documented an inverse relationship between the laterality index and FTD severity: the more pronounced the FTD-related language impairment, the smaller the ratio between the size of the left and right STG. Apart from attenuations in the L > R asymmetry, a reversal in the PT lateralization has been observed in severely thought disordered patients, too (Shapleske *et al.*, 1999).

Although the majority of studies reported an association of reduced gray matter volume of the *left* temporal gyrus and the amount of FTD (Rossi *et al.*, 1994; Shenton *et al.*, 1992), volume reductions in chronic schizophrenia patients (Ohnishi *et al.*, 2006) as well as negative correlations between incoherence of speech and gray matter density in high-risk male adolescents (Spencer *et al.*, 2007) have recently been found in the contralateral, *right* middle temporal gyrus (MTG).

Altogether, the degree of FTD seems to be inversely correlated with a decrease in leftward lateralization of the STG and PT, in particular. This structure–symptom relationship belongs to the most robust finding in the field of schizophrenia research despite inconsistent methodological approaches. Across studies, differences are apparent in the way FTD symptomatology has been assessed, in the quality and spatial resolution of the structural data, and the definition of anatomical boundaries of the relevant structures (Shapleske *et al.*, 1999).

However, beside strong evidence for a correlation between structural STG anomalies and the degree of FTD, it is premature to draw a causal inference between the two factors alone without having looked at functional correlations (see below).

Metabolic changes of the STG in patients with FTD

Apart from reports on structural changes in brain regions relevant for language processing, studies using positron emission tomography (PET) or single photon emission computed tomography (SPECT) in patients with schizophrenia and FTD detected abnormalities in the cerebral metabolism. Most frequently, regional cerebral blood flow (rCBF) has been correlated with severity of disorganization (i.e., mainly positive FTD) and measured during resting state, i.e., while the patient was instructed to "not think of anything".

Investigating the relationship between cerebral metabolism and the disorganization syndrome, the left superior temporal cortex has been identified as a key region: Liddle and colleagues (1992) observed positive correlations between disorganization and rCBF in the left superior temporal sulcus, Friston and collaborators (1992) have associated this syndrome to metabolic activity in the left STG and Kaplan and co-workers (1993) reported a negative correlation between disorganization and relative glucose metabolism in the left superior temporal and inferior parietal region. Besides the left temporal cortices, other brain regions have also been implicated in the aberrant metabolism of disorganized patients, such as the medial temporal and prefrontal lobes (Friston *et al.*, 1992; Kawasaki *et al.*, 1996; Liddle *et al.*, 1992).

Summing up, the results of PET and SPECT studies indicate that the STG is affected in patients of the disorganized subtype, which is reflected in either hypo- or hypermetabolic activity in this area. However, compared to volumetric investigations metabolic studies are rare and the data are more heterogeneous. A major methodological issue is that in these studies FTD has not been isolated from the global disorganization syndrome, which might have skewed the results. Furthermore, the neural activity of the brain's resting state is hard to control for since it is dependent on the patient's cognitive processes during "resting". Less arbitrary in this context is the correlation of specific symptoms or cognitive functions to brain regions in patients with FTD using functional imaging during the production of the symptom in question or the "on line" monitoring of cognitive processes.

Functional lateralization anomalies in patients with FTD during language processing

The core feature in the psychopathology of patients with FTD is a pronounced impairment in the linguistic domain, which is supposed to be provoked by an aberrant lateralization of brain areas relevant for intact speech and word processing, i.e., mainly the STG bilaterally. Over the last two decades, functional magnetic resonance imaging (fMRI) and electrophysiological investigations, e.g., event-related potentials (ERP), have been employed to study the neurobiological basis of this symptom, thus providing empirical evidence for lateralization anomalies in the brains of patients with FTD during language tasks. Hereby, two basic methodological approaches have emerged: FTD can either be measured *directly* e.g., during the expression of disorganized speech, or alternatively, and this is the most common approach, the neural correlates of FTD can be assessed via the patient's performance and neural activity during specific psycholinguistic tasks compared, ideally, to a patient control group without this symptom. Either way, these studies aim to relate the linguistic anomalies observed in patients as they occur to localized brain activity. Basically we will see that, on the functional level, deviations from the L > R asymmetry of language processes in the temporal lobes have been found during both productive (e.g., Kircher *et al.*, 2002) and perceptive speech tasks (e.g., Ngan *et al.*, 2003). In an ultimate step, the altered functional activation patterns associated with FTD-related language dysfunctions have been linked to structural changes in the brain in the same study, thus providing a more comprehensive picture of the symptom–structure–function relation (in Kasai *et al.*, 2002; McCarley *et al.*, 2002; Weinstein *et al.*, 2007).

Brain activation during language production in patients with FTD

In this approach, subjects are scanned while they are speaking overtly. For the data analysis, specific aspects of speech, such as the number of words, the syntactic complexity, or the amount of FTD and the expression of single, concrete symptoms (e.g., neologisms), are correlated with measures of brain activation. Among other regions, alterations in patients have most frequently been linked to aberrant neural response patterns in the temporal lobes (Kircher *et al.*, 2001a, 2001b, 2002, 2005; McGuire *et al.*, 1998).

In one study, natural language production processes have been assessed while patients with severe FTD spoke about Rorschach inkblots (Kircher *et al.*, 2002). Each 20-second speech epoch was assigned a specific score describing the degree of FTD that was produced during this time interval. Hereby, a correlation with blood-oxygen-level-dependent (BOLD)-signal changes revealed an inverse relationship between activity in the left posterior STG and the extent of FTD in patients with schizophrenia. The same region was found to be negatively correlated with FTD in an analogous study using PET (McGuire *et al.*, 1998). This is somewhat surprising, since the patients scanned, the stimuli used, the time frames of analysis, and, particularly, the scanning technique applied, were different, arguing for the robustness of the results. Classically, dysfunctions in the left STG have been associated with semantic anomalies and incoherences observed in patients with Wernicke aphasia who suffer from lesions in this part of the temporal cortex. Comparable semantic impairments are found in the speech of thought disordered patients with schizophrenia, which implies that FTD might be evoked by a temporary "functional lesion" in the STG.

Apart from reductions in BOLD-response, a reversal of lateralized brain activity in temporal lobes has also been reported in patients with FTD (Kircher *et al.*, 2001b, 2002). A positive correlation was observed between the speech rate (number of words spoken per 20-second epoch) of healthy control subjects and neural activity in the left STG (Kircher *et al.*, 2002). In contrast, enhanced BOLD-responses in the opposite hemisphere, i.e., in the right lateral temporal cortex, co-occurred with increasing speech rate in patients with FTD. This inverse left–right asymmetry in patients during speech production might be the consequence of a reversed access to the left and right mental lexica in patients with FTD during speaking. Hemifield and neglect studies investigating the contribution of each hemisphere to word comprehension separately, have shown that the semantic fields of words differ in such a way, that very narrow semantic fields have been attributed to the left, and broader, more diffuse semantic fields to the right temporal cortex (see for the local–global dichotomy Beeman *et al.*, 1994). According to this model, the semantic incoherences observed in FTD can be explained by an increased access to or use of the right mental lexicon, which, on the neural level, is reflected in abnormal BOLD-enhancements in the corresponding right STG.

Besides impairments on the semantic level, reduced temporal activation in patients with FTD compared to healthy controls has been observed during syntactic manipulations e.g., the production of syntactically simple vs. complex sentences during spontaneous speech (Kircher *et al.*, 2005). Hereby, right middle temporal BOLD-attenuation was accompanied by decreases in left superior frontal activity, which together might have accounted for the expression of a significantly lower number of complex sentences in patients with FTD compared to the control group during speaking.

Formal thought disorder has also been linked to functions operating on the single sentence level where isolated linguistic elements (words) needed to be integrated into a coherent, overall context (sentence). In a word production paradigm cued by sentence stems ("The letter was sent without a xxxx"), patients with FTD displayed *left* middle and inferior temporal activity compared to a healthy control group and schizophrenia subjects without FTD (Kircher *et al.*, 2001a). The opposite comparison, i.e., where patients with FTD exhibited weaker BOLD-signals than the two other groups, revealed brain activity in the contralateral hemisphere, i.e., the right STG. The observed lack of right temporal engagement in patients with FTD has been related to deficits in the online integration and utilization of context information during online speech production.

Finally, temporal anomalies at the level of overt single word production have also been shown (Kircher *et al.*, 2008). While patients with schizophrenia formed spontaneous associations in response to a cue word (e.g., cue: dog, association: bone), a negative correlation between the amount of FTD and the right MTG and lingual gyrus was identified which strengthened the relevance of the temporal lobe in the pathophysiology of FTD.

In sum, the language production abnormalities seen in patients with FTD have been attributed to losses or reversals of lateralized neural activity in the temporal lobes.

Language comprehension deficits in patients with FTD

Impairments in the comprehension of speech or written content have been associated with the pathogenesis of schizophrenia in general, including deficits at the stages of simple speech (e.g., phonemes) and non-speech sound comprehension as well as deficits during higher-order semantic processes at the word, single sentence, or discourse level. In the following sections we will show that these impairments can be specifically associated with FTD. They will be integrated into the framework of an abnormal temporal lateralization of basic auditory and more complex language functions, respectively.

Deficits of simple speech and non-speech sound processing

Patients exhibit dysfunctions already at the very lowest level of acoustic perception (including non-linguistic and linguistic). Particularly, studies with ERP have found impairments in early auditory processing, expressed in altered P50 and mismatch negativity (MMN) potentials. The former is thought to index sensory gating functions whereas the latter is likely to reflect preattentive short-term sensory memory (for reviews see Kasai *et al.*, 2002; Mathiak & Fallgatter, 2006; Potter *et al.*, 2006; Youn *et al.*, 2002). In a combined magnetoencephalography (MEG) and fMRI study on MMN, it could be shown that there was a lateralization deficit in the magnetic as well as the BOLD response in the group of schizophrenia patients compared to a healthy control group. It could also be shown directly that the MMN signal was generated in the STG (Kircher *et al.*, 2004). Despite the tremendous amount of ERP-studies on schizophrenia in general, correlations between specific clinical symptoms and these components are rare (see, for a review on the P50, Potter *et al.*, 2006). One study detected an inverse relationship between the severity of positive symptoms and the MMN asymmetry coefficient, which was strongest for the hallucinatory syndrome (Youn *et al.*, 2002). Another study reported an inverse relationship between the severity of FTD and one measure of the P50 but not the global component (Baker *et al.*, 1987). Certainly, more research needs to be conducted in order to make confident statements about correlations between early auditory (lateralization) deficits and the language dysfunctions observed in patients with FTD in particular.

More promising are the results of studies on the P300, which indexes controlled and effortful rather than automatic processes (Kasai *et al.*, 2002). The P300 indicates the attentional resources allocated to a stimulus or allocated to the process of context updating and is reduced in patients with schizophrenia (e.g., Kasai *et al.*, 2002). It seems to be specifically dependent on the severity of positive symptoms (e.g., Higashima *et al.*, 2003) and, most importantly, associated with the degree of FTD (Frodl *et al.*, 2002; Higashima *et al.*, 1998; Iwanami *et al.*, 2000; Kirihara *et al.*, 2005). All studies reported a negative correlation between P300 amplitude and increasing FTD ratings. This is of particular interest since reductions in P300 amplitude in schizophrenia have been preferably seen over the left hemisphere (or more specifically the left temporal lobe), a key region in the pathogenesis of FTD, and been even linked to volumetric changes of this structure (Craven, 2002). Kirihara and colleagues (2005) strengthened the role of a reduced leftward lateralization when they observed a more pronounced negative correlation between FTD and the left compared to the right temporal region.

Evidence of functional anomalies in the temporal cortices, particularly in FTD patients, was further provided in a study by Ngan and colleagues (2003) who employed an oddball target-detection task, using fMRI. Subjects were required to respond via button press to deviant sounds (speech vs. non-speech stimuli), which were randomly embedded into a series of regular background noise. An abnormally stronger BOLD-signal was observed for patients compared to controls in the left temporo-parietal junction, but most importantly in the right STG, when speech and non-speech sounds were compared. This right-sided hyperactivation was interpreted in favor of an aberrant lateralization of early speech processes to the non-dominant, right hemisphere in schizophrenia. With respect to FTD, a positive correlation was found in the left temporo-parietal cluster with symptom severity.

Altogether, these results imply a fundamental auditory processing deficit in schizophrenia, which seems to be particularly related to patients with FTD and their underlying neurophysiological changes in the temporal cortices.

Impaired comprehension at the word level

Evidence for an aberrant semantic network on the single word level has been provided in behavioral studies using semantic priming paradigms (e.g., Manschreck *et al.*, 1988; Spitzer *et al.*, 1993). In these behavioral studies, FTD was associated with a decrease in reaction time to words that were preceded by semantically related (e.g., lion – tiger) compared to unrelated (e.g., lion – pencil) words (Manschreck *et al.*, 1988). The same fast response pattern was recorded for indirectly related word pairs (e.g., lion – stripes) where the semantic association can only be established by an invisible mediator (e.g., lion – (tiger) – stripes) (Spitzer *et al.*, 1993, Weisbrod *et al.*, 1998). Neither healthy control subjects nor patients without FTD displayed that behavior. Hyperpriming for indirectly related words at the automatic processing stage (i.e., prime-target presentation interval below 300 ms) in patients with FTD are well replicated (see, for a review on priming, Minzenberg *et al.*, 2002).

A reversal of left–right asymmetry in the semantic network (see also Kircher *et al.*, 2002) has been provided by several behavioral priming studies, which presented word pairs in either the left (LVF) or right visual field (RVF) (Minzenberg *et al.*, 2002). For example, in the hemifield study by Weisbrod and colleagues (1998), thought disordered patients with schizophrenia showed indirect priming effects to words presented to the LVF and RVF (i.e., the right and left hemisphere) whereas controls and patients without FTD responded to indirectly related word pairs in the LVF (i.e., the right hemisphere) only. According to the local–global dichotomy (Beeman *et al.*, 1994) it could be argued that access to the mental lexicon seems to be disturbed in patients with FTD.

However, it should be noted that alternative approaches exist in order to explain the semantic deficits in patients with schizophrenia (Bullen & Hemsley, 1987; Cohen & Servan-Schreiber, 1992; Frith, 1979; Goldberg *et al.*, 1998; Titone *et al.*, 2000). Nonetheless, priming paradigms have been successful in explaining many of the semantic language deficits in schizophrenia and in associating them with FTD in particular (see, for a review, Minzenberg *et al.*, 2002). Recent fMRI studies reported increased brain activity in the fronto-temporal language network during semantic priming tasks in patients with schizophrenia compared to controls (Han *et al.*, 2007; Kuperberg *et al.*, 2007). Particularly, a positive correlation was found between activation of the ventral temporal cortex bilaterally and severity of FTD during semantic priming (Kuperberg *et al.*, 2007). Similarly, Han and colleagues (2007) observed a positive correlation between the SAPS items illogicality, distracted speech, and incoherence and activation in the left middle/superior temporal lobe. The authors interpreted the results in favor of an aberrant functionality of the semantic system(s) located in the left and right temporal cortices in patients with FTD (see also Kircher *et al.*, 2002).

Electrophysiologically, the N400 is a marker for semantic processes because it is known to reflect the demand of integrating a word into its previous context (Kutas & Hillyard, 1980). Hereby, higher N400 amplitudes for unrelated compared to related words are observed during priming. This modulation of N400 amplitude is diminished in patients with schizophrenia and has often been specifically associated with semantic impairments in patients with FTD (see, for a review, Kumar & Debruille, 2004). Using an ERP priming paradigm, Kostova and colleagues (2005) observed an inverse correlation between symptom severity of FTD and the N400 effect: the more impaired the patients, the higher the N400 amplitude for related words and, thus, the lower the difference in N400 amplitude between the unrelated to the related condition.

To conclude, deviations from the regular L > R asymmetry of brain activation in the temporal lobes have been associated with disturbances in the semantic network in patients with FTD during single word comprehension.

Impaired sentence/discourse comprehension

An impairment in the understanding of isolated (i.e., single sentence comprehension) or connected (i.e., discourse comprehension) sentences in patients with schizophrenia is a phenomenon possibly resulting from a failure in the build-up and utilization of contextual information during on-line comprehension (Cohen & Servan-Schreiber, 1992). Pronounced impairments are particularly seen in patients with FTD supported by an increase of aberrant neural or electrophysiological activation patterns with enhanced symptom severity. Most frequently, patients' performances have been analyzed in response to sentences with semantic anomalies, but deficits were also observed on the level of pragmatic or syntactic violations (Kuperberg *et al.*, 2000). Although difficulties in proverb, metaphor, or joke interpretations, clinically referred to as "concretism", have been consistently reported in patients with FTD, neuroimaging studies are rare. In one study, Kircher and colleagues (2007) observed significantly lower brain activity in the right middle and superior temporal gyrus (and the precuneus) in schizophrenia patients compared to healthy control subjects during the comprehension of metaphorical sentences. Patients, on the other hand, exhibited stronger BOLD-signals than controls in the left inferior frontal gyrus (BA 44). Activation in close proximity to this area (BA 45) correlated negatively with the extend of the "concretism" item in the PANSS scale. This study emphasizes the role of the left lateral prefrontal cortex in "concretism" in schizophrenia patients.

Electrophysiologically, the N400 has been considered again to be a useful tool in identifying semantic processing deficits during sentence/discourse comprehension. In schizophrenia, several ERP-studies replicated reductions in the N400 effect (see above) during on-line comprehension to different kinds of semantic manipulations (see, for a review, Kumar & Debruille, 2004). Specific correlations between N400 abnormalities and FTD symptom severity have also been detected (see, for a review, Kumar & Debruille, 2004; Adams *et al.*, 1989; Andrews *et al.*, 1993). For example, Salisbury and colleagues (2000) manipulated the integration process of words into their context by introducing homonyms, i.e., words with different meanings. The sentences were neutral (i.e., not biased towards one or the other meaning) until the point of disambiguation, i.e., the sentence-final word, where the N400 was recorded. For example, the sentence "The bank was closed" provoked the selection of the more frequent, dominant meaning of *bank* whereas "The bank was steep" favored the subordinate meaning referring to the river side. A positive correlation was found between the N400 amplitude in sentences triggering the subordinate meaning and the degree of FTD. Integrating the word into its context became more difficult with increasing symptom severity for patients with FTD. In the latest investigation, Ditman and Kuperberg (2007) observed a reduced N400 effect in patients with schizophrenia during the comprehension of highly related and unrelated discourse excerpts. Higher scores of FTD were related to decreasing N400 effects, implying that especially patients with FTD have problems in building discourse coherences from the contextual information provided by the sentences.

Evidence for a disturbed left–right asymmetry during natural language comprehension in patients with schizophrenia was provided by an fMRI study by Weinstein and colleagues (2006). Although not statistically significant, left superior and middle temporal BOLD-enhancement surfaced in patients but not in the healthy control group during listening to English compared to Mandarin text. Statistically reliable, on the other hand, was the correlation between FTD and increased activity in the left posterior superior temporal sulcus and middle temporal gyrus. Considering that discourse comprehension is primarily subserved by the right hemisphere, the results speak in favor of a reversed lateralization of language comprehension functions in the temporal cortices.

Taken together, the findings of sentence and discourse comprehension on the electrophysiological and neuroimaging level support a problem in the build-up of an overall meaning from sentence or discourse context.

Structure–function relationships in patients with FTD

Considering the amount of FTD-specific changes in neural structure and brain activity during simple auditory and more complex semantic processing tasks, several attempts have been made to establish a link between the anatomical (i.e., reduced STG volume) and functional (i.e., aberrant activation patterns) substrates of FTD. It has been hypothesized that specific brain responses might be the direct result of macroscopic morphological changes in the STG in schizophrenia (e.g. Craven, 2002).

First evidence for a structure–function relationship in patients with schizophrenia has been provided by electrophysiological studies investigating the P300 during standard oddball tasks. Investigating a single schizophrenia patient with pronounced volume reductions in the left temporal lobe and severe FTD, Shenton and colleagues (1993) demonstrated a reduction in P300 amplitude during an oddball task. The authors suggested a connection between the three components (1) structural and (2) functional anomalies and (3) the expression of FTD. More recent studies reported correlations between P300 abnormalities and gray matter volume changes of the left STG in schizophrenia patients but did not link these results to specific clinical symptoms such as FTD (e.g., McCarley et al., 2002; also see for a review on neuroanatomy and neurophysiology in schizophrenia Kasai et al., 2002). By analyzing structure–function relationships, evidence for an abnormal lateralization of the temporal cortices in patients with schizophrenia has also been provided. In their two publications (McCarley et al., 1993, 2002), the research group reported a correlation between volume deficits in the PT and reversed P300 asymmetry, indicating smaller amplitudes on the left than on the right temporal region in patients with schizophrenia. Unfortunately, associations with clinical symptoms have been ignored.

A combined MRI/ERP study filled the gap and addressed this issue (Meisenzahl et al., 2004). The correlation between the degree of FTD, P300 amplitude at the left temporal electrode site (T3), and gray matter volume of the left PT was investigated. The results replicated the reliable negative correlation between P300 amplitude at T3 and FTD symptom severity. Contrary to their expectations though, volume reductions in the left PT were neither related to P300 amplitude nor FTD. In general, altered P300 amplitude and reductions in the STG were not apparent in their schizophrenia patients compared to healthy controls in this study, which might have accounted for the unexpected results with respect to FTD. The authors made the state of their patients (medicated, stabilized, few positive symptoms) in contrast to previous investigations and the difficulty in establishing reliable PT borders across studies responsible for their negative findings.

With respect to higher-order language processes, Weinstein and colleagues (2007) documented that the relationship between gray matter volume reduction in the left PT and severity of FTD was mediated by brain activation in the left posterior middle temporal gyrus in their fMRI study. The latter region was chosen because it was engaged during the respective language task (i.e., passive story comprehension) and positively correlated with FTD. The authors suggested that due to a compromised left PT, which is engaged in early auditory (speech) processes, later linguistic (e.g., semantic) processing components had to compensate for this deficiency. Hereby, the middle temporal gyrus became more activated dependent on the expression of FTD in each patient.

Despite the low number of investigations, the finding of these studies already indicate that it is important to simultaneously investigate both, anatomical and functional, aspects in order to yield a comprehensive picture of the underlying pathophysiology of FTD. Further research, particularly in the field of semantic language impairments, should be conducted since these deficits are hallmark features of the FTD symptom.

Conclusion

Positive FTD in schizophrenia has been related to impairments in semantic and executive components during language processing, among others. Deviations from the cerebral lateralization of language functions in the lateral temporal lobes, reaching from simple passive tone listening to metaphor and discourse comprehension, have been associated with schizophrenia and in particular with FTD. The relevance of a deficient left–right asymmetry for the pathophysiology of perceptive (e.g., "concretism") and expressive (FTD) language-related symptoms of schizophrenia has been highlighted by numerous anatomical, metabolic, and functional investigations. To which extent the volume reductions in the STG and the aberrant neural activity in temporal cortices and other brain areas are related to etiological factors such as genetic liability or environmental factors, and in which way they contribute to the expression of FTD needs to be clarified in future investigations.

REFERENCES

Adams, J., Faux, S., McCarley, R. W., Marcy, B. & Shenton, M. (1989). *The N400 and language processing in schizophrenia. Proceedings of the Ninth International Conference on Event Related Potentials of the Brain (EPIC IX Congress).* Noordwijk, the Netherlands, pp. 12–13.

Andrews, S., Shelley, A. M., Ward, P. B. *et al.* (1993). Event-related potential indices of semantic processing in schizophrenia. *Biol Psychiatry*, **34**, 443–58.

Baker, N., Adler, L. E., Franks, R. D. *et al.* (1987). Neurophysiological assessment of sensory gating in psychiatric inpatients: comparison between schizophrenia and other diagnoses. *Biol Psychiatry*, **22**, 603–17.

Barrera, A., McKenna, P. J. & Berrios, G. E. (2005). Formal thought disorder in schizophrenia: an executive or a semantic deficit? *Psychol Med*, **35**, 121–32.

Beeman, M., Friedman, R. B., Grafman, J. *et al.* (1994). Summation priming and coarse semantic coding in the right hemisphere. *J Cogn Neurosci*, **6**, 26–45.

Bullen, J. G. & Hemsley, D. R. (1987). Schizophrenia: a failure to control the contents of consciousness? *Br J Clin Psychol*, **26**, 25–33.

Cohen, J. D. & Servan-Schreiber, D. (1992). Context, cortex and dopamine: a connectionist approach to behavior and biology in schizophrenia. *Psychol Rev*, **99**, 45–77.

Craven, R. (2002). Lateral thinking. *Nature Rev Neurosci*, **3**, 414.

DeLisi, L. E., Hoff, A. L., Neale, C. & Kushner, M. (1994). Asymmetries in the superior temporal lobe in male and female first-episode schizophrenic patients: measures of the planum temporale and superior temporal gyrus by MRI. *Schizophr Res*, **12**, 19–28.

Ditman, T. & Kuperberg, G. (2007). The time course of building discourse coherence in schizophrenia: an ERP investigation. *Psychophysiology*, **44**(6), 991–1001.

Friston, K. J., Liddle, P. F., Frith, C. D., Hirsch, S. R. & Frackowiak, R. S. J. (1992). The left medial temporal region and schizophrenia. *Brain*, **115**, 367–82.

Frith, C. D. (1979). Consciousness, information processing and schizophrenia. *Br J Psychiatry*, **134**, 225–35.

Frodl, T., Meisenzahl, E. M., Muller, D. *et al.* (2002). P300 subcomponents and clinical symptoms in schizophrenia. *Int J Psychophysiol*, **43**, 237–46.

Goldberg, T. E., Aloia, M. S., Gourovitch, M. L. *et al.* (1998). Cognitive substrates of thought disorder, I: the semantic system. *Am J Psychiatry*, **155**(12), 1671–6.

Goldberg, T. E. & Weinberger, D. R. (2000). Thought disorder in schizophrenia: a reappraisal of older formulations and an overview of some recent studies. *Cogn Neuropsychiatry*, **5**, 1–19.

Han, S. D., Nestor, P. G., Hale-Spencer, M. *et al.* (2007). Functional neuroimaging of word priming in males with chronic schizophrenia. *Neuroimage*, **35**, 273–82.

Higashima, M., Nagasawa, T., Kawasaki, Y. *et al.* (2003). Auditory P300 amplitude as a state marker for positive symptoms in schizophrenia: cross-sectional and retrospective longitudinal studies. *Schizophr Res*, **59**, 147–57.

Higashima, M., Urata, K., Kawasaki, Y. *et al.* (1998). P300 and the thought disorder factor extracted by factor-analytic procedures in schizophrenia. *Biol Psychiatry*, **44**, 115–20.

Iwanami, A., Okajima, Y., Kuwakado, D. *et al.* (2000). Event-related potentials and thought disorder in schizophrenia. *Schizophr Res*, **42**, 187–91.

Kaplan, R. D., Szechtman, H., Franco, S. *et al.* (1993). Three clinical syndromes of schizophrenia in untreated subjects: relation to brain glucose activity measured by positron emission tomography (PET). *Schizophr Res*, **11**, 47–54.

Kasai, K., Iwanami, A., Yamasue, H. *et al.* (2002). Neuroanatomy and neurophysiology in schizophrenia. *Neurosci Res*, **43**, 93–110.

Kawasaki, Y., Maeda, Y., Sakai, N. *et al.* (1996). Regional cerebral blood flow in patients with schizophrenia: relevance of symptom structures. *Neuroimaging*, **67**, 49–58.

Kerns, J. G. & Berenbaum, H. (2002). Cognitive impairments associated with formal thought disorder in people with schizophrenia. *J Abnor Psychol*, **111**, 211–34.

Kircher, T. T., Bulimore, E. T., Brammer, M. J. *et al.* (2001a). Differential activation of the temporal cortex during sentence completion in schizophrenic patients with and without formal thought disorder. *Schizophr Res*, **50**, 27–40.

Kircher, T. T., Leube, D. T., Erb, M., Grodd, W. & Rapp, A. M. (2007). Neural correlates of metaphor processing in schizophrenia. *Neuroimage*, **34**, 281–9.

Kircher, T. T., Liddle, P. F., Brammer, M. J. *et al.* (2001b). Neural correlates of formal thought disorder in schizophrenia. *Arch Gen Psychiatry*, **58**, 769–74.

Kircher, T. T., Liddle, P. F., Brammer, M. J. *et al.* (2002). Reversed lateralization of temporal activation during speech production in thought disordered patients with schizophrenia. *Psychol Med*, **32**, 439–49.

Kircher, T. T., Oh, T. M., Brammer, M. J. & McGuire, P. K. (2005). Neural correlates of syntax production in schizophrenia. *Br J Psychiatry*, **186**, 209–14.

Kircher, T. T., Rapp, A., Grodd, W. *et al.* (2004). Mismatch responses in schizophrenia: a combined fMRI and whole-head MEG study. *Am J Psychiatry*, **161**, 294–304.

Kircher, T. T., Whitney, C., Krings, T., Huber, W. & Weis, S. (2008). Hippocampal dysfunction during free word association in male patients with schizophrenia. *Schizophr Res*, **101** (1–3), 242–55.

Kirihara, K., Araki, T., Kasai, K. *et al.* (2005). Confirmation of a relationship between reduced auditory P300 amplitude and thought disorder in schizophrenia. *Schizophr Res*, **80**, 197–201.

Kostova, M., Passerieux, C., Laurent, J. P. & Hardy-Bayle, M. C. (2005). N400 anomalies in schizophrenia are correlated with the severity of formal thought disorder. *Schizophr Res*, **78**, 285–91.

Kumar, N. & Debruille, J. B. (2004). Semantics and N400: insights for schizophrenia. *J Psychiatry Neurosci*, **29**, 89–98.

Kuperberg, G. R. & Caplan, D. (2003). Language dysfunction in schizophrenia. In: R. B. Schiffers, S. M. Rao & B. S. Fogel (eds.) *Neuropsychiatry*, 2nd edn Philadelphia: Lippincott Williams and Wilkins, pp. 444–66.

Kuperberg, G. R., Deckersbach, T., Holt, D., Goff, D. & West, W. C. (2007). Increased temporal and prefrontal activity to semantic associations in schizophrenia. *Arch Gen Psychiatry*, **64**, 138–51.

Kuperberg, G., McGuire, P. K. & David, A. S. (2000). Sensitivity to linguistic anomalies in spoken sentences: a case study approach to understanding thought disorder in schizophrenia. *Psychol Med*, **30**, 345–57.

Kutas, M. & Hillyard, S. A. (1980). Event-related brain potentials to semantically inappropriate and surprisingly large words. *Biol Psychol*, **11**, 99–116.

Landre, N. A. & Taylor, M. A. (1995). Formal thought disorder in schizophrenia. Linguistic, attentional, and intellectual correlates. *J Nerv Ment Dis*, **183**, 673–80.

Leeson, V. C., Simpson, A., McKenna, P. J. & Laws, K. R. (2005). Executive inhibition and semantic association in schizophrenia. *Schizophr Res*, **74**, 61–7.

Liddle, P. F., Friston, K. J., Frith, C. D. *et al.* (1992). Patterns of cerebral blood flow in schizophrenia. *Br J Psychiatry*, **160**, 179–86.

Liddle, P. F., Ngan, E. T. C., Caissie, S. L. *et al.* (2002). Thought and Language Index: an instrument for assessing thought and language in schizophrenia. *Br J Psychiatry*, **181**, 326–30.

Manschreck, T. C., Maher, B. A., Milavetz, J. J. *et al.* (1988). Semantic priming in thought disordered schizophrenic patients. *Schizophr Res*, **1**, 61–6.

Mathiak, K. & Fallgatter, A. J. (2006). Combining magnetoencephalography and functional magnetic resonance imaging. *Int Rev Neurobiol*, **68**, 121–48.

McCarley, R. W., Salisbury, D. F., Hirayasu, Y. *et al.* (2002). Association between smaller left posterior superior temporal gyrus volume on magnetic resonance imaging and smaller left temporal P300 amplitude in first-episode schizophrenia. *Arch Gen Psychiatry*, **59**, 321–31.

McCarley, R. W., Shenton, M. E., O'Donnell, B. F. *et al.* (1993). Auditory P300 abnormalities and left posterior superior temporal gyrus reduction in schizophrenia. *Arch Gen Psychiatry*, **50**, 190–7.

McGuire, P. K., Quested, D. J., Spence, S. A. *et al.* (1998). Pathophysiology of "positive" thought disorder in schizophrenia. *Br J Psychiatry*, **173**, 231–5.

Meisenzahl, E. M., Frodl, T., Muller, D. *et al.* (2004). Superior temporal gyrus and P300 in schizophrenia: a combined ERP/ structural magnetic resonance imaging investigation. *J Psychiatr Res*, **38**, 153–62.

Menon, R. R., Barta, P. E., Aylward, E. H. *et al.* (1995). Posterior superior temporal gyrus in schizophrenia: grey matter changes and clinical correlates. *Schizophr Res*, **16**, 127–35.

Minzenberg, M. J., Ober, B. A. & Vinogradov, S. (2002). Semantic priming in schizophrenia: a review and synthesis. *J Int Neuropsy Soc*, **8**, 699–720.

Mitchell, R. L. C. & Crow, T. J. (2005). Right hemisphere language functions and schizophrenia: the forgotten hemisphere? *Brain*, **128**, 963–78.

Ngan, E. T. C., Vouloumanos, A., Cairo, T. A. *et al.* (2003). Abnormal processing of speech during oddball target detection in schizophrenia. *Neuroimage*, **20**, 889–97.

Ohnishi, T., Hashimoto, R., Mori, T. *et al.* (2006). The association between the Val158Met polymorphism of the catechol-0-methyl transferase gene and morphological abnormalities of the brain in chronic schizophrenia. *Brain*, **129**, 399–410.

Pearlson, G. D. & Marsh, L. (1999). Structural brain imaging in schizophrenia: a selective review. *Biol Psychiatry*, **46**, 627–49.

Potter, D., Summerfelt, A., Gold, J. & Buchanan, R. W. (2006). Review of clinical correlates of P50 sensory gating abnormalities in patients with schizophrenia. *Schizophr Bull*, **32**, 692–700.

Rajarethinam, R., DeQuardo, J. R., Miedler, J. *et al.* (2001). Hippocampus and amygdala in schizophrenia: assessment of the relationship of neuroanatomy to psychopathology. *Psychiatry Res*, **108**, 79–87.

Rossi, A., Serio, A., Stratta, P. *et al.* (1994). Planum temporale asymmetry and thought disorder in schizophrenia. *Schizophr Res*, **12**, 1–7.

Salisbury, D. F., O'Donnell, B. F., McCarley, R. W., Nestor, P. G. & Shenton, M. E. (2000). Event-related potentials elicited during a context-free homograph task in normal versus schizophrenic subjects. *Psychophysiology*, **37**, 456–63.

Shapleske, J., Rossell, S. L., Woodruff, P. W. & David, A. S. (1999). The planum temporale: a systematic, quantitative review of its structural, functional and clinical significance. *Brain Res Brain Res Rev*, **29**, 26–49.

Shenton, M. E., Dickey, C. C., Frumin, M. & McCarley, R. W. (2001). A review of MRI findings in schizophrenia. *Schizophr Res*, **49**, 1–52.

Shenton, M. E., Kikinis, R., Jolesz, F. A. *et al.* (1992). Abnormalities of the left temporal lobe and thought disorder in schizophrenia. A quantitative magnetic resonance imaging study. *N Engl J Med*, **327**, 604–12.

Shenton, M. E., O'Donnell, B. F., Nestor, P. G. *et al.* (1993). Temporal lobe abnormalities in a patient with schizophrenia who has word-finding difficulty: use of high-resolution magnetic resonance imaging and auditory P300 event-related potentials. *Harvard Rev Psychiatry*, **1**, 110–17.

Spencer, M. D., Moorhead, T. W. J., McIntosh, A. M. *et al.* (2007). Grey matter correlates of early psychotic symptoms in adolescents at enhanced risk of psychosis: a voxel-based study. *Neuroimage*, **35**, 1181–91.

Spitzer, M., Braun, U., Hermle, L. & Maier, S. (1993). Associative semantic network dysfunction in thought-disordered schizophrenic patients: direct evidence from indirect semantic priming. *Biol Psychiatry*, **34**, 864–77.

Stirling, J., Hellewell, J., Blakey, A. & Deakin, W. (2006). Thought disorder in schizophrenia is associated with both executive dysfunction and circumscribed impairments in semantic function. *Psychol Med*, **36**, 475–84.

Subotnik, K. L., Bartzokis, G., Green, M. F. & Nuechterlein, K. H. (2003). Neuroanatomical correlates of formal thought disorder in schizophrenia. *Cogn Neuropsychiatry*, **8**, 81–8.

Titone, D., Levy, D. L. & Holzman, P. S. (2000). Contextual insensitivity in schizophrenic language processing: evidence from lexical ambiguity. *J Abnorm Psychol*, **109**, 761–7.

Vita, A., Dieci, M., Giobbio, G. M. *et al.* (1995). Language and thought disorder in schizophrenia: brain morphological correlates. *Schizophr Res*, **15**, 243–51.

Weinstein, S., Werker, J. F., Vouloumanos, A., Woodward, T. S. & Ngan, E. T. (2006). Do you hear what I hear? Neural correlates of thought disorder during listening to speech in schizophrenia. *Schizophr Res*, **86**, 130–7.

Weinstein, S., Woodward, T. S. & Ngan, E. T. C. (2007). Brain activation mediates the association between structural abnormality and symptom severity in schizophrenia. *Neuroimage*, **36**, 188–93.

Weisbrod, M., Maier, S., Harig, S., Himmelsbach, U. & Spitzer, M. (1998). Lateralised semantic and indirect semantic priming effects in people with schizophrenia. *Br J Psychiatry*, **172**, 142–6.

Youn, T., Park, H.-J., Kim, J.-J., Kim, M. S. & Kwon, J. S. (2002). Altered hemispheric asymmetry and positive symptoms in schizophrenia: equivalent current dipole of auditory mismatch negativity. *Schizophr Res*, **59**, 253–60.

13

LRRTM1: a maternally suppressed genetic effect on handedness and schizophrenia

Clyde Francks

Summary

The molecular, developmental, and evolutionary bases of human brain asymmetry are almost completely unknown. Genetic linkage and association mapping have pin-pointed a gene called LRRTM1 (leucine-rich repeat transmembrane neuronal 1) that may contribute to variability in human handedness. Here I describe how LRRTM1's involvement in handedness was discovered, and also the latest knowledge of its functions in brain development and disease. The association of LRRTM1 with handedness was derived entirely from the paternally inherited gene, and follow-up analysis of gene expression confirmed that LRRTM1 is one of a small number of genes that are imprinted in the human genome, for which the maternally inherited copy is suppressed. The same variation at LRRTM1 that was associated paternally with mixed-/left-handedness was also over-transmitted paternally to schizophrenic patients in a large family study.

LRRTM1 is expressed in specific regions of the developing and adult forebrain by post-mitotic neurons, and the protein may be involved in axonal trafficking. Thus LRRTM1 has a probable role in neurodevelopment, and its association with handedness suggests that one of its functions may be in establishing or consolidating human brain asymmetry.

LRRTM1 is the first gene for which allelic variation has been associated with human handedness. The genetic data also suggest indirectly that the epigenetic regulation of this gene may yet prove more important than DNA sequence variation for influencing brain development and disease.

Intriguingly, the parent-of-origin activity of LRRTM1 suggests that men and women have had conflicting interests in relation to the outcome of lateralized brain development in their offspring.

Background

Structural and functional asymmetry are found in many vertebrate central nervous systems. Asymmetrical brain function and morphology are particularly pronounced in humans, and much of our behavior, cognition, and emotion is based on asymmetrical neuronal circuitry, with one or the other hemisphere having a dominant role for particular processes.

Roughly 90% of humans are right-handed. This is the strongest population-level bias in handedness for any primate. Left-handedness in humans is associated with reductions or reversals of the normal brain asymmetries (Mevorach *et al.*, 2005), particularly of cerebral cortical areas related to language perception and production (see Chapter 4 in this volume). Data from family studies suggest that this association is likely to be partly genetic in causation (Geschwind *et al.*, 2002; Anneken *et al.*, 2004). Handedness and complex cognition in humans may therefore be related developmentally and evolutionarily, although the nature and extent of these relationships remain undetermined.

Schizophrenia is a heterogeneous neuropsychiatric disorder affecting approximately 1% of the adult human population. Post-mortem and magnetic resonance imaging studies have shown associations between schizophrenia and abnormal asymmetrical morphologies of diverse brain structures, including the medial temporal lobe, superior temporal gyrus, planum temporale, and the overall brain anterior–posterior torque (DeLisi *et al.*, 1997; Shenton *et al.*, 2001). Schizophrenia is also associated with an elevated rate of mixed- or left-handedness (DeLisi *et al.*, 2002b; Orr *et al.*, 1999).

Language Lateralization and Psychosis, ed. Iris E. C. Sommer and René S. Kahn. Published by Cambridge University Press.
© Cambridge University Press 2009.

Crow highlighted the association of abnormal brain asymmetry with schizophrenia-like psychoses (Berlim *et al.*, 2003), and has studied a human-specific re-arrangement of the sex chromosomes and a putative candidate gene there, Protocadherin X-Y (Williams *et al.*, 2006). However, this gene has not yet been shown to be associated with asymmetry, language, or psychosis within any human population.

Great strides have been made in understanding the genetic and molecular basis of vertebrate visceral asymmetry over the last decade (Speder *et al.*, 2007). In contrast, human brain asymmetry remains almost entirely uncharacterized at a molecular level. While human brain asymmetry appears to develop independently from visceral asymmetry, visceral development does highlight some important principles that are likely to hold also in the brain. Following an initial asymmetry-breaking event in the early embryo, a downstream cascade is initiated that involves asymmetrical activity of a host of diverse proteins, that act in concert to determine differentiation of the left–right visceral axis (Speder *et al.*, 2007). Disruptions of many components in this cascade have been shown to cause altered asymmetrical development in animal models.

It is therefore reasonable to consider that a multi-component developmental program also operates in the human brain to determine asymmetry, and one recent study has identified some potentially important proteins in this developmental pathway (Sun *et al.*, 2005). There are likely to be multiple opportunities for genetic and environmental factors to influence the outcome of asymmetrical brain development. Although monogenic models have been fitted adequately to the segregation of left-handedness in human families (Annett, 1972; McManus, 1985), these models require strongly reduced penetrance in order to fit with the complex segregation of the trait, such that they are quite flexible and therefore difficult to refute. Risch and Pringle (1985) found that a monogenic model did not provide a better fit to family data than a polygenic, complex-trait model for handedness. However, one strength of single gene models may be in their common conception that some loss-of-function alleles cause a loss of directional asymmetry during development, such that the outcome of asymmetrical development

can become randomized to either right or left (as observed for visceral asymmetry in the presence of mutations in the DNAH5 or DNAH11 genes) (Speder *et al.*, 2007). This idea may carry through as we begin to understand the molecular underpinnings of human brain asymmetry and handedness.

Regarding schizophrenia, it is clear that the bulk of genetic epidemiological, linkage and association data, together with data on environmental influences, indicate that this is a complex and heterogeneous trait (Sullivan *et al.*, 2003), but one which may be partly related to abnormalities of asymmetry during neuro-development. In searching for genetic effects on handedness and schizophrenia, it is therefore reasonable to approach these traits as multi-factorial, and to apply relatively model-free methods developed for human complex-trait genetics. An important corollary of this approach is that we do not expect any single genetic effect to determine the overall genetic epidemiology of either trait, but merely to act as contributory factors with various degrees of importance at a population level.

Linkage mapping and replication

Our genetic studies of handedness began with a sample of 191 sibling pairs from 89 independent nuclear families, which formed the first sub-sample of an on-going study of the genetics of dyslexia, and in which a full genome-wide linkage screen for dyslexia was performed previously (Fisher *et al.*, 2002; Francks *et al.*, 2002). The families were recruited clinically through at least one reading-disabled (RD) proband, with a requirement for evidence of reading problems in at least one sibling of the proband.

Relative hand skill was assessed for all probands and all available siblings and parents in each nuclear family, using Annett's peg moving task. The task involved measuring the time taken, with each hand, to move a row of pegs from one location on a board to another. Relative hand skill was then derived as $(L - R)/((L + R)/2)$ i.e., the difference between mean left and right hand times (over five trials per hand), adjusted for overall hand skill. This continuous measure of relative hand skill has a roughly normal population distribution with a positive mean that reflects the preponderance of right-handedness in unselected populations, and which was correlated strongly with handedness as defined by writing hand (Francks *et al.*, 2002). The relative hand skill measure showed a significant sib–sib correlation that gave a familiality estimate of 38% for this measure in this sample, some or all of which was potentially heritable. The RD siblings scored as an unselected population for relative hand skill, and we found that relative hand skill was not correlated with reading ability, reading-related cognition, or overall motor coordination in this sample (Francks *et al.*, 2003c).

Genome-wide quantitative genetic linkage analysis demonstrated that a locus on chromosome 2p12-q11 influenced relative hand skill (Figure 13.1), such that sibling pairs who had higher identity-by-descent sharing across this chromosomal region were also more similar for their relative hand skill. The 2p12-q11 locus showed the strongest linkage to relative hand skill in our genome-wide screen ($P = 0.00007$, genome-adjusted $P \approx 0.05$) (Francks *et al.*, 2002). No other locus approached significance when adjusted for multiple testing across the entire genome. This remains the only well-powered genome-wide screen performed so far for a measure related to handedness. (There was no linkage of reading-related measures to 2p12-q11.)

We failed to replicate the 2p12-q11 linkage to relative hand skill in a separate sample of RD siblings that had been assessed in the same way, but we then replicated the linkage using the same phenotypic measure in an independent sample of 105 pairs of adult left-handed brothers ($P = 0.0009$) (Francks *et al.*, 2003a). This new linkage mapped extremely closely to the first (Figure 13.1). The existence of the 2p12-q11 quantitative-trait-locus (QTL) was therefore confirmed, although the overall pattern of results suggests that relative hand skill has a multi-factorial etiology. Of note, our second RD sib-pair sample that failed to support the linkage had shown a weaker sib–sib correlation, which may have been due to increased noise in the measure arising from the lower age of the siblings in this sample (mean age 11 years compared to 14.5 years in the first study sample).

Parent-of-origin effect on handedness

In the sample of RD siblings that we used for the genome-wide scan, we observed that the relative hand skill of the siblings was correlated more strongly with their fathers' than their mothers' relative hand skill (Francks *et al.*, 2003b). Correlations for relative hand skill in this sample were: Father:Child $r = 0.19$, SE $= 0.08$, Mother:Child $r = 0.07$, SE $= 0.08$, Sib:Sib $r = 0.24$, SE $= 0.09$. Thus the Mother:Child correlation was not significant, while the paternal correlation was significant and roughly equalled the sibling correlation, suggesting that paternal transmission was primarily responsible for the familial clustering of the trait in this sample (Francks *et al.*, 2003b).

Since 2p12-q11 had shown the strongest linkage to relative hand skill anywhere in the genome, we reasoned that this locus may partly or wholly explain the paternal transmission within this sample, and we therefore re-analysed 2p12-q11 in this sample under parent-of-origin linkage models. This analysis was based on separating the paternal allele sharing from the maternal allele sharing, within the sib pairs, by use of parental genotype data (Francks *et al.*, 2003b). Sib-pair regression analysis yielded a peak paternal linkage $t = -4.67$, $P = 0.0000037$, to a locus within chromosome band 2p12 that corresponds to the position of marker D2S139 (Fig. 13.1). In contrast to this strong paternal linkage, there was no significant linkage of relative hand skill across this entire genomic region to the maternally inherited locus (all $t > -0.83$, $P > 0.20$).

Maximum likelihood variance-components modeling, with independent paternal and maternal QTL effects, also yielded an estimate of the paternal effect roughly five times that of the maternal effect at the peak of linkage (Francks *et al.*, 2003b). This model did not provide a significantly better fit ($P > 0.1$) than a paternal-only effect model, i.e., a model with the maternal effect constrained to zero. Under the paternal-only effect model, the peak linkage LOD score was 2.65, within 2cM from the peak identified with regression analysis. We saw an LOD score as high or higher than this in only three out of 100 000 simulations under the null hypothesis of no linkage, and we could therefore assign an approximate significance level $P = 0.00003$ under this analysis.

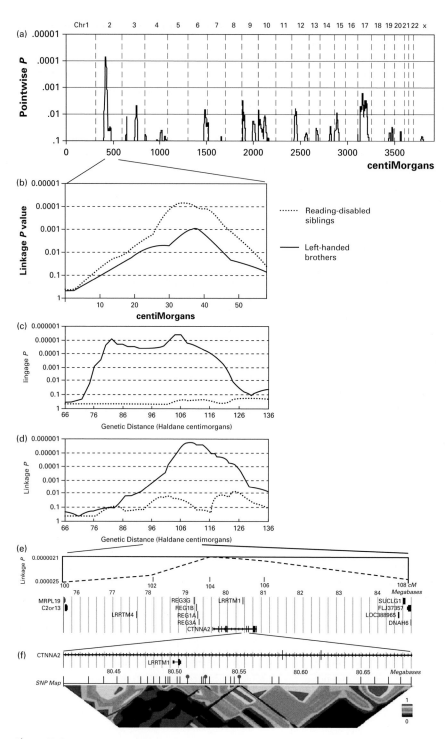

Figure 13.1 See caption opposite.

The paternal linkage of 2p12-q11 to relative hand skill in our RD sample was in accord with the stronger father–child than mother–child correlation for this trait in this sample. However, epidemiological studies of left-handedness have tended to find a slightly stronger mother–child than father–child association (McManus & Bryden, 1992), which suggests that the 2p12-q11 effect is just one of a multi-factorial range of influences on handedness that does not dominate the overall genetic epidemiology (see the Background section above). This being said, no large-scale genetic epidemiological studies have so far analyzed a continuous measure of relative hand skill.

A multi-factorial etiology for relative hand skill is further suggested by our second sample of reading-disabled sibling pairs (see above), which failed to show linkage of 2p12-q11 to this trait in standard analysis, and continued to show no significant linkage under parent-of-origin analysis. This second sample also showed very weak parent–child and sib–sib correlations (which we noted above may be due to increased noise arising from the lower age of the siblings in this sample (Francks et al., 2003b). We had no parental data available for the sample of left-handed brothers (Francks et al., 2003a), so we were not able to assess that data set with parent-of-origin analysis.

The parent-of-origin linkage on 2p12-q11 led us to propose in 2003 that the causative gene, when identified, would be imprinted, and inactivated or down-regulated on the maternally inherited chromosome (Francks et al., 2003b). Imprinted genes are unusual in that their activity depends on their parental origin (Reik & Walter, 2001), and they comprise only a tiny minority of all genes. We hypothesized that maternal suppression of gene expression would result in variation within the causative gene having phenotypic consequences only when inherited paternally (Francks et al., 2003b).

A matching parent-of-origin effect on schizophrenia

DeLisi and colleagues (2002a) performed a genome-wide linkage screen with 382 affected sibling pairs drawn from 294 families with at least two siblings affected with schizophrenia or schizoaffective disorder. An association between schizophrenia and non-right-handedness was found previously in this sample. The

Figure 13.1 Mapping of an imprinted genetic effect on human handedness to LRRTM1. (a) Genome-wide multipoint linkage analysis of relative hand skill (from Francks et al., 2002, with permission). Cumulative distance in Haldane centi morgans is shown along the X-axis, with chromosome identities along the top. Evidence for linkage is given (Y-axis) as pointwise empirically derived significance, calculated under a Variance Components framework. The QTL on chromosome 2p11.2–12 yielded a pointwise peak $P = 0.00007$, suggesting a positive relationship between sibling phenotypic and genetic similarity at this locus. (b) Comparison of linkage to relative hand skill across 2p16-q14 in RD siblings (Francks et al. 2002, with permission) and left-handed brothers (from Francks et al., 2003a, with permission). X-axis; genomic interval with markers shown: Y-axis; pointwise significance of linkage. (c) Paternal linkage of relative hand skill to chromosome 2p12-q11 in 191 reading-disabled sibling pairs (from Francks et al., 2003b, with permission). X-axis; chromosome region spanning 2p21-q14 (given as genetic distance from marker D2S2259). Y-axis; significance of linkage under regression analysis. Solid curve; paternal linkage. Punctate curve; maternal linkage. (d) Linkage of schizophrenia to 2p12-q11 in 241 affected sibling pairs (from Francks et al., 2003b, with permission). Solid curve; paternal linkage. Punctate curve; maternal linkage. (e) Top: Pointwise significance of linkage derived from paternal sharing across 8 centimorgans of chromosome 2p12-q11 (from Francks et al., 2007, with permission). This corresponds roughly to a 1-LOD unit support interval for the QTL. Significance of linkage is shown on a logarithmic scale. Bottom: Known genes within the region (adapted from UCSC Genome Browser). Note LRRTM1 (transcribed proximal to distal (right to left)) sited within an intron of CTNNA2 (transcribed distal to proximal). (f) Close-up of 286 kilobases around LRRTM1 (from Francks et al., 2007, with permission). Two exons of CTNNA2 are also visible. The final SNP map that we used in this region is shown, and the three SNPs that showed the initial paternal-specific haplotype associations are highlighted by pink circles (rs1446109-rs1007371-rs723524). Pairwise intermarker LD (Cramer's V) is shown at the bottom. (See color plate section.)

second strongest linkage in that genome screen was centered on 2p12, LOD = 2.99, point-wise $P = 0.00021$, although this did not achieve statistical significance when adjusted for multiple testing in a genome-wide context. However, the investigators had found the LOD score to be higher, and to reach genome-wide significance, if only those siblings with a narrower phenotype of chronic schizophrenia were considered as affected (Lynn DeLisi; personal communication). In addition, some independent and weaker linkages to schizophrenia have been reported (DeLisi *et al.*, 2002a) around the centromeric region of chromosome 2, and a meta-analysis of 20 genome-wide linkage screens for schizophrenia, that included the sample of DeLisi and colleagues (2002a), found that 2p12-q22 showed the strongest evidence for linkage in the genome (Lewis *et al.*, 2003). Indeed, 2p12-q22 was the only location to reach significance when adjusted for genome-wide testing in that meta-analysis of 20 studies.

In 2003 we re-analyzed the schizophrenia sib-pair data set of DeLisi and colleagues (2002a) with an updated genetic marker map (Francks *et al.*, 2003b). In affected-sib-pair analysis of schizophrenia and schizoaffective disorder (376 affected sibling pairs with data available for chromosome 2), the LOD score was 3.71 at a location in 2p11, 2cM from our peaks of linkage to relative hand skill that we had observed in dyslexic sibs and left-handed brothers. This linkage to schizophrenia was 0.72 LOD units higher than that reported by DeLisi and colleagues (2002a) (reported LOD = 2.99), and we attributed this difference to our use of a more recent genetic marker map, together with a different linkage analytical package, and genotype error checking routines (Francks *et al.*, 2003b). The linkage evidence on 2p11 increased to a highly significant LOD = 5.13 when we excluded the individuals affected with schizoaffective disorder and performed affected-sib-pair analysis with the schizophrenia-only phenotype (241 pairs in 196 independent nuclear families) (Francks *et al.*, 2003b).

Our parent-of-origin findings on relative hand skill then led us to re-analyze 2p12-q11 in relation to schizophrenia, using the affected sib-pair family sample of DeLisi and colleagues (2002a), but this time under parent-of-origin methods (Francks *et al.*, 2003b). Again,

this was based on distinguishing paternal and maternal allele sharing within the sib pairs, by use of parental genotype data. We found that the peak paternal LOD was 4.72 ($P = 0.0000016$) at a location on 2p11 near to marker D2S417, 3–5 cM from the peaks of paternal linkage to relative hand skill (Fig. 13.1). In contrast, the evidence for maternal linkage across the region was weak or non-significant, and ambiguous in location (Fig. 13.1) (LOD = 0.6, $P = 0.048$, at the locus corresponding to the maximally linked paternal peak). When the schizoaffective individuals were also included, a similar albeit less striking pattern emerged, with paternal LOD = 3.12, maternal LOD = 1.06, again at different locations (Francks *et al.*, 2003b).

As parent-of-origin effects are unusual in the genome (Reik & Walter, 2001), and no imprinted genes were known within the region of linkage that we had identified, we predicted in 2003 that a single paternally expressed gene would be found to be responsible for the linkages of 2p12-q11 to handedness and schizophrenia (Francks *et al.*, 2003b).

Mapping of the 2p12-q11 effect to LRRTM1

We returned to our original dyslexic sib-pair sample that had shown strong parent-of-origin linkage to relative hand skill at 2p12-q11. We genotyped 87 single nucleotide polymorphisms (SNPs) in these siblings and their parents, within the region of paternal-specific linkage to relative hand skill (Fig. 13.1) (Francks *et al.*, 2007). The SNPs were targeted within four positional and functional candidate genes on 2p12-p11 (LRRTM4, CTNNA2, LRRTM1, DNAH6). Following from our parent-of-origin linkage data, we tested for quantitative association of paternally inherited SNP alleles with relative hand skill. The principle of the test was to detect an effect of the alleles on the mean relative hand skill of the siblings, while controlling for the linkage signal across the region (Francks *et al.*, 2007). Four SNPs in distinct locations, which were not in significant linkage disequilibrium (LD) with one another, showed nominally significant paternal-specific association with relative hand skill ($0.05 > P > 0.01$). This was no more than the expected false positive rate.

We then aimed to interrogate underlying haplotype structure by testing haplotypes for association, that were constructed in "sliding windows" representing all sets of three consecutive SNPs (disregarding any instances where SNPs were not in significant linkage disequilibrium) (Francks *et al.*, 2007). Significance levels for paternal-specific association were all $P > 0.05$, except for haplotypes derived from the SNPs rs1446109-rs1007371-rs723524 ($P = 0.00002$), and the overlapping window rs1007371-rs723524-rs1025947 ($P = 0.0007$) (Francks *et al.*, 2007). These SNPs are on 2p12 within a region of strong inter-marker linkage disequilibrium that spans at least the first exon and 137 kilobases upstream of the gene LRRTM1, which is located within an intron of another gene, CTNNA2 (Fig. 13.1). There was no significant maternal haplotype association at any location (all $P > 0.05$).

The rs1446109-rs1007371-rs723524 haplotype 2-2-2 (where 2 is the minor allele of each SNP) was responsible primarily for the paternal-specific association observed with haplotypes derived from these three SNPs. The 2-2-2 haplotype had 9% frequency, and was associated with a mean shift of 1.1 SD towards left-handedness in the relative hand skill distribution (Francks *et al.*, 2002, 2003c) when inherited paternally, compared to all other haplotypes. Genotyping of 32 more SNPs, including 12 within 137 kb upstream of LRRTM1, confirmed that rs1446109-rs1007371-rs723524 haplotype 2-2-2 represents a distinct haplotype clade for at least 76 kb upstream of, and including, the predicted promoter of LRRTM1.

We screened the first two exons and predicted promoter of LRRTM1 for polymorphisms in 26 left-handers from the RD sample by denaturing high performance liquid chromatography and sequencing, but we did not detect any polymorphisms that tagged rs1446109-rs1007371-rs723524 haplotype 2-2-2, or that had overt disruptive effects on the predicted LRRTM1 protein (entirely coded within exon 2). We therefore speculated that variation upstream of LRRTM1 was likely to affect its regulation and expression (Francks *et al.*, 2007).

We analyzed the SNPs rs1007371 and rs723524, which together can be used to construct a close proxy to the "risk" haplotype described above, in a sample of normal twin-based sibships from Brisbane, Australia,

that was derived from 215 independent families. However, we found no significant evidence for paternal association of the risk haplotype with our quantitative measure of human handedness ($P > 0.1$) (Francks *et al.*, 2007).

LRRTM1 is the first gene to be implicated in human handedness by genetic mapping. As we detected an effect of LRRTM1 on handedness in dyslexic siblings, but not in normal twin-based sibships, we considered that LRRTM1 may influence behavioral lateralization more strongly in clinically selected populations for psychiatric/neurodevelopmental dysfunctions, than in the general population (Francks *et al.*, 2007). This would suggest an interactive, non-additive effect of LRRTM1 with other genetic and/or environmental effects that predispose to neuropsychiatric dysfunction, such that the effect of LRRTM1 depends on other risk factors in order to manifest fully. However, it is also possible that the failure to replicate the association with handedness was due to low power in the Australian sample. It is a well-described statistical feature of genetic association analysis that follow-up samples should usually be much larger than initial samples to provide adequate power, as the genetic effect in the initial sample is typically inflated (Ioannidis *et al.*, 2001).

LRRTM1 is confirmed as an imprinted gene

No imprinted genes were known previously on chromosome 2p. We found that human LRRTM1 is imprinted (paternal-only expression) in hybrid A9 cells (Kugoh *et al.*, 1999) (mouse cell lines containing single human chromosomes of known parental origin) (Fig. 13.2) (Francks *et al.*, 2007). Mouse A9 cells have been used for the reliable identification and verification of human imprinted genes (Kugoh *et al.*, 1999).

We also used transcribed polymorphisms to show mono-allelic LRRTM1 expression in tissue samples from a minority of unrelated post-mortem human brains (3 out of 18) by RT-PCR and sequencing or restriction digestion (Francks *et al.*, 2007). However, bi-allelic expression was found in 15 out of 18 brains. These results suggest that imprinting of LRRTM1 is either variable between individuals, as for the

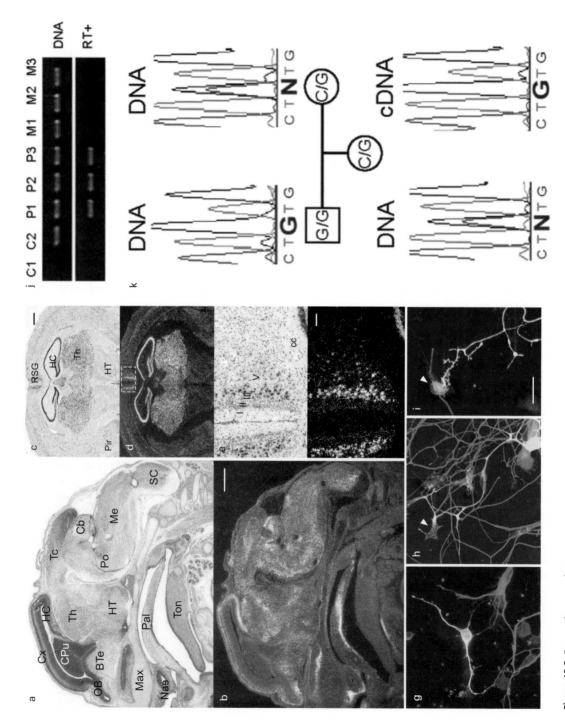

Figure 13.2 See caption opposite.

imprinted genes IMPT1 or IGF2 (Sakatani *et al.*, 2001), and/or variable between different brain regions or cell/tissue types, as for UBE3A (Yamasaki *et al.*, 2003).

We also found mono-allelic paternal expression of LRRTM1 in four out of four unrelated EBV-transformed human lymphoblastoid cell lines that were heterozygous for a transcribed SNP (Fig. 13.2) (Francks *et al.*, 2007). Thus our determination of LRRTM1 imprinting, and maternal suppression, was confirmed in three different experimental settings and designs.

We tested CTNNA2 (the surrounding gene of LRRTM1) for mono-allelic expression in ten post-mortem brain samples from normal, unrelated individuals, by use of a transcribed SNP in exon 12, but expression was always bi-allelic, in contrast to LRRTM1 (Francks *et al.*, 2007). We did not detect CTNNA2 expression in the A9 hybrids, or in human lymphoblastoid cell lines. The first CTNNA2 exon is over 750 kilobases from LRRTM1 (Fig. 13.1), and several LD blocks away, further suggesting that the regulation of these genes is distinct. There are no other genes within 1.13 megabases of LRRTM1, and the next closest gene expressed in the forebrain (expression data available via the UCSC genome browser) is over 2.75 megabases distally (LRRTM4; Fig. 13.1).

Of a total of approximately 35 000 human genes, only roughly 40 were known previously to be imprinted, and the total number is unlikely to exceed this greatly (Imprinted Gene Catalogue http://igc.otago.ac.nz/home.html, 2006; Morison *et al.*, 2005; Reik & Walter, 2001). The finding that LRRTM1 is imprinted, and maternally suppressed, was a confirmation of the parent-of-origin genetic data that led to this locus, because the a priori probability that LRRTM1 would be imprinted was very low (roughly 1 in 1000). Our association data suggested that allelic variation upstream of LRRTM1, which may affect the gene's expression, is relevant functionally for brain asymmetry when inherited on the active paternal chromosome, but not on the relatively inactive maternal chromosome, at certain locations and time points during human brain development.

However, the "risk" haplotype that we identified at LRRTM1 can not explain the majority of the paternal-specific linkage across the genomic region of 2p12 (Fig. 13.1), and therefore additional genetic or

Figure 13.2 Developmental increase of Lrrtm1 mRNA expression in mouse thalamus, hippocampus, and retrosplenial cortex, and localization of LRRTM1 in neurons (from Francks *et al.*, 2007, with permission). *In situ* hybridization analysis in sagittal sections of E15 mouse embryos (a, b) and coronal sections of adult mouse brain (c–f) Shown are bright-field images counterstained with hematoxylin (a, c, e) and corresponding dark-field autoradiographs (b, d, f) The white signal in the dark-field images indicates Lrrtm1 expression. (e, f) Higher magnification of the retrosplenial granular cortex (boxed area in (d) shows a high level of Lrrtm1 expression in layer III-IV neurons. (g–i) Myc-LRRTM1 was transfected into E17 mouse cortical neurons (g) and nucleofected into rat P18 dorsal root ganglion neurons (h, i) and detected 40 hours later with anti-myc antibody. Neurons were visualized with anti-beta-tubulin antibody. LRRTM1 is localized to the cell soma and in the neurites; in neurites it is also localized to lamellipodia of the growth cones (arrowheads in (h, i)). BTe, basal telencephalon; Cb, cerebellum; cc, corpus callosum; CPu, caudate-putamen; Cx, cerebral cortex; HC, hippocampus; HT, hypothalamus; Max, maxilla; Me, medulla; Nas, nasal cavity; OB, olfactory bulb; Pal, palatine; Pir, piriform cortex; Po, pons; RSG, retrosplenial granular cortex; Sc, Spinal cord; Tc, tectum; Th, thalamus; Ton, tongue. Scale bar is 500 μm in (a–d), 100 μm in (e, f), and 20 μm in (g–i).

(j) LRRTM1 expression is down regulated maternally in humans (from Francks *et al.*, 2007, with permission). Data are shown from A9 cells that each contain a single human chromosome 2 of known parental origin. Products are shown from PCR using primers specific for human LRRTM1. *Upper panel*: The human gene is present in genomic DNA (labelled "DNA") from all cell lines tested, apart from C1 (mouse A9 cell line containing no human chromosome). *Lower panel*: The human gene is only expressed (detected by RT-PCR) in three cell lines containing paternally derived human chromosome 2s (P1, P2, P3), and not in three cell lines containing maternally derived human chromosome 2s (M1, M2, M3). (C2 is a human fibroblast cell line). (k) Mono-allelic paternal expression of LRRTM1 in a human EBV-transformed lymphoblastoid cell line. Sequence traces derived from genomic DNA (labeled "DNA") surrounding a C/G SNP are shown for a father, mother, and child. The child is heterozygous, but the cDNA prepared from mRNA showed expression of only the paternally inherited G allele of LRRTM1. (See color plate section.)

epigenetic variability at LRRTM1, or neighboring genes, may also be responsible partly for the linkages of handedness and schizophrenia to 2p12 (Francks *et al.*, 2003b). Although we found evidence that LRRTM1 is variably imprinted in the post-mortem adult human brain (as is the imprinted gene 5HT2A) (Bunzel *et al.*, 1998), we can not conclude directly, on the basis of our data, that variability in imprinting of LRRTM1 is involved in individual differences in human handedness, and schizophrenia liability. Our data indicate a role for the 2-2 haplotype in handedness variability and susceptibility to schizophrenia, in European populations, while the data on imprinting are consistent with the paternal-specific nature of this effect.

Methylation of CpG dinucleotides is the primary mechanism by which some genes are imprinted. Methylation is a form of epigenetic chemical modification of DNA that affects its chromatin state, and the ability to bind cofactors necessary for transcriptional activity (Reik & Walter, 2001). We analyzed methylation within 2 CpG islands that correspond to the predicted promoter and coding exon of LRRTM1, and a third island roughly 18 kb upstream of LRRTM1, in 17 lymphoblastoid cell lines and 17 human post-mortem brain samples, but we did not find evidence that these CpG islands are differentially methylated regions that would be supportive of imprinting (Francks *et al.*, 2007). However, recent unpublished data from the Human EpiGenome Project indicate that LRRTM1 has tissue-specific methylation at the transcription start-site, just upstream of the first CpG island where we had scanned (S. Beck; personal communication). Also, the second exon of LRRTM1 shows extensive methylation in placenta, which is again supportive of the imprinting of this gene. We therefore recommended that the mechanism of imprinted regulation at this locus should be investigated as a priority, as epigenetic mis-regulation of LRRTM1 may have clinical relevance and could underlie much of the paternal linkage of 2p12 to schizophrenia.

Functions of LRRTM1 in brain development

LRRTM1 is one of a four-member family of type I transmembrane proteins containing leucine-rich repeat (LRR) domains, which are commonly involved in protein–protein interactions. Leucine-rich repeat domains are present in the Slits and Nogo-receptor (Fournier *et al.*, 2002; Lauren *et al.*, 2003) involved in axonal pathfinding. Each LRRTM member has a specific, dynamically regulated regional brain expression distribution (Lauren *et al.*, 2003).

By use of *in situ* hybridization in the mouse, we found that Lrrtm1 is expressed predominantly in the nervous system by post-mitotic neurons, but also in some non-neuronal tissues (Fig. 13.2) (Francks *et al.*, 2007). Expression is upregulated in the mouse brain during embryonic development and early post-natally. In adult brain, Lrrtm1 expression is most prominent in the forebrain, particularly in the thalamus (in most or all nuclei), and in cortical areas including hippocampus, piriform, and posterior cingulate (Fig. 13.2).

In Northern blot analysis of the adult human brain, LRRTM1 also showed predominant expression in forebrain regions including thalamus and cerebral cortex (Francks *et al.*, 2007). By *in situ* hybridization in coronal sections of the post-mortem developing human brain (14–16 weeks' gestation), strong expression was observed in anterior sections throughout the cortical plate and in septum, caudate, and putamen (Francks *et al.*, 2007). The absence of signal in the subventricular zone argued against a direct involvement in neurogenesis. Transcript distribution was similar in more caudal sections with the addition of signal in dorsolateral thalamus. More caudal still, thalamic signal shifted ventrally to a structure consistent with the lateral geniculate body.

When comparing expression between human and mouse, it seemed that there is a striking absence of signal in caudate and putamen in mouse, at least at e15 and in adult (Francks *et al.*, 2007). Also, expression within the fetal human thalamus is more restricted as compared to the mouse, with staining in the human relatively limited to dorsomedial regions. Interestingly, the dorsolateral thalamus has been implicated in schizophrenia (Andrews *et al.*, 2006; Harrison & Weinberger, 2004).

No consistent asymmetric expression was observed in any of three human developing brains examined by *in situ* hybridization (14–16 weeks' gestation), regardless of whether cerebral hemispheres were analyzed in aggregate or cortical sub-regions were examined in isolation (dorsolateral, temporal, ventrolateral, or cingulate) (Francks *et al.*, 2007). Similarly to embryonic brain, LRRTM1 was expressed at similar levels (i.e., symmetrically) in all analyzed regions of left and right adult human cerebral cortex (several different cortical regions from five individuals were analyzed by quantitative PCR). We also quantified left- and right-brain Lrrtm1 mRNA expression levels in rats and embryonic mice, but did not detect evidence for asymmetrical expression in rodents (Francks *et al.*, 2007). In addition, we tested cerebral cortex, cerebellum, brain stem, olfactory bulb, thymus, heart, lung, liver, intestine, pancreas, spleen, kidney, muscle, and testis of two reciprocal crossed F1 mice between C57BL/6J and JF1 strains for allele-specific expression. Each of the F1 mice was 30 weeks old. Expression of Lrrtm1 was detected in cerebral cortex, cerebellum, and brain stem, but it was bi-allelic (Francks *et al.*, 2007).

In rodent primary sensory (DRG) and cortical neurons (Fig. 13.2), and in cerebellar granular neurons, over-expressed LRRTM1 localized to the cell soma, neurites, and lamellipodia of growth cones, suggesting a function in axon guidance and/or synaptogenesis. Unexpectedly, in transfected MRC5, Cos-7, and Neuro-2a cells, LRRTM1 co-localized with endoplasmic reticulum markers (Francks *et al.*, in press). Live-cell staining for over-expressed LRRTM1 in DRG neurons revealed that the protein is not accessible on the plasma membrane under conditions that allowed surface detection of a related member of the LRR protein super-family, Lingo1 (Francks *et al.*, 2007). These results suggest that endogenous LRRTM1 may have a role in intracellular trafficking within axons. However, it remains possible that LRRTM1 is localized to plasma membrane in cells expressing an unidentified LRRTM1 chaperone or co-receptor protein that promotes its processing and/or transport.

In summary, by use of several gene-functional approaches, we found that LRRTM1 is likely to play a role during the development of specific forebrain structures by influencing neuronal differentiation and connectivity, with a possible role in intracellular trafficking in axons. Thus, LRRTM1 is an ideal candidate gene for

having an involvement in subtle developmental abnormalities of the central nervous system.

We found no evidence for overtly asymmetrical expression of LRRTM1 in the developing or adult brain of rodents or humans, using *in situ* hybridization and/or quantitative PCR (Francks *et al.*, 2007). However, we can not rule out a subtle asymmetry of function or expression at some restricted time point during human brain development, as for the transcription factor LMO4 (Sun *et al.*, 2005). It remains possible that LRRTM1 is important in the establishment, consolidation, or elaboration of the left–right axis during human brain growth and development, particularly prior to 14 weeks' gestation, which was the earliest stage that we were able to analyze in human. (Population-level morphological asymmetries of the cerebral cortex are already noticeable shortly after this time, and are visible by ultrasound in normal fetuses at 20–22 weeks' gestation (Hering-Hanit *et al.*, 2001).) Therefore, detailed studies of the roles of LRRTM1 and the pathways in which it functions in mammalian brain development are warranted, particularly at developmental time points earlier than 14 weeks in humans, that may reveal critical new insights into the establishment and/or maintenance of normal and abnormal human brain function and asymmetry.

LRRTM1 and schizophrenia

We studied the SNPs rs1446109 and either rs723524 or rs718466 (the latter are equivalent tagging SNPs according to international HapMap data) in four family samples of white European descent that included individuals with schizophrenia or poor outcome schizoaffective disorder (Francks *et al.*, 2007). These comprised a subset of the New York/Oxford sample (DeLisi *et al.*, 2002a) (226 families), an Irish "high density" sample (Thiselton *et al.*, 2004) (236 families), a sample collected in Montreal (Xiong *et al.*, 2005) (124 families), and an Afrikaner sample (Abecasis *et al.*, 2004) (416 families). The 2-2 haplotype defined by the rare alleles of these SNPs is equivalent to the risk haplotype for left-handedness described above. The 2-2 haplotype varied in frequency between 7.6% and 12.1% in the four sample sets (Francks *et al.*, 2007). We found that haplotype 2-2 was over-transmitted paternally to affected individuals in a combined analysis of the four samples, $P = 0.0014$, (one-tailed test, 38 transmissions to 16 non-transmissions). This was a specific hypothesis test that required no statistical adjustment. There was no significant paternal over-transmission of any other haplotype, nor was there maternal over-transmission of any haplotype. The paternal 2-2 result was derived roughly equally from three of the four samples (Francks *et al.*, 2007).

We genotyped rs1446109 (almost tagging for the risk haplotype), in two case-control collections of European descent (461 cases and 459 controls from Munich, Germany, and 429 cases and 428 controls from Scotland. All cases had DSM-IV diagnoses of schizophrenia, and both sample sets were recruited according to the same protocol (Van den Oord *et al.*, 2006). As the parental origin of the alleles could not be established and the paternal and maternal alleles were confounded, we expected this analysis to be low-powered to detect an imprinted effect. Nonetheless, this SNP showed a trend towards association ($P = 0.09$) when tested under a genotypic 2-d.f. logistic regression model using covariates for gender and the collection site (Francks *et al.*, 2007). The additive component of this model was significant at $P = 0.036$, and the direction of allelic effect was the same as in the family samples. When we repeated the analysis using only those cases (151) who reported a positive family history of schizophrenia or bipolar disorder, with the aim of removing sporadic environmental cases, rs1446109 showed significant association with $P = 0.013$, and the additive component of the model showed $P = 0.0038$, again in the expected direction. We also tested for association in a sample of 270 Han Chinese families (Takahashi *et al.*, 2003) but we found no significant bias in paternal or maternal transmission of any haplotype to schizophrenia patients (there were 65 paternal transmissions to 78 paternal non-transmissions of the 2-2 haplotype).

The frequency of the 2-2 risk haplotype was somewhat higher in the Han Chinese, at 18%, than in the Europeans. The failure to replicate may nonetheless be related to modest power in the Chinese sample of 270 families. Alternatively, the non-replication in the

Chinese may indicate that the 2-2 haplotype does not carry risk variation in this population; it may also be relevant that native Chinese speakers show some morphological differences to English-speakers in language-related areas of the brain (Kochunov *et al.*, 2003). A further study in a larger Chinese sample will be required to distinguish these possibilities, together with identification of the functional variants in European populations.

Taken together, our data published in Francks *et al.*, (2007) suggest that a subtype of schizophrenia, linked to mis-regulation of human LRRTM1, may have its origins in fetal neurodevelopment. Since LRRTM1 appears to underlie the strongest linkage to schizophrenia in the genome, as identified by a meta-analysis of 20 genome-wide linkage scans (Lewis *et al.*, 2003), it is possible that LRRTM1 dysfunction causes a major, common subtype of schizophrenia. Assessing the frequency of this subtype will require studies in further clinical and epidemiological samples, together with a better definition of the functional genetic and epigenetic variation at the LRRTM1 locus. This information may have a substantial impact on pharmacogenetic studies and the development of new treatments for schizophrenia, by allowing patient heterogeneity to be accounted for in clinical trial studies. The receptor-like structure of LRRTM1 also suggests that it may be a drug-tractable target in its own right.

LRRTM1 evolution

Humans have the strongest population-level bias in handedness of any primate (Rogers & Andrew, 2002; Hugdahl & Davidson, 2003), and LRRTM1 is a candidate for having had a role in the evolution of this trait. As the human and mouse predicted LRRTM1 proteins are 96% identical, and the human and chimpanzee proteins are 100% identical, any potential human-specific properties of LRRTM1 may involve the spatiotemporal control of its imprinted expression. It is interesting that recent analysis of conserved non-coding elements demonstrated that a sequence element 130 kb downstream of LRRTM1 displays accelerated evolution in the human lineage, which may be important for the gene's regulation (Prabhakar *et al.*, 2006).

We detected only bi-allelic, non-imprinted expression of LRRTM1 in cerebral cortex, cerebellum, and brain stem from two 30-week-old reciprocal crossed F1 mice between C57BL/6J and JF1 strains, and only bi-allelic expression in the post-mortem brains of two adult chimpanzees (Francks *et al.*, 2007). Larger sample sizes will be needed to test whether imprinting of LRRTM1 is found only in humans. There is a high level of discordance in imprinting between humans and mice (Morison *et al.*, 2005); the gene DLX5 is an example (Kimura *et al.*, 2004). It will also be interesting to compare the regulation of LRRTM1 longitudinally during development of humans and other species, as the imprinted regulation may be restricted to certain developmental periods (Sun *et al.*, 2005). In addition, human genetic variation at this locus in non-clinical populations could be analyzed with dense marker genotyping, to test for evidence of selection, particularly with regard to the risk haplotype.

Genomic imprinting can arise when the optimal level of maternal resource investment in offspring differs between the two parental sexes, in polygamous mating systems (Reik & Walter, 2001; Wilkins & Haig, 2003). Paternally inherited alleles of imprinted genes often sequester more maternal resources than do maternally inherited alleles, especially when influencing growth in utero (Reik & Walter, 2001; Wilkins & Haig, 2003). The imprinting of LRRTM1 in humans therefore suggests an intriguing evolutionary scenario, in which the parental sexes have conflicting interests in relation to the outcome of lateralized brain development in their offspring, which underlies much of human cognition and behavior. This may relate conceivably to the extremely protracted period of postnatal care that is demanded by human children before they develop cognitive and behavioral independence, compared to other mammals. Further study of the neural systems and behaviors that LRRTM1 influences will be required to understand the selective forces that drove LRRTM1 to be imprinted.

Future directions

The epigenetic regulation of LRRTM1 should now be characterized in detail, and attempts made to relate abnormalities of the epigenetic state to cognitive and psychiatric variation in human cohorts. It may be that the epigenetic state at this locus will prove more important for schizophrenia and brain-asymmetrical development than allelic DNA variation, although the two may interact. This is because the allelic association that we have identified (Francks *et al.*, 2007) does not explain all of the paternal-specific linkage to schizophrenia in sib pairs across this genomic region. One possibility is that the paternal linkage in sib pairs may result from incomplete erasure of the maternal imprint at LRRTM1 during spermatogenesis.

It may now prove possible to use LRRTM1 as a route into understanding asymmetrical development of the human brain at a molecular level. The molecular basis of this is almost completely unknown. We propose that pathway expansion work should begin for LRRTM1, using yeast-2-hybrid screening and/or co-immunoprecipitation. It will also be necessary to characterize this gene's role in the developing and adult mouse brain using knockout technology, followed by detailed histopathological, behavioral, and electrophysiological characterization. Such research will also be expected to drive further genetic studies in humans. For example, interacting partners of LRRTM1 may be investigated for effects on psychiatric variation, and the mouse work will indicate brain regions and structures that can be investigated in human imaging-genetic studies.

In humans there are microanatomical asymmetries between left and right cerebral cortices, including asymmetries of cortical columnar widths, and the degree of dendritic branching of some neuronal classes (Hutsler & Galuske, 2003). These differences may underlie the different specializations of the two cerebral hemispheres in normal right-handers, who have left-hemisphere language dominance. The neuronal circuitry of the left hemisphere may indeed support a class of operations that involve sequential and motor processing, as opposed to more holistic processing in the right hemisphere (Hutsler & Galuske, 2003). Although mice do not have noticeable asymmetries of the cerebral cortex, it may still prove possible to model the human conditions in mice via perturbation of the LRRTM1 pathway, and characterization of the micro-anatomical and eletrophysiological properties that arise.

The imprinting of LRRTM1 appears to be human- or primate-specific based on preliminary data. This suggests an intriguing evolutionary scenario, in which there has been a conflict between the parental sexes over the outcome of lateralized brain development in their offspring, which relates to much of human thought and emotion. Through relating variability at LRRTM1 to variability in human cognition, behavior, and brain development, it may be possible to understand the selective forces that have acted to cause LRRTM1 to become imprinted. This may shed light on the evolutionary origins of complex human cognition. There is also strong evidence (unpublished) of positive selection directly upstream of LRRTM1 in the European population, with the disease-protective haplotype having apparently undergone positive selection in relatively recent history (D. Davison, J. Marchini; personal communication).

In addition to schizophrenia, other neurodevelopmental disorders including bipolar disorder, autism, and language impairment have shown evidence for associations with left-handedness and/or abnormal asymmetrical brain structure/function (Hugdahl & Davidson, 2003; Csernansky *et al.*, 2004; De Fosse *et al.*, 2004; DeLisi *et al.*, 1997; Herbert *et al.*, 2002; Paulesu *et al.*, 2001; Shenton *et al.*, 2001; Sommer *et al.*, 2002). LRRTM1 is therefore also a candidate for involvement in these traits. The LRRTMs are a four-member gene family first described in 2003, and it is interesting to note that LRRTM3 has recently been proposed as a susceptibility factor for late-onset Alzheimer's disease (Majercak *et al.*, 2006). We therefore recommend that the whole LRRTM gene family is investigated in relation to psychiatric and neurological disorders.

ACKNOWLEDGMENTS

This chapter uses extracts and figures from: Francks *et al.*, 2002, 2003a, 2003b, 2003c, 2007. With permission.

I am indebted to over forty scientists from around the world who have made critical contributions to this research program over several years: Shinji Maegawa, Juha Laurén, Brett S. Abrahams, Antonio Velayos-Baeza, Sarah E. Medland, Stefano Colella, Matthias Groszer, Erica Z. McAuley, Tara M. Caffrey, Tõnis Timmusk, Priit Pruunsild, Indrek Koppel, Penelope A. Lind, Noriko Matsumoto-Itaba, Jérôme Nicod, Lan Xiong, Ridha Joober, Wolfgang Enard, Benjamin Krinsky, Eiji Nanba, Alex J. Richardson, I. Laurence MacPhie, Angela J. Marlow, Steve H. Laval, Judith E. Rue, Sarah H. Shaw, Kathleen E. Taylor, Brien P. Riley, Nicholas G. Martin, Stephen M. Strittmatter, Hans-Jürgen Möller, Dan Rujescu, David St. Clair, Pierandrea Muglia, J. Louw Roos, Simon E. Fisher, Richard Wade-Martins, Guy A. Rouleau, John F. Stein, Maria Karayiorgou, Daniel H. Geschwind, Jiannis Ragoussis, Kenneth S. Kendler, Matti S. Airaksinen, Mitsuo Oshimura, Lynn E. DeLisi and Anthony P. Monaco. In particular I wish to thank Shinji Maegawa for studies of LRRTM1 imprinting; Juha Laurén for gene-functional work; Brett Abrahams for *in situ* hybridization work with human brain, Lynn DeLisi for access to patient samples and her founding and continued support; Simon Fisher for his key involvement in our first genome-wide scan for handedness; Tony Monaco for supporting this program in his laboratory for several years. I have been supported on this project by the Wellcome Trust, the Schizophrenia Research Fund, and NARSAD (National Alliance for Research on Schizophrenia and Depression). Most of the data described in this chapter were first presented in the journal articles cited throughout the text.

REFERENCES

Abecasis, G. R., Burt, R. A., Hall, D. *et al.* (2004). Genomewide scan in families with schizophrenia from the founder population of Afrikaners reveals evidence for linkage and uniparental disomy on chromosome 1. *Am J Hum Genet*, **74**(3), 403–17.

Andrews, J., Wang, L., Csernansky, J. G., Gado, M. H. & Barch, D. M. (2006). Abnormalities of thalamic activation and cognition in schizophrenia. *Am J Psychiatry*, **163**(3), 463–9.

Anneken, K., Konrad, C., Dräger, B. *et al.* (2004). Familial aggregation of strong hemispheric language lateralization. *Neurology*, **63**, 2433–5.

Annett, M. (1972). The distribution of manual asymmetry. *Br J Psychol*, **63**, 343–58.

Berlim, M. T., Mattevi, B. S., Belmonte-de-Abreu, P. & Crow, T. J. (2003). The etiology of schizophrenia and the origin of language: overview of a theory. *Compr Psychiatry*, **44**(1), 7–14.

Bunzel, R., Blumcke, I., Cichon, S. *et al.* (1998). Polymorphic imprinting of the serotonin-2A (5-HT2A) receptor gene in human adult brain. *Mol Brain Res*, **59**(1), 90–2.

Csernansky, J. G., Schindler, M. K., Splinter, N. R. *et al.* (2004). Abnormalities of thalamic volume and shape in schizophrenia. *Am J Psychiatry*, **161**(5), 896–902.

De Fosse, L., Hodge, S. M., Makris, N. *et al.* (2004). Language-association cortex asymmetry in autism and specific language impairment. *Ann Neurol*, **56**(6), 757–66.

DeLisi, L. E., Sakuma, M., Kushner, M. *et al.* (1997). Anomalous cerebral asymmetry and language processing in schizophrenia. *Schizophr Bull*, **23**(2), 255–71.

DeLisi, L. E., Shaw, S. H., Crow, T. J. & *et al.* (2002a). A genome-wide scan for linkage to chromosomal regions in 382 sibling pairs with schizophrenia or schizoaffective disorder. *Am J Psychiatry*, **159**(5), 803–12.

DeLisi, L. E., Svetina, C., Razi, K. *et al.* (2002b). Hand preference and hand skill in families with schizophrenia. *Laterality*, **7**(4), 321–32.

Fisher, S. E., Francks, C., Marlow, A. J. *et al.* (2002). Independent genome-wide scans identify a chromosome 18 quantitative-trait locus influencing dyslexia. *Nat Genet*, **30**(1), 86–91.

Fournier, A. E., GrandPre, T., Gould, G., Wang, X. & Strittmatter, S. M. (2002). Nogo and the Nogo-66 receptor. *Prog Brain Res*, **137**, 361–9.

Francks, C., DeLisi, L. E., Fisher, S. E. *et al.* (2003a). Confirmatory evidence for linkage of relative hand skill to 2p12-q11. *Am J Hum Genet*, **72**(2), 499–502.

Francks, C., DeLisi, L. E., Shaw, S. H. *et al.* (2003b). Parent-of-origin effects on handedness and schizophrenia susceptibility on chromosome 2p12-q11. *Hum Mol Genet*, **12**(24), 3225–30.

Francks, C., Fisher, S. E., MacPhie, I. L. *et al.* (2002). A genome-wide linkage screen for relative hand skill in sibling pairs. *Am J Hum Genet*, **70**(3), 800–5.

Francks, C., Fisher, S. E., Marlow, A. J. *et al.* (2003e). Familial and genetic effects on motor coordination, laterality, and reading-related cognition. *Am J Psychiatry*, **160**(11), 1970–7.

Francks, C., Maegawa, S., Laurén, J. *et al.* (2007). LRRTM1 on chromosome 2p12 is a maternally suppressed gene that is associated paternally with handedness and schizophrenia. *Mol Psychiatry*, **12**(12), 1129–39.

Geschwind, D. H., Miller, B. L., DeCarli, C. & Carmelli, D. (2002). Heritability of lobar brain volumes in twins supports genetic models of cerebral laterality and handedness. *Proc Natl Acad Sci USA*, **99**(5), 3176–81.

Harrison, P. J. & Weinberger, D. R. (2004). Schizophrenia genes, gene expression, and neuropathology: on the matter of their convergence. *Mol Psychiatry*, **10**(1), 40–68.

Herbert, M. R., Harris, G. J., Adrien, K. T. *et al.* (2002). Abnormal asymmetry in language association cortex in autism. *Ann Neurol*, **52**(5), 588–96.

Hering-Hanit, R., Achiron, R., Lipitz, S. & Achiron, A. (2001). Asymmetry of fetal cerebral hemispheres: in utero ultrasound study. *Arch Dis Child Fetal Neonatal Ed*, **85**(3), F194–F196.

Hugdahl, K. & Davidson, R. J. (eds.) (2003). *The Asymmetrical Brain*. Cambridge, Massachusetts: MIT Press.

Hutsler, J. & Galuske, R. A. (2003). Hemispheric asymmetries in cerebral cortical networks. *Trends Neurosci*, **26**(8), 429–35.

Imprinted Gene Catalogue http://igc.otago.ac.nz/home.html. Web. 20-11-2006.

Ioannidis, J. P. A., Ntzani, E. E., Trikalinos, T. A. & Contopoulos-Ioannidis, D. G. (2001). Replication validity of genetic association studies. *Nat Genet*, **29**(3), 306–9.

Kimura, M. I., Kazuki, Y., Kashiwagi, A. *et al.* (2004). Dlx5, the mouse homologue of the human-imprinted DLX5 gene, is biallelically expressed in the mouse brain. *J Hum. Genet*, **49**(5), 273–7.

Kochunov, P., Fox, P., Lancaster, J. *et al.* (2003). Localized morphological brain differences between English-speaking Caucasians and Chinese-speaking Asians: new evidence of anatomical plasticity. *Neuroreport*, **14**(7), 961–4.

Kugoh, H., Mitsuya, K., Meguro, M. *et al.* (1999). Mouse A9 cells containing single human chromosomes for analysis of genomic imprinting. *DNA Res*, **6**(3), 165–72.

Lauren, J., Airaksinen, M. S., Saarma, M. & Timmusk, T. (2003). A novel gene family encoding leucine-rich repeat transmembrane proteins differentially expressed in the nervous system. *Genomics*, **81**(4), 411–21.

Lewis, C. M., Levinson, D. F., Wise, L. H. *et al.* (2003). Genome scan meta-analysis of schizophrenia and bipolar disorder, Part II: schizophrenia. *Am J Hum Genet*, **73**(1), 34–48.

Majercak, J., Ray, W. J., Espeseth, A. *et al.* (2006). LRRTM3 promotes processing of amyloid-precursor protein by BACE1 and is a positional candidate gene for late-onset Alzheimer's disease. *PNAS*, **103**(47), 17967–72.

McManus, I. C. (1985). Handedness, language dominance and aphasia: a genetic model. *Psychological Medicine*, Monograph Supplement 8.

McManus, I. C. & Bryden, M. P. (1992). *The Genetics of Handedness, Cerebral Dominance and Lateralization*. Amsterdam: Elsevier.

Mevorach, C., Humphreys, G. W. & Shalev, L. (2005). Attending to local form while ignoring global aspects depends on handedness: evidence from TMS. *Nat Neurosci*, **8**(3), 276–7.

Morison, I. M., Ramsay, J. P. & Spencer, H. G. (2005). A census of mammalian imprinting. *Trends Genet*, **21**(8), 457–65.

Orr, K. G., Cannon, M., Gilvarry, C. M., Jones, P. B. & Murray, R. M. (1999). Schizophrenic patients and their first-degree relatives show an excess of mixed-handedness. *Schizophr Res*, **39**(3), 167–76.

Paulesu, E., Demonet, J. F., Fazio, F. *et al.* (2001). Dyslexia: cultural diversity and biological unity. *Science*, **291**(5511), 2165–7.

Prabhakar, S., Noonan, J. P., Paabo, S. & Rubin, E. M. (2006). Accelerated evolution of conserved noncoding sequences in humans. *Science*, **314**, 786.

Reik, W. & Walter, J. (2001). Genomic imprinting: parental influence on the genome. *Nat Rev Genet*, **2**(1), 21–32.

Risch, N. & Pringle, G. (1985). Segregation analysis of human hand preference. *Behav Genet*, **15**(4), 385–400.

Rogers, L. J. & Andrew, R. (eds.) (2002). *Comparative Vertebrate Lateralization*. Cambridge, UK: Cambridge University Press.

Sakatani, T., Wei, M., Katoh, M. *et al.* (2001). Epigenetic heterogeneity at imprinted loci in normal populations. *Biochemical and Biophysical Research Communications*, **283**(5), 1124–30.

Shenton, M. E., Dickey, C. C., Frumin, M. & McCarley, R. W. (2001). A review of MRI findings in schizophrenia. *Schizophr Res*, **49**(1–2), 1–52.

Sommer, I. E., Ramsey, N. F., Mandl, R. C. & Kahn, R. S. (2002). Language lateralization in monozygotic twin pairs concordant and discordant for handedness. *Brain*, **125** (12), 2710–18.

Speder, P., Petzoldt, A., Suzanne, M. & Noselli, S. (2007). Strategies to establish left/right asymmetry in vertebrates and invertebrates. *Curr Opin Genet Dev*, **17**(4), 351–8.

Sullivan, P. F., Kendler, K. S. & Neale, M. C. (2003). Schizophrenia as a complex trait: evidence from a meta-analysis of twin studies. *Arch Gen Psychiatry*, **60**(12), 1187–92.

Sun, T., Patoine, C., Abu-Khalil, A. *et al.* (2005). Early asymmetry of gene transcription in embryonic human left and right cerebral cortex. *Science*, **308**(5729), 1794–8.

Takahashi, S., Cui, Y. H., Kojima, T. *et al.* (2003). Family-based association study of markers on chromosome 22 in schizophrenia using African-American, European-American, and Chinese families. *Am J Med Genet B Neuropsychiatr Genet*, **120**(1), 11–17.

Thiselton, D. L., Webb, B. T., Neale, B. M. *et al.* (2004). No evidence for linkage or association of neuregulin-1 (NRG1) with disease in the Irish study of high-density schizophrenia families (ISHDSF). *Mol Psychiatry*, **9**(8), 777–83.

Van den Oord, E. J. C. G., Rujescu, D., Robles, J. R. *et al.* (2006). Factor structure and external validity of the PANSS revisited. *Schizophr Res*, **82**(2–3), 213–23.

Wilkins, J. F. & Haig, D. (2003). What good is genomic imprinting: the function of parent-specific gene expression. *Nat Rev Genet*, **4**(5), 359–68.

Williams, N. A., Close, J. P., Giouzeli, M. & Crow, T. J. (2006). Accelerated evolution of Protocadherin11X/Y: a candidate gene-pair for cerebral asymmetry and language. *Am J Med Genet B Neuropsychiatr Genet*, **141**(6), 623–33.

Xiong, L., Rouleau, G. A., DeLisi, L. E. *et al.* (2005). CAA insertion polymorphism in the 3′UTR of Nogo gene on 2p14 is not associated with schizophrenia. *Mol Brain Res*, **133**(1), 153–6.

Yamasaki, K., Joh, K., Ohta, T. *et al.* (2003). Neurons but not glial cells show reciprocal imprinting of sense and antisense transcripts of Ube3a. *Hum Mol Genet*, **12**(8), 837–47.

Index